Tim Leiner

Mathias Goyen

Martin Rohrer

Stefan Schönberg (Eds.)

Clinical Blood Pool MR Imaging

Tim Leiner
Mathias Goyen
Martin Rohrer
Stefan Schönberg (Eds.)

Clinical Blood Pool MR Imaging

With 331 Figures and 26 Tables

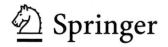
Springer

Tim Leiner
Department of Radiology
Maastricht University Medical Center
Peter Debijelaan 25
6229 HX Maastricht
The Netherlands

Martin Rohrer
Bayer Schering Pharma AG
European Business Unit Diagnostic Imaging
Muellerstrasse 178
13353 Berlin
Germany

Mathias Goyen
University Medical Center
Hamburg-Eppendorf
Martinistrasse 52
20251 Hamburg
Germany

Stefan O. Schoenberg
Department of Clinical Radiology and Nuclear Medicine
University Hospital Mannheim
Medical Faculty Mannheim – University of Heidelberg
Theodor-Kutzer-Ufer 1-3
68167 Mannheim
Germany

Clinical Blood Pool MR Imaging
The Vasovist® Product Monograph

Marketing Approval Number EU1.DI.06.2008.0017

ISBN 978-3-540-77860-8 Springer Medizin Verlag Heidelberg

Bibliografische Information der Deutschen Bibliothek
The Deutsche Bibliothek lists this publication in Deutsche Nationalbibliographie;
detailed bibliographic data is available in the internet at http://dnb.ddb.de.

Springer Medizin Verlag
springer.com
© Springer Medizin Verlag Heidelberg 2008

Design: deblik Berlin
Typesetting: TypoStudio Tobias Schaedla, Heidelberg
Cover illustrations: courtesy of Dr. Alexander Huppertz, Imaging Science Institute, Charité, Berlin, Germany, Dr. Henrik Michaely, Medical Faculty Mannheim, University of Heidelberg, Germany and Dr. Regina Beets-Tan, Maastricht University Medical Center, The Netherlands
Printer: Grosch! Druckzentrum GmbH, Heidelberg

SPIN: 12215607

18/5135 – 5 4 3 2 1 0

Foreword

Magnetic resonance angiography has made great strides, with continuing improvements in hardware, pulse sequencing, and know-how allowing ever-increasing speed, resolution, and suppression of artifacts. However, an inherent physical barrier has always been limited SNR. Gadolinium contrast agents help to increase SNR by facilitating T1 relaxation, but they can be injected only at a finite rate and at a limited molar dose, and there is a rapid drop in concentration following the brief arterial phase due to redistribution into the extracellular fluid compartment. With its sixfold increase in T1 relaxivity, blood pool distribution, and longer serum half-life, Vasovist® represents a new breakthrough which promises to revolutionize MRA image quality once again.

This excellent treatise on Vasovist®, created by a team of exceptional faculty who are pioneers in MR angiography, covers the basic techniques, safety, efficacy, image processing, and pharmacoeconomic details, to successfully implement a new level of MRA image quality with this new contrast agent. In addition to improving all the usual arterial phase MRA applications, the blood pool distribution opens up new possibilities, including detecting internal bleeding and imaging stent graft endoleaks, which are reviewed in detail. In the complex, competitive field of cardiovascular imaging, this book articulates the cutting edge in imaging vascular disease.

Martin R. Prince, MD, PhD
Professor of Radiology
Weill Medical College of Cornell University
Columbia College of Physicians and Surgeons
New York, NY, USA

Foreword

Almost two decades ago, Martin Prince was able to demonstrate that the limitations of non-contrast MRA techniques could be overcome by injection of contrast agent. Subsequently, contrast-enhanced-MRA established itself in clinical practice as the standard for non-invasive depiction of almost all blood vessels. MR manufacturers have addressed the demands for faster acquisition speed to allow higher resolution imaging during the finite and relatively short imaging window of first pass MRA by a combination of faster gradients, parallel imaging techniques, and novel K-space sampling strategies. However, a perceived limit for improvement in spatial resolution, coupled with the negative impact of faster acquisition on contrast-to-noise ratios, has led to the development of »Vasovist®«, the first contrast agent »tailored« to the vascular tree.

With its high relaxivity and unique pharmacokinetics, Vasovist® opens up new horizons in vascular diagnostics with a prolonged imaging window, enhanced topographic information, and unrivaled new visualization options. The editors and authors have made groundbreaking contributions towards establishing MR angiography in various investigative settings, rendering it more precise and applying it for diverse indications. The work presented here is founded upon the extensive experience of the editors, and it includes a broad range of experience from other scientific working groups.

This book presents the applications of Vasovist®-enhanced angiography; its potential advantages, such as the change in signal-to-noise ratio and intravascular distribution, are discussed systematically, thus giving a comprehensive overview of the basic principles and imaging techniques. Presentation of the various clinical fields is well-structured and is illustrated with excellent image material that addresses the essential questions concerning vascular diagnostics. This includes imaging of the intracranial and supra-aortic vessels and visualization of the coronary arteries, as well as of the renal and visceral vessels. Key chapters cover MR angiography of the aortoiliac and peripheral vessels. Whole-body MR angiography represents a special challenge for angiography. The new options offered by Vasovist®-enhanced MR angiography are also discussed. All in all, this monograph presents the ideal opportunity to gain relevant information, read either as a review or as a detailed account of the increasing scientific potential offered by this method of vascular MR diagnosis.

What can we predict for the future? Two decades following Dr. Prince's (then) heretical thesis that contrast-agent injection was required for dramatically improved MRA, we are now equipped with a tailored vascular contrast agent. This development parallels improvements in scanner performance, satisfies a demand for higher spatial resolution, and opens up a whole new perspective on the benefit of additional information available from the steady state images as a routine part of the study.

Prof. Dr.Dr.h.c. Maximilian F. Reiser
Department of Clinical Radiology
Director of the Department
Ludwig-Maximilians-University of Munich
Marchioninistr. 15
81377 Munich
Germany

Introduction

The successful introduction of extracellular gadolinium-based contrast agents for contrast-enhanced MR angiography, and their wide acceptance today, raise the question of what part an intravascular contrast agent might play in diagnostic imaging. The answer lies in the capacity of an intravascular agent to give us high-level diagnostic information from first pass arterial imaging and, at the same time, to yield additional diagnostic value by allowing delayed imaging from the same contrast injection.

Clinical experience gathered since the introduction of Vasovist® (Gadofosveset) appears to provide the answer »yes«: not only is Vasovist® useful for first pass arterial imaging, but it also provides high intravascular enhancement that lasts much longer and is significantly greater than that afforded by conventional extracellular agents. Taking advantage of this effect, one can now acquire additional high-resolution images in the steady state which lead to much better delineation of vessel pathology. Steady state imaging offers the possibility of depicting the entire vascular system without relevant extravasation of the contrast medium from the intravascular space.

The extended diagnostic window of Vasovist® makes the examination more convenient because it is less dependent upon bolus dynamics. Imaging of a Gadofosveset bolus missed in the first pass examination does not require an additional injection of contrast agent. For these reasons, Vasovist® may enable physicians to detect systemic vascular disease earlier and to optimize the evaluation of therapeutic options, including percutaneous intervention and vascular surgery. In addition, imaging of the vascular system and surrounding tissues in the delayed phase appears to promise new contrast mechanisms that may improve the detection of inflammatory or malignant changes.

In summary, Vasovist® has the potential to open new horizons in diagnostic MR angiography by increasing the spatial resolution and the robustness of MRA examinations and facilitating the examination of multiple vascular beds. Vasovist® was first approved in 2005, and we are now looking at an expanded spectrum of clinical applications that has rapidly evolved and addresses the majority of clinical questions in vascular medicine and related fields. Therefore, this monograph is subdivided into chapters on technology, followed by a detailed review of the clinical fields for MR angiography with Vasovist®. With this steady increase of applications and clinical experience it is necessary to review not only the technical feasibility and reliability of the method, but also the potential additional benefit for the patient. Therefore, aspects of patient management are also analyzed, with the aim of deriving more effective and comprehensive imaging standards.

We would like to thank all of the authors for their valuable contributions and dedicated collaboration, which made this current compilation of essential aspects of Vasovist®-enhanced MR imaging possible. Also, we gratefully acknowledge the contributions of our publisher, Springer, and Mr. Eric Henquinet for his constructive, friendly and patient collaboration.

Tim Leiner (Maastricht University Hospital, The Netherlands),
Mathias Goyen (University Medical Center Hamburg-Eppendorf, Germany),
Martin Rohrer (Bayer Schering Pharma AG, Berlin, Germany),
Stefan Schönberg (University Hospital Mannheim, Germany)

Table of Contents

Foreword V

Foreword VII

Introduction IX

Part I   Contrast Agent Properties and Technical Aspects

1   MRI Contrast Media – Introduction and Basic Properties of the Blood
    Pool Agent Vasovist® 3
    Martin Rohrer

2   Contrast Enhanced MRA – First Pass and Steady State 17
    Harald H. Quick

Part II   Safety and Efficacy

3   Risks and Safety Issues Related to Radiological Imaging, in Particular MRI.......... 35
    Gunnar Brix

4   Summary of Safety of Vasovist® at 0.03 mmol/kg Body Weight Dose –
    Clinical Data.. 43
    Matthias Voth and Andrea Löwe

5   Efficacy of Vasovist®: Overview of the Clinical Development Program 51
    Mathias Goyen

Part III   Blood Pool Agents in MRA: Indications, Clinical Applications and Benefits

6   Head and Neck MRA... 59
    Marco Essig

7   Pulmonary MRA... 69
    Christian Fink, Ulrike Attenberger, and Konstantin Nikolaou

8   Abdominal MRA... 81
    Henrik Michaely

9   MRA of the Peripheral Vasculature 93
    Tim Leiner and Jeffrey H. Maki

10 Magnetic Resonance Venography 115
    Giles Roditi

Part IV   New Horizons in Vascular Diagnostics

Part V   Image Processing

Part VI   Pharmacoeconomic Impact

List of Contributors

Ulrike Attenberger
Department of Clinical Radiology
Grosshadern Campus
Ludwig-Maximilians-University of
Munich
Marchioninistrasse 15
81377 Munich
Germany

Lambertus W. Bartels
Image Sciences Institute, QS.459
University Medical Center Utrecht
Heidelberglaan 100
3584 CX Utrecht
The Netherlands

Geerard L. Beets
Department of Surgery
University Hospital Maastricht
PO Box 5800
6202 AZ Maastricht
The Netherlands

Regina G.H. Beets-Tan
Department of Radiology
Maastricht University Medical Center
Peter Debijelaan 25
6229 HX Maastricht
The Netherlands

Karsten Bergmann
Bayer Schering Pharma AG
Global Medical Affairs Diagnostic
Imaging
Müllerstrasse 178
13353 Berlin
Germany

Michael Bock
German Cancer Research Center (dkfz)
Department of Medical Physics in
Radiology
Im Neuenheimer Feld 280
69120 Heidelberg
Germany

Gunnar Brix
Department of Medical Radiation
Hygiene and Dosimetry
Federal Office for Radiation Protection
Ingolstädter Landstrasse 1
85764 Oberschleißheim
Germany

Sandra A.P. Cornelissen
Department of Radiology/Image
Sciences Institute, E01.132
University Medical Center Utrecht
Heidelberglaan 100
3584 CX Utrecht
The Netherlands

R. Bert Jan de Bondt
Department of Radiology
Maastricht University Medical Center
Peter Debijelaan 25
6229 HX Maastricht
The Netherlands

Sanne M.E. Engelen
Department of Radiology
Maastricht University Medical Center
Peter Debijelaan 25
6229 HX Maastricht
The Netherlands

Marco Essig
Department of Radiology
German Cancer Research Center (dkfz)
Im Neuenheimer Feld 280
69120 Heidelberg
Germany

Christian Fink
Department of Clinical Radiology and
Nuclear Medicine
University Medical Center Mannheim
Medical Faculty Mannheim - University
of Heidelberg
Theodor-Kutzer-Ufer 1-3
68167 Mannheim
Germany

Clemens Fitzek
Neuroradiological Centre
ASKLEPIOS Fachklinikum Brandenburg
Anton-Saefkow-Allee 2
14772 Brandenburg
Germany

Michael Forsting
Department of Diagnostic and
Interventional Radiology and
Neuroradiology
University Hospital Essen
Hufelandstrasse 55
45147 Essen
Germany

Frederik L. Giesel
German Cancer Research Center (dkfz)
Department of Radiology
Im Neuenheimer Feld 280
69120 Heidelberg
Germany

Mathias Goyen
University Medical Center Hamburg-
Eppendorf
Martinistrasse 52
20251 Hamburg
Germany

Joachim Graessner
Siemens AG
Healthcare Sector
MED ES BMG MR
Lindenplatz 2
20099 Hamburg
Germany

Gerald F. Greil
King's College London
Division of Imaging Sciences
The Rayne Institute,
4th Floor, Lambeth Wing, St. Thomas'
Hospital
London SE1 7EH
United Kingdom

Dariusch R. Hadizadeh
Department of Radiology
University of Bonn
Sigmund-Freud-Strasse 25
53105 Bonn
Germany

Christoph U. Herborn
Medical Prevention Center Hamburg
(MPCH)
University Medical Center Hamburg-
Eppendorf
Falkenried 88
20251 Hamburg
Germany

Sebastian Kelle
German Heart Institute Berlin
Department of Internal Medicine
Division of Cardiology
Augustenburger Platz 1
13353 Berlin
Germany

Susanne Kienbaum
Bayer Schering Pharma AG
Global Health Economics, Outcomes &
Reimbursement
Diagnostic Imaging
Muellerstrasse 178
13353 Berlin
Germany

Harald Kramer
Institute for Clinical Radiology
University Hospitals Munich –
Grosshadern
Marchioninistr. 15
81377 Munich
Germany

Max J. Lahaye
Department of Radiology
Maastricht University Medical Center
Peter Debijelaan 25
6229 HX Maastricht
The Netherlands

Tim Leiner
Department of Radiology
Maastricht University Medical Center
Peter Debijelaan 25
6229HX Maastricht
The Netherlands

Andrea Löwe
Bayer Schering Pharma AG
Global Medical Affairs Diagnostic
Imaging
Müllerstrasse 178
13353 Berlin
Germany

Joachim Lotz
Magnetic Resonance Imaging
Department of Radiology
Hannover Medical School
Carl-Neuberg-Strasse 1
30625 Hannover
Germany

Jeffrey H. Maki
Department of Radiology
Puget Sound Veterans
Adminstration Health Care System
Seattle, Washington,
USA

Henrik J. Michaely
Department of Clinical Radiology and
Nuclear Medicine
University Medical Center Mannheim
Medical Faculty Mannheim - University
of Heidelberg
Theodor-Kutzer-Ufer 1-3
68167 Mannheim
Germany

Eike Nagel
King's College London
Division of Imaging Sciences
The Rayne Institute, 4th Floor Lambeth
Wing
St. Thomas' Hospital
London SE1 7EH
UK

Konstantin Nikolaou
Department of Clinical Radiology
Grosshadern Campus
Ludwig-Maximilians-University of
Munich
Marchioninistrasse 15
81377 Munich
Germany

Mathias Prokop
Department of Radiology, E01.132
University Medical Center Utrecht
Heidelberglaan 100
3584 CX Utrecht
The Netherlands

Harald H. Quick
Department of Diagnostic and
Interventional Radiology and
Neuroradiology
University Hospital Essen
Hufelandstrasse 55
45122 Essen
Germany

Reza Razavi
King's College London
Division of Imaging Sciences
Floor 5 Thomas Guy House
Guy's Hospital
London SE1 9RT
UK

Giles Roditi
Department of Radiology
Glasgow Royal Infirmary
16 Alexandra Parade
Glasgow G31 2ER
UK

Martin Rohrer
Bayer Schering Pharma AG
European Business Unit Diagnostic
Imaging
Muellerstrasse 178
13353 Berlin
Germany

Carsten Schwenke
SCO:SSiS
Zeltinger Strasse 58g
13465 Berlin
Germany

Stefan O. Schoenberg
Department of Clinical Radiology and
Nuclear Medicine
University Hospital Mannheim
Medical Faculty Mannheim - University
of Heidelberg
Theodor-Kutzer-Ufer 1-3
68167 Mannheim
Germany

Hence J.M. Verhagen
Department of Vascular Surgery
Suite H-993
Erasmus University Medical Center
PO Box 2040
3000 CA Rotterdam
The Netherlands

Joan C. Vilanova
Department of Magnetic Resonance
& CT
Clínica Girona
Lorenzana, 36
17002 Girona
Spain

Matthias Voth
Bayer Schering Pharma AG
Global Medical Affairs Diagnostic
Imaging
Muellerstrasse 178
13353 Berlin
Germany

Frank Wacker
Charité, Campus Benjamin Franklin
Radiology and Nuclear Medicine
Hindenburgdamm 30
12200 Berlin
Germany

Klaus Wasser
Department of Clinical Radiology and
Nuclear Medicine
University Hospital Mannheim
Medical Faculty Mannheim - University
of Heidelberg
Theodor-Kutzer-Ufer 1-3
68167 Mannheim
Germany

Winfried A. Willinek
Department of Radiology
University of Bonn
Sigmund-Freud-Strasse 25
53105 Bonn
Germany

List of Abbreviations

2D	Two-dimensional	ECG	Electrocardiogram
3D	Three-dimensional	EMEA	European Medicines Agency
3D FFT	3D Fast Fourier Transform	EMF	Electromagnetic field
SSFP	Steady state free precession	ECS	Extracellular space
ADC	Apparent diffusion coefficient	EUS	Endoluminal ultrasonography
ALARA	As low as reasonably achievable	EVAR	Endovascular aortic aneurysm repair
AngioSURF	Angiographic System for Unlimited Rolling Field-of-views	F/P	First pass
		FDA	US Food and Drug Administration
APAOD	Atherosclerotic peripheral arterial occlusive disease	FDG	^{18}Fluorodeoxyglucose
		FFT	Fast Fourier-transformation
ASSET	Array Spatial Sensitivity Encoding Technique	FLAIR	Fluid attentuated inversion recovery
		FLASH	Fast low-angle shot
AVF	Arteriovenous fistulae	FMD	Fibromuscular Dysplasia
BBB	Blood-brain barrier	FNAC	Fine-needle aspiration cytology
BOLD	Blood oxygenation level-dependent	FOV	Fields-of-view
BPCAs	Blood-pool contrast agents	GBCA	Gd-based contrast agent
CA	Contrast agents	GCP	Good clinical practice
CAD	Coronary artery disease	Gd	Gadolinium
CE	Contrast-enhanced	GI	Gastrointestinal
CE-MRA	Contrast-enhanced magnetic resonance angiography	GRAPPA	Generalized Autocalibrating Partially Parallel Acquisitions
CENTRA	Contrast-enhanced timing robust angiography	GRE	Gradient recalled echo
		H&E	Histological examination
CFA	Common femoral artery	HIFU	High-intensity focused ultrasound
CIS	Clinically isolated syndrome	HNSCC	Head and neck squamous cell carcinoma
CKD	Chronic kidney disease	HSA	Human serum albumin
CLI	Critical limb ischemia	HTA	Health technology assessment
CM	Contrast medium	IA-DSA	Intra-arterial X-ray-based digital subtraction angiography
CMR	Cardiovascular MR		
CNR	Contrast-to-noise ratio	IC	Intermittent claudication
CNS	Central nervous system	ICH-GCP	International Conference on Harmonisation on Good-Clinical-Practice
CSF	Cerebrospinal fluid		
CT	Computed tomography	ICNRIP	International Commission on Non-ionizing Radiation Protection
CTA	Computed tomography angiography		
CTEPH	Chronic thromboembolic pulmonary hypertension	IEC	International Electrotechnical Commission
		iPAT	Integrated Parallel Acquisition Techniques
CVC	Central venous catheters	IVC	Inferior vena cava
cVR	Color volume rendering	IVUS	Intravascular ultrasound
d	Diameter	KTWS	Klippel-Trenaunay-Weber syndrome
Da	Daltons	LAVA	Liver acquisition with volume acquisition
DCE-MRI	Dynamic contrast-enhanced MRI	LGIB	Lower GI bleeding
DEALE	Declining Exponential Approximation of Life Expectancy	LITT	Laser-induced thermal therapy
		LNT	Linear non-threshold
DKG-NT	Deutsche Krankenhausgesellschaft Nebenkostentarif	MAPCAs	Major aorto-pulmonary collateral arteries
		MBF	Myocardial blood flow
DOR	Diagnostic odds ratio	MDCT	Multidetector computed tomography
DSA	Digital subtraction angiography	MIP	Maximum intensity projection
DVT	Deep venous thrombosis	MPR	Multiplanar reconstructions
E/P	Equilibrium phase	MR	Magnetic resonance
ECCM	Extracellular contrast media	MRA	Magnetic resonance angiography

MRCA	Magnetic resonance coronary angiography		TIPS	Transjugular intrahepatic portosystemic shunts
MRI	Magnetic resonance imaging		TOF	Time-of-flight
MRV	Magnetic resonance venography		TR	Repetition Time
MS	Multi-slice		TREAT	Time-resolved echoshared angiography technique
mSENSE	Modified SENSE		TTP	Time-to-peak
MSI	Maximal-signal-intensity		UGIB	Upper GI bleeding
MTT	Mean-transit-time		USg-FNAC	Ultrasound-guided fine-needle aspiration cytology
NSF	Nephrogenic systemic fibrosis			
PAD	Peripheral artery disease		USPIO	Ultrasmall super paramagnetic iron oxide
PAH	Pulmonary arterial hypertension		VESPA	Venous-emhanced substracteed peak arterial
PAOD	Peripheral arterial obstructive disease			
PAT-factor	Parallel acquisition technique factor		VIBE	Volumetric interpolated breath-hold examination
PC	Phase-contrast			
PE	Pulmonary embolism		VQ scan	Ventilation-perfusion scintigraphy
PET	Positron emission tomography		VRT	Volume rendering technique
PR	Perfusion reserve		VSOP	Very small superparamagnetic iron oxide
PTA	Percutaneous transluminal angioplasty		XRA	X-ray angiography
QALY	Quality-adjusted-life-year		τm	Average time
RARE	Rapid acquisition with relaxation enhancement			
RAS	Renal artery stenosis			
RES	Reticuloendothelial system			
RF	Radiofrequency			
R-factor	Acceleration factor			
RIME	Receptor-induced magnetization enhancement			
RVT	Renal vein thrombosis			
SAE	Serious adverse events			
SAR	Severe adverse reactions			
SENSE	Sensitivity encoding			
SI	Signal intensity			
SLE	Systemic lupus erythematosus			
SLN	Sentinel lymph node			
SMA	Superior mesenteric artery			
SMASH	Simultaneous acquisition of spatial harmonics			
SNR	Signal-to-noise ratio			
SPECT	Single photon emission computed tomography			
SPGR	Spoiled gradient recalled echo			
SPIO	Superparamagnetic iron oxide particles			
SR	Surface rendering			
SSD	Surface-shaded display			
SSFP	Steady state free precession			
STD	Standard deviation			
STIR	Short tau inversion recovery			
SWI	Susceptibility-weighted imaging			
T1-SE	T1-spin echo			
T2-FSE	T2-fast spin echo			
TAO	Thromboangiitis obliterans			
TE	Echo time			
THRIVE	T1-weighted high-resolution isotropic volume imaging			

Part I   Contrast Agent Properties and Technical Aspects

1.1 Introduction

Twenty years ago, the first MRI contrast medium (MRI-CM) was introduced to the market: in 1988, Gd-DTPA (Magnevist®, Bayer Schering Pharma AG, Berlin, Germany) received market approval for clinical use in the United States, Europe and Japan. In the years to follow, application of MRI-CM became a widely established, powerful tool in MRI for improved diagnosis in approximately 30% of all MRI examinations worldwide [1,2,3,4,5].

During these two decades, only a few novel contrast media concepts have successfully stepped out of research laboratories to undergo clinical development and eventually to receive market approval. These include:

– Coated iron oxide nanoparticles, often referred to as SPIO (superparamagnetic iron oxide particles) with an average core particle size in the nanometer range. The SPIO-based MRI-CM Ferumoxide (Feridex®, Bayer HealthCare Pharmaceuticals, Wayne, NJ, USA) and Ferucarbotran Resovist® (Ferucarbotran, Bayer Schering Pharma AG, Berlin, Germany) are taken up predominantly by the reticuloendothelial system (RES) in the liver.

– Tissue-specific Gd- or Mn-based approaches. Marketed products are the liver-specific MRI-CM Gd-EOB-DTPA (Primovist®, Bayer Schering Pharma AG, Berlin, Germany), Gd-BOPTA (MultiHance®, Bracco, Milan, Italy) and Mn-DPDP (Teslascan®, GE Healthcare, Chalfont St. Giles, U.K.).

– Highly concentrated contrast media solutions, such as the 1.0 molar Gd-concentrated Gadobutrol (Gadovist 1.0®, Bayer Schering Pharma AG, Berlin, Germany).

Most recently, another class of MRI contrast agents has been introduced to the market, mainly to overcome current limitations of MR angiography (MRA): highly intravascular, slow-clearing blood pool contrast agents for MRI. Vasovist® (Gadofosveset, Bayer Schering Pharma AG, Berlin, Germany) – the first intravascular contrast agent approved for use with MRA in the European Union – is based on non-covalent transient protein binding, which leads to both an extended imaging window and strongly decreased Gd-dosage requirements.

1.1.1 Basic Mode of Action of MRI Contrast Media

Contrast media for MRI are well-known to strongly influence proton spin relaxation times, represented in vivo mainly by the vastly available hydrogen nuclei from water molecules in organic liquids and tissues.

The tissue-specific longitudinal (T_1) and transverse ($T_2^{(*)}$) relaxation times are – besides the less important local proton density – the most important physical parameters in MRI to obtain spatially resolved differences in signal intensity (SI) and hence the prerequisites for any soft-tissue and other contrasts in MRI. Taking effect at this most basic level, the option to additionally enhance contrast in MRI by introducing T_1- and $T_2^{(*)}$-shortening contrast media has made contrast-enhanced MRI such an important and often indispensable diagnostic tool.

Furthermore, not only does the use of MRI-CM provide an exclusive opportunity to directly modulate contrasts at the most basic biophysical level of MRI; because MRI-CM significantly shortens relaxation times, e.g. in T_1-weighted MRA, there is another important and basic advantage of contrast media use compared with unenhanced MRI procedures: contrast-enhanced MRI allows not only for additional contrasting with a minimum of artifacts, but also for substantially accelerated data acquisition due to much shorter repetition times (TR) and ultimately shorter scan times at a given spatial resolution. This is particularly the case for MRA, where the T_1 shortening achieved by contrast media reduces the native longitudinal relaxation time (T_1) of blood from over 1 sec down to the millisecond range, as will be discussed below in more detail.

For all classes of MRI-CM, shortening of proton spin relaxation times is achieved by the paramagnetic properties of the contrast media. Paramagnetism is based on unpaired electrons, resulting in strong and fluctuating local magnetic field distortions in the vicinity of the contrast medium molecules. These local magnetic field distortions are capable of destroying the much weaker proton spin order in the external, static magnetic field. Consequently, shortening of spin-lattice (T_1) and spin-spin (T_2) relaxation times is obtained in the tissue or liquid containing a sufficiently high concentration of contrast medium molecules. A more detailed and quantitative explanation of these effects is provided in Sect. 4.2.

1.1.2 Metal Complexes (Gd-Chelates)

As a result of their high number of unpaired electron spins, ions of transition metals and of lanthanides have been found to be well-suited as paramagnetic atoms in MRI-CM. The Gd^{3+} cation with seven unpaired electron spins (S = 7/2) and its large magnetic moment became the most important atom for use in MRI-CM. To assure the stability and biodistribution required for safety, Gd^{3+} ions are chelated in different chemical complexes, which also modulate their magnetic and pharmacokinetic properties to some extent. (Please also refer to the chapters in this book related to safety.) The interaction between the unpaired electron spins of the metal ion and the nuclear spins of protons from the surrounding water molecules is dominated by the short-distance, anisotropic dipol-dipol hyperfine interaction, as well as by contributions from the isotropic Fermi-contact interaction. Longitudinal and transverse relaxation times are comparably affected, leading to ratios r_2/r_1 between 1 and 2 [6].

1.1.3 Iron Oxide Nanoparticles

As mentioned above, so-called superparamagnetic particles have also been shown to be suitable as MRI-CM. They are often referred to as superparamagnetic iron oxide particles (SPIO) and have been investigated with different coatings (e.g. carboxydextran or dextran), different core particle diameters, and hydrodynamic size distributions. Their basic magnetic properties are determined not only by the interactions of nuclear spins with single paramagnetic ions in a chelate, but also by the bulk effects of the much larger spin ensembles of the unpaired electrons from the Fe_2O_3 and Fe_3O_2 molecules in the iron oxide nanoparticles. For the larger SPIO particles and for SPIO clusters in particular, these effects add up to almost macromolecular conditions and local ferromagnetic properties (»superparamagnetism«). Consequently, depending on SPIO core diameters or SPIO clustering effects, their influence on proton spin relaxation times applies over larger distances and is characterized by strong susceptibility effects and larger-scale magnetic field inhomogeneities. Naturally, the transverse relaxation processes dominate, which makes the SPIOs often better suited for T_2 and T_2^*-weighted MRI sequences. Resulting r_2/r_1 ratios can be up to the order of one hundred.

1.2 Blood Pool Contrast Media for MRI

Several classes of MRI contrast media have been briefly introduced in the previous section. This section takes a closer look at the characteristic properties of blood pool contrast media for MRI.

Intravascular contrast agents show less extravasation into the interstitium than conventional extracellular contrast agents. Depending on their mode of action, they also have a longer retention time in the vascular system due to slower blood clearance. Both characteristics can be realized only with special physicochemical and biochemical properties. For this reason, these properties, as well as the resulting typical pharmacokinetics, will be examined first in general, and then specifically for Vasovist®.

If we take a closer look, additional subgroups within the class of intravascular MR contrast agents can be distinguished, and it becomes clear that the terms »intravascular« and »blood pool« do not have to be synonyms in the strictly literal sense. According to the dominant effect – reduced extravasation, decelerated resorption, or glomerular excretion – and the resulting pharmacokinetics, the terms »intravascular« and »blood pool« will be used differently.

According to a proposal by Bogdanov and Weissleder [7,8], the components circulating in the blood vessel system may be divided into the following three groups:
1. Cellular components (predominantly erythrocytes)
2. Water
3. Proteins (mainly albumin as the most common plasma protein)

1.1.4 Overview of Currently Marketed MRI Contrast Media

◼ Table 1.1. Contrast media for MRI with market approval in at least either Europe, Japan or the USA

Short name or internal development code	Generic name (INN)[1]	Trade name(s)	Company
Gd-DTPA	Gadopentetate dimeglumine	MAGNEVIST®	Bayer Schering Pharma AG
Gd-DO3A-butrol	Gadobutrol	GADOVIST®	Bayer Schering Pharma AG
MS-325	Gadofosveset trisodium	VASOVIST®	Bayer Schering Pharma AG
Gd-EOB-DTPA	Gadoxetic acid, disodium	PRIMOVIST®	Bayer Schering Pharma AG
SH U 555 A	Ferucarbotran	RESOVIST®	Bayer Schering Pharma AG
AMI-25	Ferumoxide	FERIDEX® / ENDOREM®	Bayer Healthcare / Guerbet
Gd-HP-DO3A	Gadoteridol	PROHANCE®	Bracco
Gd-BOPTA	Gadobenate dimeglumine	MULTIHANCE®	Bracco
Gd-DTPA-BMA	Gadodiamide	OMNISCAN®	General Electric Healthcare
Mn-DPDP	Mangafodipir trisodium	TESLASCAN®	General Electric Healthcare
Gd-DOTA	Gadoterate meglumine	DOTAREM®	Guerbet
Gd-DTPA-BMEA	Gadoversetamide	OPTIMARK®	Tyco Healthcare

[1]) International Nonproprietary Name

Quite analogously, the optional modes for intravascular contrast agents may be presented according to these target components.

1.2.1 Cellular Target Component: Erythrocyte-bound or Liposomal Systems

So far it has not been possible to advance research strategies on intravascular MR contrast agents based on direct coupling or on cytoplasmatic »loading« of erythrocytes through to clinical development, owing to the excessive quantities of contrast agent that were required [9]. However, a vascular circulation pattern similar to that in natural cells has been observed in liposomal, cell-like systems, whereby liposomes could be formed with compartments separated by a double lipid layer similar to a cell membrane. Iron, manganese, or gadolinium complexes could be trapped in their aqueous inner space and thus transported into the circulatory system. However, the compounds investigated so far were not stable over a long period and became rapidly metabolized by the reticuloendothelial system (RES) [10].

1.2.2 Aqueous Target Component: Macromolecules – Polymers, Iron-oxide Particles and Covalently Bound Metal Complexes

The systems within this subcategory are characterized by their inherent or, in the case of covalently bound systems, their effective macromolecular size, which is why they are subject to extravasation to only a small degree, if at all. Only large Gd-based systems and coated iron-oxide particles are discussed here, as some of these compounds are currently undergoing preclinical or clinical development, respectively. An example of the first group is Gadomer [11], a dendritic macromolecule, in which 24 Gd^{3+} ions are bound. Its molecular weight is approximately 17 kDa. This was the origin of the previous name, Gadomer-17, for this dendrimeric concept developed by Bayer Schering Pharma AG. The investigational drug successfully underwent preclinical evaluation for various indications, such as coronary angiography [12] and lymphography [13]. Another example is gadomeritol (Vistarem®, P792, Guerbet) [14], whose intravascular properties are also based on molecular size. Gadomeritol also shows rapid clearance through glomerular filtration [15]. Gadomer and gadomeritol are highly intravascular contrast agents in the strict sense with limited blood pool characteristics (fast- clearing intravascular contrast agents).

In terms of very small superparamagnetic iron oxide particles (*ultrasmall superparamagnetic iron oxide (USPIO), very small superparamagnetic iron oxide (VSOP)*), reference is made to VSOP-C184 (Ferropharm GmbH) [16], ferumoxtran-10 (Sinerem®, Guerbet, Combidex®, Advanced Magnetics) [17,18], and Ferucarbotran (Supravist®, SH U 555 C, Bayer Schering Pharma AG) [19,20]. These compounds are partially also being investigated for other than MRA indications, such as lymphography.

1.2.3 Proteins as Target Component: Non-covalently Bound Metal Complexes

This group of innovative MR contrast agents includes Gadofosveset (Vasovist®) as the only blood pool contrast agent currently (January 2008) approved in the 27 member states of the European Union and several other countries, including Switzerland, Norway, Turkey, Canada and Australia. An increase in retention time in the vascular system is achieved by reversible binding of the magnetically active metal complex specifically to the most prevalent albumin [human serum albumin (HSA)] in the plasma. An essential feature is the non-covalent type of binding between the contrast agent molecule and the plasma protein, which distinguishes this type of intravascular contrast agent from those molecules which bind permanently to large proteins or cells. Nevertheless, a high fraction of binding can be achieved with this concept, and both a significantly longer retention time and greatly reduced extravasation combined with generally good tolerance are therefore ensured [21].

For the bound fraction in blood, the concentration of the contrast agent molecule is observed to be largely independent of the relative concentrations of proteins in the dynamic equilibrium, which is quickly attained after venous injection. This and other characteristics will be examined in detail below, based on the example of Gadofosveset.

1.3 Molecular Structure and Physicochemical Properties

The molecular structure of Gadofosveset is shown in ◻ Fig. 1.1 and in a 3-D model in ◻ Fig. 1.2. The molecule can be divided into two functional entities. The first, MR-active, part is formed by the stable chelate structure of the gadolinium acid, gadolinium diethylenetriaminepentaacetic acid, Gd-DTPA [22]. The cation Gd^{3+} bound within this structure and the dipole-dipole interactions of its unpaired electron spin (S = 7/2) lead to strong decreases in

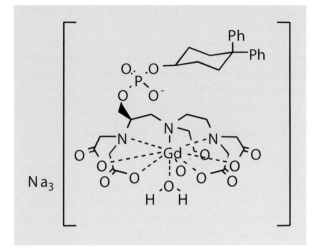

Fig. 1.1. Molecular structure of Gadofosveset

nuclear spin relaxation times, especially of proton spins ($I = \frac{1}{2}$) of the H_2O in the immediate molecular vicinity.

The innovative, additional properties of Vasovist®, on the other hand, are achieved by the second functional entity, a diphenylcyclohexyl group covalently bound with the Gd complex via a phosphate diester bridge. This enhances the hydrophilic character of the molecule and allows reversible, non-covalent binding of the molecule with albumin.

Further properties are provided in **Table 1.2** [6,23].

The active substance consists of the metal complex as described (stable up to 282°C), which, as a white powder, has a low solubility for organic solvents but a very high water solubility.

The administered formula of Vasovist® consists of a 250-mM (244 mg/ml) aqueous solution of the active substance with a 0.1% excess (by mass) of the ligand.

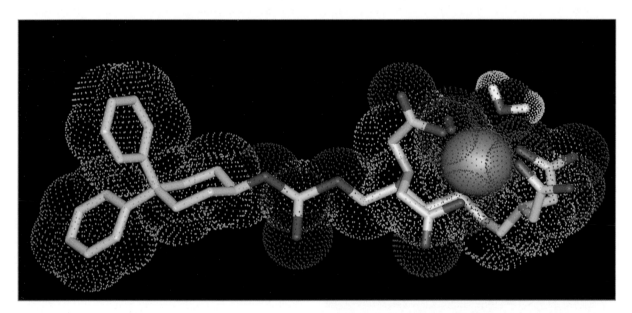

Fig. 1.2. Three-dimensional model of the active substance of Gadofosveset. The chelate structure with the Gd^{3+} atom (gray) may be seen on the right.

Table 1.2. Physicochemical properties of Vasovist®

Viscosity	at 20°C	3.0 mPa·s
Density	at 25°C	1.12 g/ml
Osmolarity	at 37°C	825 mOsm/kg
pH	Ready-to-use solution	6.5–8.0
Relaxivity r_1 in H_2O	at 37°C, 1.5 T, 0.5 mM	(5.2 ± 0.3) l mmol^{-1} s^{-1}
Relaxivity r_1 in bovine plasma	at 37°C, 1.5 T, 0.5 mM	$(19 \pm)$ l mmol^{-1} s^{-1}

1.4   Biophysical Properties – Reversible Protein Binding

As described in the previous section, the diphenylcyclohexyl group (linked to the Gd complex via a phosphate diester bridge) leads to the specific, reversible binding of the molecule to albumin [22,23].

A spatial depiction of the molecule reversibly bound to a protein binding site is shown in ▢ Fig. 1.3. It is not a chemical process in the strict sense; rather the temporary link is based on structural molecular properties and on the formation of weak hydrogen bridges between the protein and the diphenylcyclohexyl group from the contrast agent molecule.

The key effects of these unique binding properties on the contrast agent effects are well-known phenomenologically: they are first to be found in modified pharmaco*kinetics* compared with conventional extracellular contrast agents, which result in a significantly longer retention time for the active substance in blood circulation. In the bound state, the contrast agent is not subject to glomerular filtration in the kidneys, i.e. only a small part – according to the non-bound fraction at the time – is filtered out of circulation in the kidneys. Extravasation is also largely reduced, as this is limited to the non-bound fraction of the active substance in the blood.

The second key effect lies in the influence on pharmaco*dynamics* and consists essentially of a considerably increased relaxivity compared with conventional extracellular contrast agents. This principle of increasing relaxivity through reversible protein binding was first described

under the title *Receptor-induced magnetization enhancement (RIME)* [24].

The special characteristics of the pharmacokinetics and pharmacodynamics are interdependent owing to their common origins via protein binding, which is described in the following section.

1.4.1   Pharmacokinetics – Prolonged Retention Time

Different retention times are shown schematically in ▢ Fig. 1.4 for both a conventional extracellular and a slow-clearing intravascular contrast agent with extended retention time in the vascular system. The representation qualitatively illustrates that an initial bolus phase exists in both cases; in the case of an intravascular contrast agent with extended retention time, this is followed by an »equilibrium phase« or »steady state«.

Let us take a closer look at the special pharmacokinetics of Gadofosveset: Following injection, there is initially a high local concentration of Gadofosveset in blood. Due to its specific binding affinity to albumin, the fraction of the bound Gadofosveset molecules depends both on the local albumin concentration and on the local Gadofosveset concentration. At very high Gadofosveset concentrations (»excess Gadofosveset«), the binding fraction is, of course, lower than at low Gadofosveset concentrations (»excess albumin«). This is shown in ▢ Fig. 1.5 for plasma solutions under different example conditions [25]: Accordingly, below the respective minimum concentrations there is a plateau range with an almost constant fraction of bound molecules.

For the pharmacokinetics in the initial phase after injection this means that the relative binding share has to rise from a small initial value (with very high local Ga-

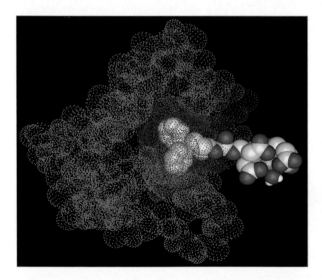

▢ **Fig. 1.3.** A binding site of a protein structure (extract from the much larger total protein) with the non-covalently bound contrast agent molecule Gadofosveset. The phosphate groups are located in the binding pocket of the protein (center of the image). The chelate structure containing the Gd ion (gray) may be seen on the right.

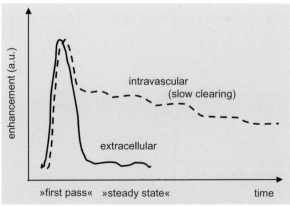

▢ **Fig. 1.4.** Schematic representation of the available signal enhancements for conventional extracellular (*solid line*) and slow-clearing intravascular contrast agents (*dashed line*).

dofosveset concentration) to an equilibrium state. This is shown in ▣ Fig. 1.6 with measurements from a preclinical investigation in primates [26], especially well-suited for illustration purposes due to the relatively high dose used of 0.1 mmol/kg. The initial rise in the albumin-bound percentage fraction and the arrival at the plateau at approximately 80–85% for this species can be clearly seen.

Obviously, the time course of the protein-bound fraction has a direct influence on the pharmacokinetics: Because only the unbound fraction is subject to renal filtration, elimination from the vascular system is faster at first until an approximately homogeneous distribution is attained in the total blood volume. Furthermore, the un-

bound fraction is subject to extravasation, into the interstitial space or by passage of a defect blood-brain barrier.

The two half-lives $t_{1/2\alpha}$ and $t_{1/2\beta}$ must be taken into consideration for an accurate, quantitative description of the pharmacokinetics of Gadofosveset; these characterize the typical initial ($t_{1/2\alpha} = 0.48 \pm 0.11$ h) and the subsequent time course ($t_{1/2\beta} = 16.3 \pm 2.6$ h) of the Gadofosveset concentration in blood. In ▣ Fig. 1.7 this is depicted on the basis of the results of a clinical licensing study over a period of 48 h after injection [27]. From the logarithmic scale of the parameter axes (plasma concentration in mmol/l) the typical, averaged half-lives $t_{1/2\alpha}$ and $t_{1/2\beta}$ may be recognized in the early and the later time points, respectively.

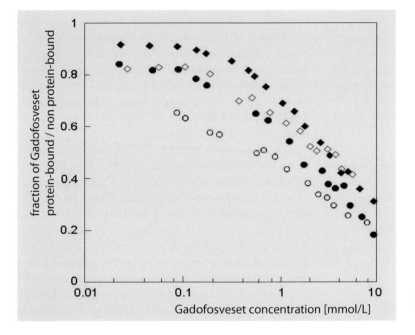

▣ **Fig. 1.5.** Fraction of protein-bound Gadofosveset as a function of concentration in serum albumin from different species: ◆ Human, ● Rabbit, ◊ Pig, ○ Rat. Derived from [25]

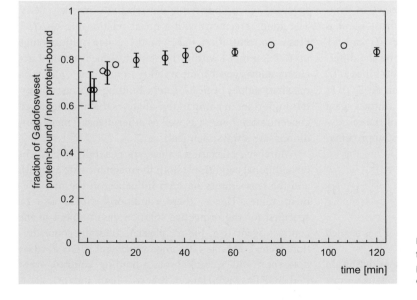

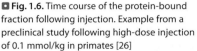

▣ **Fig. 1.6.** Time course of the protein-bound fraction following injection. Example from a preclinical study following high-dose injection of 0.1 mmol/kg in primates [26]

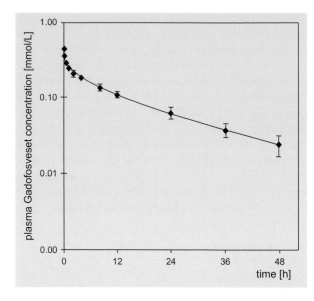

Fig. 1.7. Logarithmic presentation of the bi-exponential pharmacokinetics of Gadofosveset. Early time points can be assigned to the initial distribution phase ($t_{1/2\alpha}$), whereas the much longer distribution phase ($t_{1/2\beta}$) is reflected by the straight section of the graph

The half-life labeled here with disposition phase and characterized by ($t_{1/2\beta}$) is also known as the (terminal) plasma elimination time. It has to be distinguished from the terminal elimination time $t_{1/2term}$, with which the active substance is eliminated not only from the vascular system, but also from the organism. For Vasovist® this is $t_{1/2term}$ = 18.5 ±3 h [27].

1.4.2 Pharmacodynamics – Relaxivity

The reduction in the longitudinal (T_1) and transversal (T_2) relaxation times of the proton spin detected by magnetic resonance imaging with an MR contrast agent is quantitatively described by relaxivity values (r_1 and r_2). The definition of r_i (with i = 1, 2) is given by the difference in the relaxation rates (inverse relaxation times $1/T_i$) of a solution with and without contrast agent ($1/T_{i(0)}$). In the definition, there is also division by the contrast agent concentration, which yields independence of the relaxivity values from the concentration in the first approximation [28]:

$$r_i = \left(\frac{1}{T_i} - \frac{1}{T_{i(0)}} \right) \cdot \frac{1}{[CM]} \quad i = 1, 2 \qquad \text{Eq. (1)}$$

The contrast medium concentration (in mmol/l) is termed [CM].

Equation (1) is obviously a very expedient definition for the relaxivities, especially for conventional contrast

agents, which have little or no interaction with plasma proteins. The difference in the relaxation rates ($1/T_i$ – $1/T_{i(0)}$) is often abbreviated as $\Delta 1/T_i$. $\Delta 1/T_i$ represents the actual observed reduction in relaxation times under the given conditions quantitatively and is therefore one of the most important parameters to describe contrast agent effects in MRI. The $\Delta 1/T_i$ measurement values are often entered in a graph as a function of concentration [CM]. For non-protein-binding contrast agents a good approximation to a linear fit is obtained, whose constant slope ($\Delta 1/T_i)/\Delta[CM]$ corresponds to the respective relaxivity r_i.

However, for MR contrast media which interact appreciably with proteins and whose relaxivity is influenced by protein binding – which is the case for Vasovist® and some other MR contrast agents – there is also a clear dependence of the reduction in relaxation time on the relative concentration of the respective plasma proteins as well as on the concentration of the contrast agent. The relaxivity can therefore no longer be described by a straight line over a large concentration range in this case [29,30]. This is shown in Fig. 1.8 for Vasovist® on the basis of results from a clinical study [27].

As is apparent in Fig. 1.8, the slope ($\Delta 1/T_i)/\Delta[CM]$ of the curve falls with higher concentrations as anticipated, because the relative fraction of bound molecules – as described above – is lower at higher Gadofosveset concentrations. At the same time, Fig. 1.8 also shows that the deviation from linearity in the concentration range shown is moderate overall and especially at low concentrations below 0.1 mmol/l is negligible. This means that relaxation values measured at concentrations up to 0.1 mmol/l cannot necessarily be extrapolated to very high concentrations. According to international recommendations for the nomenclature of MR contrast agent parameters [28], the concentration should also be specified when specifying the relaxivity in such cases. The good agreement with a linear relationship of $\Delta 1/T_i$ versus concentration [CM] in the concentration range up to 0.5 mmol/l within the statistical measurement accuracy allows good comparability in this range, also with relaxivity values of non-protein-binding contrast agents. It is important in comparative analyses that the measured concentration ranges, as well as other measurement conditions, are always identical.

Moreover, relaxation values are generally dependent on additional conditions: Both the magnetic field strength and the temperature have an influence on the measurement values. Hence, these conditions should also be specified for the respective solution environment of the contrast agent (e.g. blood, plasma, albumin concentration, water). Table 1.3 compares several values for Gadofosveset and a weak protein-binding contrast agent (Gd-BOPTA, MultiHance®, Bracco, Milan, Italy).

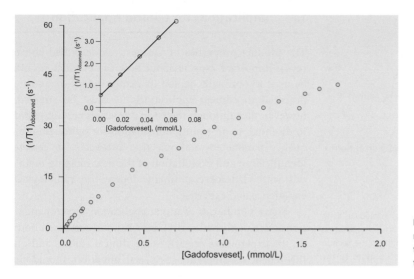

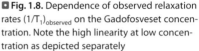

Fig. 1.8. Dependence of observed relaxation rates $(1/T_1)_{observed}$ on the Gadofosveset concentration. Note the high linearity at low concentration as depicted separately

Table 1.3. Relaxivity values[1] for Gadofosveset and a weak protein-binding MR contrast agent measured in bovine plasma at concentrations up to 0.5 mmol/l. Temperature at 1.5–4.7 T: 37°C [6]

	0.47 T [2]		1.5 T		3 T		4.7 T	
	r_1	r_2	r_1	r_2	r_1	r_2	r_1	r_2
Vasovist®	28 (27-29)	40 (38-42)	19 (18-20)	34 (32-36)	9.9 (9.4-10.4)	60 (56-64)	6.9 (6.6-7.2)	60 (57-63)
MultiHance	9.2 (8.7-9.7)	12.9 (12.2-13.6)	6.3 (6.0-6.6)	8.7 (7.8-9.6)	5.5 (5.2-5.8)	11.0 (10.0-12.0)	5.2 (4.9-5.5)	10.8 (10.1-11.5)

[1]values in l mmol^{-1} s^{-1}; [2]measured at 40 °C

1.4.3 Causes for Increased Relaxivity Due to Protein Binding

Within the theoretical framework given here, a simplified, illustrative description of the biophysical relationships is provided to make the increased relaxivity due to protein binding comprehensible. Mathematical presentations will not be offered; instead reference is made to some reviews on relaxation theory [31,32,33,34].

As with other gadolinium-based MR contrast agents, magnetic interactions take place between unpaired electron spins (= paramagnetic center) of the Gd^{3+} cation bound to the complex (S = 7/2) and unpaired nuclear spins from the solution environment of the molecule. The nuclear spins are essentially attributable to protons (hydrogen nuclei) from neighboring H_2O molecules. The known reduction in nuclear spin relaxation times arises from the much larger magnetic moment of electron spins compared with proton spins. The magnetic moment of the unpaired electrons can be viewed as a local disturbance or an additional, fluctuating, and highly inhomogeneous magnetic field for the nuclear spins.

The precise mechanisms on a molecular level are divided into contributions based on interactions with protons in direct coordination with the metal ion of the complex – inner-sphere effects – and those based on more distant protons above the second coordination level and also diffusing protons – outer-sphere effects (see **Fig. 1.9**) [31,32].

For paramagnetic metal complexes, the contributions can largely be described mathematically with the Solomon-Bloembergen-Morgan equation [35]. The magnetic interactions between electron and nuclear spins are described here with anisotropic dipole-dipole interactions and scalar Fermi-contact interactions. The contributions to longitudinal relaxation of the first coordination level (inner sphere), which usually dominate, depend on the number of transiently bound water molecules (hydration number) and their relaxation time (T_{1m}), as well as on

1

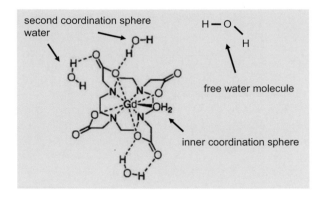

❏ **Fig. 1.9.** Representation of three classes of water molecules with regard to the Gd complex. The molecules from the first coordination level (inner sphere) are directly coordinated with Gd(III); in the second coordination level (2nd sphere) there are hydrogen bridges to the complex

the average time (τ_m) for the coordination of these water molecules with the metal ion.

The latter factor, the average time (τ_m) for the co-ordination of individual water molecules on the metal complex (which corresponds to the inverse exchange rate k_{ex}) is worthy of closer examination. Intuitively, a longer average period of presence of the directly influenced water molecule in the immediate vicinity of the Gd complex can also contribute to a more pronounced reduction in overall relaxation times. It is similarly intuitive that τ_m is influenced by the respective characteristic times of molecular movements, such as rotation, vibration and diffusion: If there are slower molecular movements (e.g., caused by Brownian motion due to lower temperature, by higher viscosity of the solution environment, and in larger molecules) the respective values for τ_m are correspondingly larger and the relaxation time reduction achieved increases.

The molecular movements are characterized by correlation times; the rotation correlation time is abbreviated by τ_r for example. The molecular dimensions of proteins, such as serum albumin, are several orders of magnitude above those of low-molecular-weight Gd complexes. Hence, the contrast agent molecule experiences a strong increase in its effective rotational correlation time of around two orders of magnitude (factor 100) as a result of protein binding. Correspondingly, the much slower motions in the protein-bound state are expressed by a *de*creased rotation rate [31]. The average period of presence τ_m of the water molecules coordinated with the Gd complex is thereby significantly increased as a consequence, accompanied by the strong increase in the relaxivity of Gadofosveset through protein binding.

1.5   Implications for Clinical Application

The product properties of Vasovist® as described above reveal important aspects about how the product should be used to optimally exploit its extraordinary diagnostic potential in clinical applications. It must be stressed, however, that although the basic properties certainly lead to essential, trend-setting information for optimizing sequence parameters and injection protocols, successive identification and exploitation of the new imaging methods with Gadofosveset finally depend on radiological experience and expertise.

Some summaries of initial application recommendations were published early [36,37,38] and are based both on the experiences of early-stage clinical studies and on theoretical considerations. Special attention should be drawn to the chapters of this book describing clinical applications as well as to the previous publications on selected studies [39,40,41], which also examine technical application aspects. However, some fundamental aspects of first pass and steady state applications are described in the following sections.

1.5.1   Relevant Implications for Application in the First Pass

As a result of its considerably higher relaxivity, a significantly lower gadolinium dosage of 0.03 mmol/kg body weight compared with conventional contrast agents could be found for MRA with Gadofosveset. This results in around one third of the standard dose of conventional contrast agents of 0.1 mmol/kg body weight. Bearing in mind the concentration of 0.25 mol/l of the ready-to-use solution (compared with 0.5 mol/l for most other contrast agents), the volume-related dose is 0.12 ml/kg body weight.

As with any other conventional contrast agent, Vasovist® can be intravenously administered manually or with an automatic injection system for first pass MRA. All the well-established techniques regarding bolus dynamics and correct timing are the same as with first pass MRA using conventional contrast agents. The situation in a patient to be examined can be determined with a test bolus of 1 ml volume prior to the measurement itself. The parameters covered here are: the individual synchronization of bolus injection, arrival time of the bolus in the target region, and the start of measurement. Alternatively, the respective manufacturer's »fluoroscopic« methods of bolus detection with fast 2D imaging of suitable target regions can be carried out in real-time (for example BolusTrack, CareBolus or SMARTprep). A saline flush following the injection is obligatory.

To obtain a comparable length of the contrast agent bolus and, at the same time, to use the tested relationship between the period of injection, scan delay, and data acquisition as established with 0.5-molar contrast agents, the Vasovist® injection rate can be adapted as follows:

Example case: A protocol using the standard dose of 0.1 mmol/kg of a 0.5-molar contrast agent has become established for a specific MRA application. For a patient with 75 kg body weight, a typical volume of 15 ml was injected at a rate of 3 ml/s over a period of 5 s. According to the standard dosage for a 75-kg patient, the Vasovist® contrast agent volume is 9 ml. To reproduce the same injection period with the lower volume, Vasovist® requires a roughly 1/3 reduced injection rate in this case. Consequently, the volume of 9 ml should be applied at 2 ml/s in 4.5 s in this case.

Comparison with the common application of a double or triple dose of conventional MR contrast agent yields even more pronounced variations. For instance, comparing the »double dose« of 0.2 mmol/kg body weight of a conventional MR contrast agent with Vasovist®, the Gd standard dose is reduced by 85% and the injection volume by 70% (9 ml instead of 30 ml).

In principle, the specific pharmacodynamics caused by protein binding (including higher relaxivity and concentration dependence) described in the last section could also be taken into account for the initial bolus phase to optimize the sequence parameters. However, the lower binding fraction in the initial bolus is offset by the very high initial concentration of Vasovist®, so that, all in all, it can be safely assumed that this *relative* effect is overcompensated by the effect of the *absolute* very high local concentration of Vasovist® to produce the actual reduction in T_1 relaxation time.

Hence, this aspect appears rather insignificant for most clinical applications and therefore adaptation of sequence parameters (e.g. flip angle) to improve image quality would not appear worthwhile in most practical cases. This is supported by quantitative estimates as well as by current experience, which shows the use of established sequence parameters with the common, fast 3D gradient echo sequences to produce excellent results in first pass MRA using Vasovist®.

1.5.2 Relevant Implications for Application in the Steady State

The situation in the later acquisition phases, i.e., advanced distribution throughout the entire vascular system, differs from the well-known first pass, as described previously. The situation in the steady state can certainly be viewed as generally far simpler and easier to calculate, as both the spatial and temporal dynamics have changed from the contrast agent bolus rapidly propagating in the vascular system with inhomogeneous concentration distribution into a now homogeneous distribution and

approximate temporal equilibrium. This applies particularly to the period of time following the actual distribution phase, whose start is very much dependent on the individual circulatory parameters of the respective patient. For patients with normal cardiovascular function, an approximately homogeneous distribution may be assumed after just a few circulation cycles within the first 3–5 min after injection, whereas in patients with cardiac insufficiency or other relevant diseases of the circulatory system, complete distribution can take up to 10 min, according to current knowledge. These precursory comments are in no way intended to imply that acquisition prior to the attainment of a homogeneous distribution should be generally avoided. Rather, it should be pointed out that, dependent on the individual circulatory parameters, relative fluctuation in arterial and venous contrast enhancement is still to be expected during the later distribution phase.

Assuming a homogeneous distribution of the protein-binding contrast agent in the entire vascular system in the steady state, the blood pool agent is generally further diluted compared with the initially higher concentration of a bolus in the first pass. This dilution effect also leads to somewhat longer relaxation times compared with the first pass, even for the very high relaxivity of Gadofosveset. The anticipated order of magnitude of T_1 is therefore estimated in the following simple example calculation [36].

Estimation of T_1 in the steady state on the basis of an example calculation:

Body weight:	*75 kg*
Total blood volume:	*5.5 l*
Vasovist® standard dose:	*0.03 mmol / kg*
Individual Gd dose:	*2.25 mmol*
Vasovist® injected concentration:	*0.25 mmol/l*
Vasovist® injected volume:	*9 ml*
Calculated maximum concentration [CM]max:	*0.45 mmol/l*
Estimated concentration following initial distribution phase 80% of [CM]max; [CM]:	*0.36 mmol/l*

Entering typical values for the non-enhanced longitudinal relaxation time in blood $T_{1(0)}$ and for the relaxivity r_1 of Vasovist® under the given standard conditions:

$T_{1(0)}^{-1} = 0.8\ s^{-1}$ (equivalent to 1.25 s = $T_{1(0)}$ of blood)
$r_1 = 19\ l\ mmol^{-1}\ s^{-1}$ (measured in whole blood at 37 °C, 1.5 T, 0.5 mM concentration) [6],

and using the general relationship between relaxivity, concentration and relaxation times (Eq. 1)

$$T_1^{-1} = T_{1(0)}^{-1} + r_1 \cdot [CM]$$

The estimated relaxation rate T_1^{-1} in blood is derived as:

$9.35 \ s^{-1} = 0.8 \ s^{-1} + 19 \ l \ mmol^{-1} \ s^{-1} \cdot 0.36 \ mmol \ l^{-1}$

and the corresponding reciprocal value for the estimated relaxation time T_1 of approx. 130 ms. Dependent on the exact time of observation and on widely varying individual physiological conditions, T_1 can be used to calculate relaxation times of approx. 100–200 ms.

In comparison, T_1 relaxation times of 20 ms and below can exist in the bolus for first pass MRA due to the higher contrast agent concentrations here. It is quite obvious that the common protocols for fast 3D gradient echo sequences established for contrast-enhanced MRA, for example, allow leeway for optimization in the steady state with Vasovist®: The sequence protocols implemented for MRI scanners are generally optimized for shorter first pass relaxation times, especially in regard to the signal intensity as a function of the parameters flip angle, echo time (TE), repetition time (TR), and relaxation times.

Accordingly, the parameter changes in the steady state tend towards smaller flip angles and longer repetition times, whereby optimization of the flip angle is calculated with the Ernst angle α:

$$\alpha = \arccos(\exp(-TR/T_1)) \qquad \text{Eq. (2)}$$

The option also arises of acquiring images with Vasovist® in the steady state over an extended period of time with a considerable increase in spatial resolution. There are different ways for 3D gradient echo sequences to achieve this without sacrificing signal-to-noise ratio. One of these is to increase the repetition time (for example in the 8- to 15-ms range), to select the flip angles smaller (approximately 15°–25°), to keep TE at the minimum, and to reduce the detection bandwidth, as appropriate. A complementary strategy would be to improve the signal-to-noise ratio by increasing the number of acquisitions, while maintaining TR short in the usual range (for example 4–7 ms), but to lower the flip angle by around 10° to account for the longer T_1. The latter method can be considered, for example, for body regions that are subject to respiratory motions, and may be applied in conjunction with respiratory triggering and advanced navigator techniques.

Specific descriptions and sequence parameters found for various regions of examination are described in the following chapters.

References

1 Claussen C, Laniado M, Schorner W, et al (1985) Gadolinium-DTPA in MR imaging of glioblastomas and intracranial metastases. AJNR Am J Neuroradiol 6:669–674
2 Weinmann H-J, Brasch RC, Press WR, et al (1984) Characteristics of gadolinium-DTPA complex: a potential NMR contrast agent. AJR Am J Roentgenol 142:619–624
3 Carr DH, Brown J, Bydder GM, et al (1984) Intravenous chelated gadolinium as a contrast agent in NMR imaging of cerebral tumours. Lancet 1:484–486
4 Runge VM, Carollo BR, Wolf CR, et al (1989) Gd DTPA: a review of clinical indications in central nervous system magnetic resonance imaging. Radiographics 9:929–958

Take home messages

- Based on unpaired electrons and their paramagnetic properties, MRI contrast media shorten proton spin relaxation times in vivo. Thereby enhancing the most important contrast mechanism in MRI, they provide a valuable option for obtaining additional diagnostic information.

- The most frequently applied class of MRI-CM consists of 0.5-molar, Gd-based metal complexes with extracellular biodistribution and fast glomerular filtration via the kidneys. Other concepts include a highly concentrated 1.0-molar contrast medium, coated superparamagnetic iron oxide (SPIO) particles, and liver-specific Gd-based MRI-CM with weak protein binding.

- Blood pool MRI-CM have been developed, but so far only godofosveset, based on non-covalent and reversible binding to serum albumin, has success-fully undergone clinical development and received market authorization.

- The mode of action of Gadofosveset is characterized basically by the two effects of the reversible protein binding: 1. significantly increased relaxivity in the protein-bound state; 2. vastly prolonged retention time in the vascular system, providing much longer imaging windows of up to 1 h (slow clearing, intravascular).

- In addition to the well-known first pass imaging, the blood pool properties and the much longer period of T1 shortening (steady state) of Gadofosveset overcome the limitations of conventional extracellular MRI-CM, for example poor resolution in peripheral MRA.

- Application of Gadofosveset for both first pass and steady state MRA is easily achieved, and is optimized in the steady state by minor protocol adaptations.

5 Knopp MV, Balzer T, Esser M, Kashanian FK, Paul P, Niendorf HP (2006) Assessment of utilization and pharmacovigilance based on spontaneous adverse event reporting of gadopentetate dimeglumine as a magnetic resonance contrast agent after 45 million administrations and 15 years of clinical use. Invest Radiol 41:491–499

6 Rohrer M, Bauer H, Mintorovitch J, Requardt M, Weinmann H-J (2005) Comparison of magnetic properties of MRI contrast media solutions at different magnetic field strengths. Invest Radiol 40:715–724

7 Bogdanov Jr. A, Lewin M, Weissleder R (1999) Approaches and agents for imaging the vascular system. Adv Drug Delivery Rev 37:279-293

8 Jacques V, Desreux JF (2002) New classes of MRI contrast agents. Top Curr Chem 221:123–164

9 Nunn AD, Liner KE, Tweedle MF (1997) Can receptors be imaged with MRI agents? Q J Nucl Med 41:155-162

10 Fossheim SL, Colet J-M, Mansson S, Fahlvik AK, Muller RN, Klaveness J (1998) Paramagnetic liposomes as magnetic resonance imaging contrast agents: assessment of contrast efficacy in various liver models. Invest Radiol 33:810–821

11 Misselwitz B, Schmitt-Willich H, Ebert W, Frenzel T, Weinmann H-J (2001) Pharmacokinetics of gadomer-17, a new dendritic magnetic resonance contrast agent. Mag Reson Materials Physics, Biol Med 12 128–134

12 Li D, Zheng J, Weinmann H-J (2001) Contrast-enhanced MR imaging of coronary arteries: comparison of intra- and extravascular contrast agents in swine. Radiology 218:670–678

13 Misselwitz B, Schmitt-Willich H, Michaelis M, Oellinger JJ (2002) Interstitial magnetic resonance lymphography T1 contrast agent: initial experience with gadomer-17. Invest Radiol 37:146–151

14 Port M, Corot C, Rousseaux O, et al (2001) P792: a rapid clearance blood pool agent for magnetic resonance imaging: preliminary results. MAGMA 12:121–127

15 Port M, Corot C, Raynal I, et al (2001) Physicochemical and biological evaluation of P792, a rapid clearance blood pool agent for magnetic resonance imaging. Invest Radiol 36:445–454

16 Taupitz M, Wagner S, Schnorr J, Kravec I, Pilgrimm H, Bergmann-Fritsch H, Hamm B (2004) Phase I clinical evaluation of citrate-coated monocrystalline very small superparamagnetic iron oxide particles as a new contrast medium for magnetic resonance imaging. Invest Radiol 39:394–405

17 Anzai Y, Prince MR, Chenevert TL, et al (1997) MR angiography with an ultrasmall superparamagnetic iron oxide blood pool agent. J Magn Reson Imaging 7:209–214

18 Kellar KE, Fujii DK, Gunther WH, et al (2000) NC100150 injection, a preparation of optimized iron oxide nanoparticles for positive-contrast MR angiography. J Magn Reson Imaging 11:488–494

19 Clarke SE, Weinmann H-J, Dai E, et al (2000) Comparison of two blood pool contrast agents for 0.5-T MR angiography: experimental study in rabbits. Radiology 214:787–794

20 Tombach B, Reimer P, Bremer C, Allkemper T, Engelhardt M, Mahler M, Ebert W, Heindel W (2004) First pass and equilibrium-MRA of the aortoiliac region with a superparamagnetic iron oxide blood pool MR contrast agent (SH U 555 C): results of a human pilot study. NMR Biomed 17:500–506

21 Steger-Hartmann T, Graham PB, Müller S, Schweinfurth H (2006) Preclinical safety assessment of Vasovist (gadofosveset trisodium), a new magnetic resonance imaging contrast agent for angiography. Invest Radiol 41:449–459

22 Farooki A, Narra V, Brown J (2004) Gadofosveset EPIX/Schering. Curr Opin Invest Drugs 5:967–976

23 Caravan P, Cloutier NJ, Greenfield MT, McDermid SA, Dunham SU, Bulte JWM, Amedio JC, Looby RJ, Supkowski RM, Horrocks WDeW, McMurry TJ, Lauffer RB (2002) The interaction of MS-325 with human serum albumin and its effect on proton relaxation rates. J Am Chem Soc 124:3152–3162

24 Lauffer RB (1991) Targeted relaxation enhancement agents for MRI. Magn Reson Med 22:339–342

25 Eldredge HB, Spiller M, Chasse JM, Greenwood MT, Caravan P (2006) Species dependence on plasma protein binding and relaxivity of the gadolinium-based MRI contrast agent MS-325. Invest Radiol 41:229–243

26 Parmelee DJ, Walovitch RC, Ouellet HS, Lauffer RB (1997) Preclinical evaluation of the pharmacokinetics, biodistribution, and elimination of MS-325, a blood pool agent for magnetic resonance imaging. Invest Radiol 32:741–747

27 Clinical Study Report MS-325-06, Clinical Summary 2.7.2. Schering AG

28 EMRF (European Magnetic Resonance Forum Foundation) (1997) Recommendations for the nomenclature of MR imaging contrast agent terms. Acta Radiol 38:5

29 Port M, Corot C, Violas X, et al (2005) How to compare the efficiency of albumin-bound and nonalbumin-bound contrast agents in vivo: the concept of dynamic relaxivity. Invest Radiol 40:565–573

30 de Haen C, Calabi L, La Ferla R (2002) The problematic determination of proton magnetic relaxation rates of protein-containing solutions. Acad Radiol 9 [Suppl 1]:S2–4

31 Lauffer RB (1987) Metal complexes as water proton relaxation agents for NMR imaging: Theory and design. Chem Rev 87:901–927

32 Caravan P, Ellison JJ, McMurry TJ, et al (1999) Gadolinium(III) Chelates as MRI contrast agents: structure, dynamics, and applications. Chem Rev 99:2293–2352

33 Banci L, Bertini I, Luchinat C (1991) Nuclear and electron relaxation: the magnetic nucleus-unpaired electron coupling in solution. Weinheim: VCH

34 Bertini I, Luchinat C (1996) NMR of paramagnetic substances. Coord Chem Rev 150:1–292

35 Bloembergen N, Morgan LO (1961) Proton relaxation times in paramagnetic solutions. Effects of electron spin relaxation. J Chem Phys 34:843–850

36 Hartmann M, Wiethoff AJ, Hentrich H-R, Rohrer M (2006) Initial imaging recommendations for Vasovist angiography. Eur Radiol Suppl 16 [Suppl 2] B15–B23

37 Goyen M, Shamsi K, Schönberg SO (2006) Vasovist-enhanced MR angiography. Eur Radiol 16[Suppl 2] B9–B14

38 Wang MS, Haynor DR, Wilson GJ, Leiner T, Maki JH (2007) Maximizing contrast-to-noise ratio in ultra-high resolution peripheral MR angiography using a blood pool agent and parallel imaging. J Magn Reson Imaging 26:580–588

39 Nikolaou K, Kramer H, Grosse C, Clevert D, Dietrich O, Hartmann M, Chamberlin P, Assmann S, Reiser MF, Schoenberg SO (2006): High-spatial-resolution multistation MR angiography with parallel imaging and blood pool contrast agent: initial experience. Radiology 241: 861–872

40 Rapp JH, Wolff SD et al (2005) Aortoiliac occlusive disease in patients with known or suspected peripheral vascular disease: safety and efficacy of gadofosveset-enhanced MR angiography – multicenter comparative phase III study. Radiology 236:71–78

41 Grist TM et al (1998) Steady state and dynamic MR angiography with MS-325: initial experience in humans. Radiology 207:539–544

Technical Aspects of Contrast Enhanced MRA – First Pass and Steady State

Harald H. Quick

2.1   Introduction

Since its introduction in the mid 1990s [1], contrast-enhanced magnetic resonance angiography (CE-MRA) has increased enormously in impact and today has replaced X-ray-based invasive catheter angiography for numerous diagnostic investigations [2]. From the beginning, MRA applications have been very demanding on the hardware requirements of MR imaging (MRI) scanners. Requiring state-of-the-art equipment, MRA has not just profited from the wide range of software and hardware developments of the recent past, but also has been a driving force behind numerous technical innovations.

In addition to superconducting magnets providing high field strength for a strong magnetization and thus a basis for high signal-to-noise ratio (SNR), the gradient system plays an important role: it must be strong enough to switch the highest possible gradient amplitudes in the shortest possible time to deliver short repetition times (TR) and echo times (TE). The radiofrequency (RF) coils have to receive the precious MRI signal with the very minimum of loss. Phased-array surface RF coil technology here provides a speed-up in acquisition time and enhanced data acquisition flexibility using parallel imaging strategies combined with whole-body surface RF coil coverage of the patient. Finally, technical developments, such as stepwise or even continuously moving table techniques in association with new image acquisition and reconstruction schemes, expand the constraints of a conventional limited field-of-view (FOV) to seamless large-FOV MRA data sets with whole-body MRA coverage.

With the clinical availability of intravascular contrast agents [3,4] such as Vasovist® (Gadofosveset, Bayer Schering Pharma AG, Berlin, Germany) [4-6], contrast-enhanced MRA now has reached another degree of flexibility. Beyond conventional first pass MRA, intravascular contrast agents with their prolonged blood retention times additionally allow for prolonged data acquisition in the steady state of the contrast agent, which potentially can be used to obtain increased spatial resolution, extended anatomic coverage, or, alternatively, to acquire MR venograms with high spatial resolution. In this chapter the general technical aspects of contrast-enhanced MRA as well as the specific aspects of MRA using intravascular contrast agents are discussed.

2.2   Hardware

The usable FOV of an MRI system in general is defined by three hardware groups and their related parameters: 1) the main magnet with its homogeneity over the imaging volume, 2) the gradient system with its linearity over the imaging volume, and 3) the radiofrequency system with its RF signal homogeneity and signal sensitivity over the imaging volume (◘ Fig. 2.1). State-of-the-art MRA imposes very specific demands on these system components of the scanner hardware.

2.2.1   Main Magnet

The magnet of a whole-body MRI scanner should have a high main magnetic field strength, B0, to provide sufficient equilibrium magnetization and therefore a high potential SNR for good image quality. MR scanners with field strengths above 1.0 Tesla or, better yet, 1.5 Tesla are currently viewed as the standard and are increasingly being supplemented with 3-Tesla systems in clinical use. The homogeneity of the basic magnetic field over the examination volume should be as high as possible to ensure low image distortion and high signal homogeneity. The homogeneous examination volume should be as large as possible and should be free of artifacts and distortions. A cylindrical design of the main magnet (solenoid) is conformant with all these requirements and therefore represents the currently most frequently occurring magnet design (◘ Fig. 2.1).

2.2.2   Gradient System

For performing contrast-enhanced MRA, two parameters of the gradient system are critical: a fast gradient slew rate (in [mT/m/ms]) combined with a high gradient amplitude (in [mT/m]) are the prerequisites for short repetition and echo times (TR and TE) and thus for fast imaging and coverage of a large examination volume in the shortest possible time and within the arterial phase of the contrast agent kinetics. This can be seen as a fundamental prerequisite for clinically acceptable examination times and for covering the large volumes of multistation or continuously moving table MRA. Attainment of a short TR is also directly coupled to achieving the highest possible T1 contrast in MRA. This results in high signal of the vasculature filled with T1-shortening contrast agent while signal from the static tissue is saturated, thus providing high vessel-to-background contrast. A high degree of gradient linearity over a large volume is required by the gradient system to keep image distortion in and around the image volume to a minimum. These requirements stated for the gradient system can also be best realized with a cylindrical design (◘ Fig. 2.1).

2.2.3   RF System

The radiofrequency (RF) system of an MRI scanner in general consists of a built-in RF transmit coil for RF

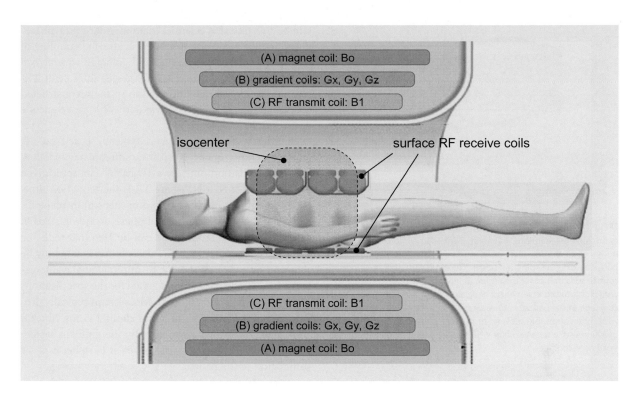

■ **Fig. 2.1A–C.** A sagittal cross-sectional view through a cylindrically shaped MRI scanner. Basically, three different cylindrically shaped sets of coils are implemented into the scanner housing: **(A)** the magnet coil producing the homogeneous static magnetic field B_0 for spin alignment; **(B)** a set of gradient coils producing the time-varying gradient fields, G_x, G_y, and G_z, for spatial encoding of the MR signals as well as **(C)** the transmit radiofrequency (RF) coil that generates an RF field (B_1) for spin excitation inside the patient's body. All three fields (B_0, G_{xyz}, and B_1) are specified such that they form an imaging volume in the isocenter of the magnet bore. Here the fields B_0 and B_1 are very homogeneous and the gradient fields G_{XYZ} are relatively linear. The MR signal response emitted from the excited spins in the patient is detected by a set of local surface RF receiver coils that are placed on above and underneath the anatomic imaging region

excitation of the spins as well as of an RF receiver coil system for receiving the weak RF signals being emitted from the patient. RF excitation of the tissue volume of interest should be as homogeneous as possible. Here it is important that the RF excitation flip angle for signal excitation remain as stable as feasible, as the image contrast is fundamentally influenced by this parameter. Large cylindrical volume transmit RF coils fitted in the cylindrical magnet tunnel are used here, as they fulfill this requirement (■ Fig. 2.1).

On the signal receive side, homogeneous RF signal reception over as large an examination volume as possible is on the list of requirements. However, homogeneity plays a lesser role here compared with signal sensitivity, as inhomogeneous reception intensity affects only the brightness distribution over the volume, but not the underlying image contrast. With regard to the homogeneous volume, the whole-body RF coil permanently fitted in the magnet tunnel also offers an advantage here. For signal reception and the maximum SNR achievable, such a large-volume coil is extremely limited, however.

Hence, diverse concepts with local RF surface coils have come into use. The aim is to receive the signal from the examination region with the highest possible SNR to achieve high image quality with good spatial resolution. Surface RF coils are placed directly over the examination region and receive signals from the immediate vicinity of the examination volume. At the same time, these coils detect the unavoidable noise from a relatively limited region so that the potentially achievable SNR with these coils is relatively high. At the same time, the disadvantage of surface coils lies in their severely restricted sensitivity range. Several coil elements of this type are required to cover larger anatomic regions; they can be combined as phased-array surface coils. Phased-array coils allow optimization of the SNR while extending the region for signal reception (■ Fig. 2.2). For imaging of large regions – up to whole-body MRA applications – a full set of dedicated local phased-array RF surface coils can be combined on state-of-the-art 1.5T and 3.0T MRI systems. A prerequisite for exploiting the advantages inherent in this type of coil technology is a large number of RF receivers to which

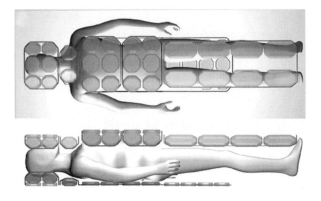

◘ **Fig. 2.2.** Modern radiofrequency (RF) surface coil technology (Siemens Medical Solutions, Erlangen, Germany). While the built-in RF body coil of the MR scanner transmits RF energy into the patient's body to excite the spins, MR signal is received with dedicated local RF surface coils that cover the region of interest. The patient can be covered with a full complement of dedicated RF surface coils. Whole-body coverage of the patient with separate RF surface coils in combination with motorized table movement permits whole-body MRA data acquisition with a relatively high SNR and the combination with parallel imaging techniques

the coil elements can be connected, either individually or in groups. This is also a basic prerequisite for the use of parallel imaging techniques.

2.3   Data Acquisition: from k-Space to MRA Images

The MR signal that is detected by the RF receiver coils in the form of image »raw data« first is collected and stored in a two-dimensional (2D) or a three-dimensional (3D) matrix also termed »k-space«. Following a mathematical operation called fast Fourier-transformation (FFT), these raw data are transformed into 2D or 3D MR images. This context is illustrated in ◘ Fig. 2.3. For 2D data acquisition a 2D matrix of complex data points with the size N_x x N_y is sampled. N_x here is the number of samples along the frequency encoding direction. During each TR interval, an echo is formed and sampled with N_x points and filled into the matrix. N_y TR intervals (phase-encoding steps) are necessary to complete the full 2D matrix. For the 3D case, N_z matrices have to be completed, where N_z is the number of phase-encoding steps in slice direction. Following data acquisition and the completion of the full 2D matrix, the resulting 2D MR image can be reconstructed with a 2D FFT. In the 3D case, k-space is reconstructed with a 3D FFT to a volume stack of 2D MR images.

For contrast-enhanced MRA it is important to synchronize the data acquisition sequence with injection of the contrast agent. For correct contrast timing and to ob-

tain best results, it is essential that the order of the phase-encoding data acquisition scheme is known. Sampling of the central lines of k-space should coincide with arrival of the contrast agent in the target vessels, since central k-space encodes contrast information in the reconstructed MR images while the peripheral parts of k-space encode spatial resolution (◘ Fig. 2.4).

Contrast-enhanced MRA is typically based on 3D gradient-echo sequences with radiofrequency spoiling [7]. The acquisition time for a 3D MRA data set is given by: $TAc = TR \times N_y \times N_z$ where TR is the repetition time, N_y is the number of phase-encoding steps in in-plane direction and N_z is the number of phase-encoding steps in slice direction [7]. From this it can be seen that reducing the acquisition time for a given resolution can simply be achieved by reducing the TR to minimal achievable values. This already has been discussed for the specifications of the gradient system. Modern MR systems typically provide minimal TRs in the range of about 2–5 ms. Shorter TRs might be limited technically by the gradient system or even physiologically by the onset of peripheral nerve stimulation of the patient.

In an effort to reduce the acquisition time with conventional Cartesian Fourier encoding even further, while maintaining the spatial resolution, one has to think about different strategies involving the reduction of phase-encoding steps. This will be discussed in the following section.

2.3.1   Parallel Imaging Strategies

Parallel imaging strategies in MRI are a technique to increase the speed of the MRI acquisition by skipping a number of phase-encoding lines in k-space during the process of MRI data acquisition. The basic idea behind this technique is to employ additional information inherent to the spatial geometry of the signal-receiving RF surface coil elements. Phased-array surface RF coils employing multiple individual coil elements are used to spatially encode the received MR signals. Thus, the time-consuming acquisition of phase-encoding steps, N_y and N_z, can be reduced by a specific reduction factor. Missing information can be reconstructed by the known spatial information provided by the individual signal-receiving coil elements. Two basic parallel imaging techniques exist: SMASH (SiMultaneous Acquisition of Spatial Harmonics) [8] and SENSE (SENSitivity Encoding) [9]. All major vendors of MRI systems to date provide parallel imaging capabilities on their systems that are, in general, based on the generic techniques SMASH and/or SENSE and that differ in their specific implementations. Parallel imaging techniques are also known under the vendor-specific acronyms: SENSE (SENSivity Encoding,

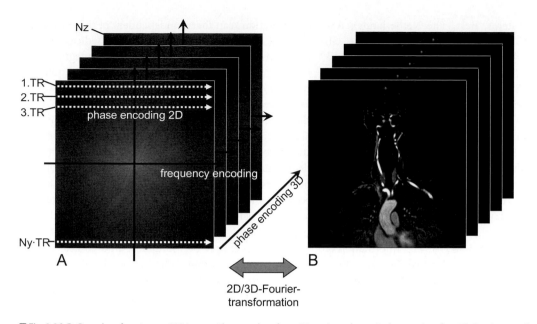

Fig. 2.3A,B. Raw data forming an MR image. The raw data for a 2D image are scanned in the form of an $N_x \times N_y$ dimensioned matrix (**A**). During each repetition time (TR) N_x complex data points are scanned in the frequency-encoding direction and thereby fill a line of the matrix with data. N_y TR times are required to fill the complete raw data matrix. A mathematical operation, fast 2D Fourier transformation (2D FFT), is used to obtain the final MRI image (**B**). In the 3D case, N_z 2D matrices are acquired and the raw data are stored in the form of a 3D-matrix, also denoted as k-space. Accordingly, a 3D FFT transforms 3D k-space into a stack of 2D images covering a 3D imaging volume

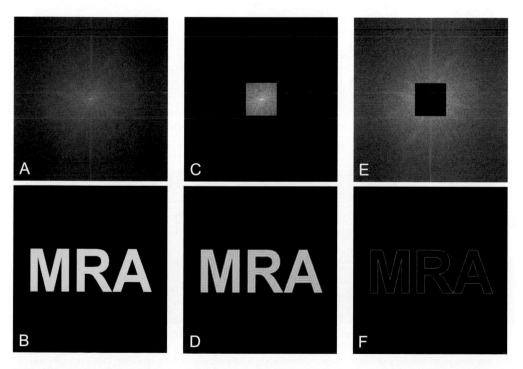

Fig. 2.4A–F. Assignment of different regions of the raw data matrix. The complete raw data matrix (**A**) is required to calculate a corresponding image (**B**). If just the very central part of the raw data matrix (**C**) is reconstructed using 2D Fourier transformation to form an image, it becomes apparent that the contrast for the final image is contained within this part of the raw data matrix (**D**). However, the image (**D**) is still blurred. Conversely, if the outer part of the raw data matrix (**E**) is reconstructed, the edges and fine detail information are obtained (**F**); the resulting image, however, does not contain contrast information and only little signal. The high-signal center of the raw data matrix is therefore of key importance for MRA. This basic knowledge is, for instance, essential for the correct synchronization of contrast agent arrival and the start of data acquisition using contrast agent-enhanced MRA

Philips Medical Systems, Best, The Netherlands); AS-SET (Array Spatial Sensitivity Encoding Technique, GE Medical Systems, Milwaukee, USA); SPEEDER (Toshiba Medical Systems, Tokyo, Japan); iPAT (integrated Parallel Acquisition Techniques, Siemens Medical Solutions, Erlangen, Germany) featuring two reconstruction algorithms mSENSE (modified SENSE) and GRAPPA (Generalized Autocalibrating Partially Parallel Acquisitions) [10,11].

With SMASH this reconstruction is performed on the raw data in k-space, while with SENSE the individual images of the individual coil elements are first reconstructed (◘ Fig. 2.5). These partial images are then added using a mathematical unfolding algorithm. In both basic parallel imaging techniques, SMASH and SENSE, information of the signal sensitivity and of the individual coil element position is used for image reconstruction. This information is obtained by performing an additional short reference or calibration scan that is independent of the subsequent imaging sequences realized by Philips Medical Systems. Alternatively, this calibration scan can be integrated into the imaging sequences by acquisition of a few additional calibration k-space data lines into the imaging sequence as realized by Siemens Medical Solutions. Depending on the number of individual RF receiving coil elements that are available for spatial encoding in a specific orientation, a specific »reduction« or »acceleration« factor (also denominated as R-factor, PAT-factor, SENSE-factor) can be achieved to reduce the acquisition time. When 3D sequences are used, parallel imaging can be performed simultaneously in two orthogonal orientations of the two phase-encoding directions. The acceleration factors in this case can simply be multiplied. In a clinical setting, however, the maximum practical acceleration factor is limited by the available SNR. If the imaging application is already limited by SNR, parallel imaging might degrade

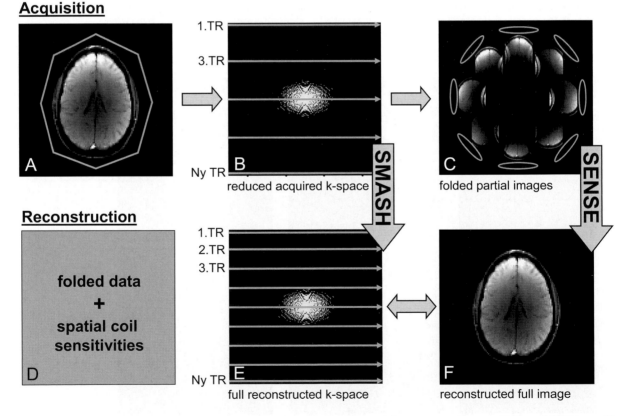

◘ **Fig. 2.5A–F.** Basic parallel MRI techniques SMASH and SENSE. In parallel MRI, data acquisition of the object (**A**) is performed using phased-array surface RF coils – here with eight independent coil elements connected to individual RF receivers. Depending on the number of RF coil elements and coil geometry, data acquisition of phase-encoding steps can be reduced (**B**) by a specific reduction or acceleration factor. In parallel MRI using SMASH, the a priori knowledge of spatial coil sensitivities (**D**) is used to reconstruct missing raw data in phase-encoding direction to a fully reconstructed k-space (**E**). Thus a full MR image (**F**) can be acquired and reconstructed in reduced time. In parallel MRI with SENSE the reduced k-space (**B**) is used to reconstruct a number of partial images that show image folding (wrap around, **C**). The knowledge of the spatial coil sensitivities (**D**) is used to unfold these folded partial images and to reconstruct a full image (**F**). Note that while SMASH reconstruction is performed in the k-space domain, SENSE reconstruction is performed in the image domain

image quality even further by adding additional noise. In cases where sufficient SNR is available, as in contrast-enhanced MRA applications, parallel imaging can be an attractive and powerful means to increase the efficiency of the administered contrast bolus [12-15]. Here parallel imaging can be used to increase volume coverage per unit time for large FOV imaging of large vessel segments, to increase the spatial resolution within a given image volume, or even to combine both effects [12-15]. Since contrast-enhanced MRA in general is performed using 3D sequences, simultaneous parallel imaging in two spatial dimensions can be used for significantly increased data acquisition volume and spatial resolution in the time window available by the administered contrast bolus [12-15].

2.4 Data Acquisition and Contrast Kinetics

With conventional contrast agents, the image acquisition window for MRA of the arteries is limited, as the concentration of contrast rapidly declines due to fast clearance of the contrast agent. This ultimately limits the achievable spatial resolution for contrast-enhanced MRA. Imaging applications that suffer the most from this time constraint are multi-station MRA of the peripheral arteries due to the bolus-chase nature of such applications, as well as MRA in regions where respiratory and/or cardiac motion compensation is necessary. Beyond performing data

acquisition during the first pass of the contrast kinetics only, MRA with Gadofosveset offers the additional possibility of acquiring MRA data during the steady state of the contrast kinetics. This opens up an additional time window in MRA for increasing the spatial resolution and/or the spatial coverage, especially in the above-mentioned applications [16].

2.4.1 First pass MRA

First pass MRA using Gadofosveset can be performed as with conventional extracellular contrast agents [17]. In order to optimize the contrast-to-tissue ratio, the flip angle has to be slightly adapted to the increased relaxivity of Gadofosveset. In general, a flip angle of approximately 35°, which is higher than the Ernst angle, is optimal for a TR of approximately 2–5 ms and an assumed blood T1 relaxation time of about 50 ms [16]. As with conventional contrast agents, the scan should be timed such that acquisition of the central k-space coincides with the peak concentration of Gadofosveset in the arterial target vessels (◘ Fig. 2.6). Fluoroscopic triggering or automatic bolus tracking should be used to determine the contrast arrival in the target vessel. Use of a small-volume test bolus is also an option, although the intravascular nature of the contrast agent may lead to minor background and venous enhancement in the actual first pass MRA scan [16].

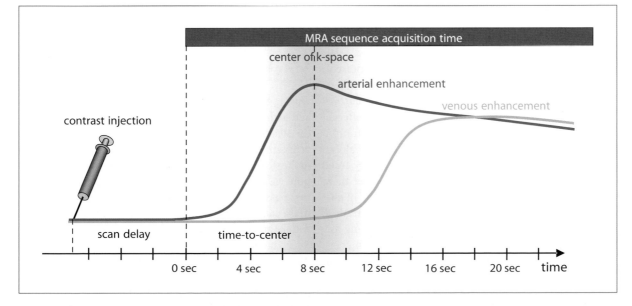

◘ **Fig. 2.6.** First pass MRA data acquisition as a function of the contrast agent kinetics. The individual circulation time was previously calculated by administration of a test bolus (scan delay). Timing and initialization of the MRA sequence is adjusted such that acquisition of the center of k-space falls into the arterial window of the contrast kinetics

2

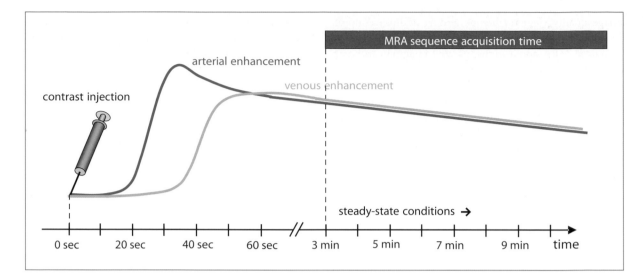

Fig. 2.7. Steady state MRA data acquisition as a function of the contrast agent kinetics. Initialization of the MRA sequence starts after the contrast agent is evenly distributed in the arterial and venous vascular system (typically 3–5 min after contrast agent injection. Data acquisition timing under steady state contrast conditions allows for a significantly prolonged data acquisition window for high-resolution MRA

2.4.2 Steady state MRA

Following contrast administration, a steady state in the contrast kinetics is reached after about 3 min or later, depending on individual physiology (■ Fig. 2.7). Due to the slow clearance from blood, imaging is possible up to 1 h after administration of Gadofosveset [16]. This significantly increases the data acquisition window for MRA applications and thus offers the possibility to acquire high-resolution MRA data sets or to use prepulses and motion-compensation schemes.

Compared with first pass imaging, where a relatively high concentration of contrast agent is present in the arterial vasculature, blood T1 shortening is less pronounced in the steady state phase of the contrast kinetics. This can be explained by the dilution effects, leading to a decreased local contrast agent concentration being distributed homogeneously in the entire blood volume. In the steady state the T1 of blood at 1.5 Tesla is about 150 ±50 ms, which is substantially shorter than the T1 of fat and vessel-surrounding tissues [6]. In the case of Gadofosveset the intravascular concentration remains relatively stable in the steady state, allowing for lengthy MRA data acquisition schemes featuring increased spatial resolution through use of larger matrices, and increasing the number of slices per volume, which ultimately results in smaller voxels (■ Fig. 2.8) [18]. Steady state MRA with Gadofosveset can be performed with standard T1-weighted fast gradient echo MRA sequences. Acquisition of isotropic voxels is recommended, as this allows for multi-planar reformation and viewing of the results.

The larger contrast window in steady state MRA can be used to increase the signal-to-noise ratio in high-resolution data sets by increasing the number of measurements and/or by deactivation of partial k-space acquisition schemes such as half Fourier imaging [16]. The optimum flip angle for maximizing blood-to-muscle contrast-to-noise ratio is approximately 6°–8° greater than the Ernst angle [19].

2.4.3 Suppression of Venous Signal

During the first pass the contrast agent is in the arteries and is then also increasingly disseminated in the veins in the steady state of the contrast kinetics. The arteries and veins are shown with a comparably high level of contrast in the steady state before the contrast agent is expelled over time via the kidneys. While MRA data acquisition in the first pass allows for pure arterial image contrast, imaging in the steady state consequently displays arteries and veins with comparable signal intensity. This can be problematic for image interpretation, since arteries and veins may be difficult to separate under certain conditions. Here new strategies for data acquisition, data reconstruction, and for data post-processing are advantageous. These will be discussed in the following chapter.

One approach for an alternative data acquisition regime is to acquire the central, contrast-encoding parts of

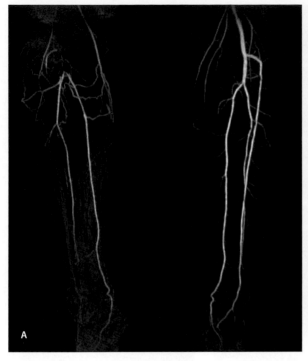

first pass MRA

steady state MRA

■ **Fig. 2.8A,B.** First pass (**A**) and steady state MRA (**B**) of the peripheral run-off arteries in the calf of a patient with severe intermittent claudication following the injection of Vasovist®. For first pass MRA, data acquisition has been timed such that the acquisition of central k-space of the MRA sequence (typically several seconds) falls into the arterial contrast window of the contrast agent in target vessels. Consequently, the maximum-intensity projection (MIP) of the first pass MRA shows only the arteries in the target region (**A**). For steady state MRA, data acquisition was started several minutes after contrast injection. Con-trast at this time point is equally distributed in the arterial and venous vessel system. Consequently, the MIP of the steady state MRA shows arteries and veins in the target region (**B**). Since the intravascular contrast agent remains in the vasculature for several more minutes, timing of steady state MRA is less critical and the increased data acquisition window (typically several minutes) can be used for acquisition of high-resolution MRA – here with an in-plane resolution of 200 μm x 200 μm. (Image examples (**A, B**) courtesy of Dr. Tim Leiner, MD, Department of Radiology, University Hospital Maastricht, The Netherlands)

k-space during first pass of the contrast agent in the arteries [20, 21] while extending data acquisition of the peripheral parts of k-space into the steady state of the contrast agent. This results in a high-resolution MRA of arteries while suppressing venous overlay to a certain extent. Segmented k-space techniques such as CENTRA (Contrast-ENhanced Time-Robust Angiography) have shown this potential for high-resolution first pass CE-MRA [22].

Another approach combining alternative data acquisition and reconstruction regimes for CE-MRA using blood pool contrast agents is displayed in ■ Fig. 2.9. During the first pass of the contrast agent through the arteries in the target region, only the central part of the raw data matrix is acquired. These data can be reconstructed to a high-contrast MR angiogram of the arteries – however, with reduced spatial resolution. During the steady state of the contrast agent, a complete high-resolution data set is acquired. The corresponding MR angiogram contains both arteries and veins with high spatial resolution. If the

central part of the first pass raw data matrix is now re-constructed together with the peripheral parts of k-space of the steady state raw data, an arterial MR angiogram with very high spatial resolution is obtained while venous superposition is avoided (■ Fig. 2.9). This data acquisition concept has been described as a proof of principle by Foo et al. [23] for multi-station peripheral MRA using a conventional contrast agent. While the technique described still has to be considered as a research application, the combination of such segmented volume acquisition with the use of intravascular contrast agents holds high potential for high-resolution MRA with venous signal suppression.

Beyond applying data acquisition and data reconstruction schemes to provide venous signal suppression in steady state MRA, this aim can also be achieved by a number of post-processing techniques for artery/vein separation [24, 25]. These techniques are examined in more detail in the chapter on post processing.

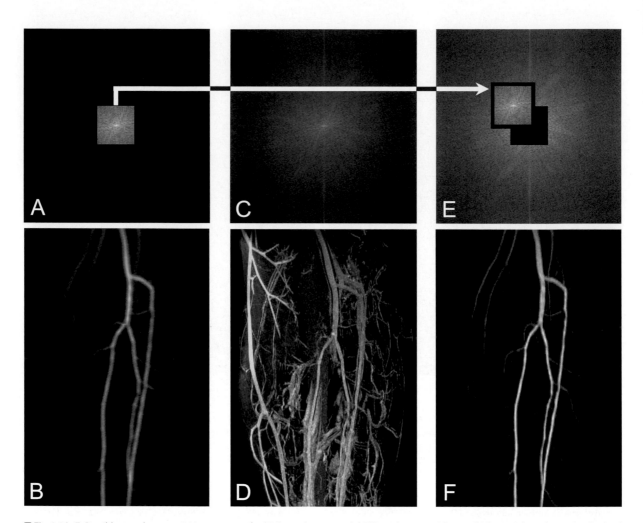

■ **Fig. 2.9A–F.** Possible raw data acquisition patterns for high-resolution MRA using a blood pool contrast agent. During the »first pass« of the contrast agent through the arteries in the target region, only the central part of the raw data matrix is acquired, which contains the contrast information (**A**). A high-contrast MR angiogram of the arteries is reconstructed, however, with reduced spatial resolution (**B**). During the »steady state« of the contrast agent, a complete high-resolution data set is acquired (**C**). The corresponding MR angiogram contains both arteries and veins with high spatial resolution (**D**). If the central part of the first pass raw data matrix is now reconstructed (**E**) from (**A**) together with the remaining steady state raw data from (**C**), an arterial MR angiogram with very high spatial resolution is obtained (**F**), however, avoiding venous superposition. As opposed to MRA with conventional extracellular contrast agent, this technique potentially can be used together with an intravascular contrast agent to increase the spatial resolution, because the contrast agent remains in the vessels during the time-consuming acquisition of the high-resolution data set. Such segmented volume data acquisition today still has to be considered as a research application. (Image examples (**B, D, F**) courtesy of Dr. Tim Leiner, MD, Department of Radiology, University Hospital Maastricht, The Netherlands)

2.5   Extending the Field-of-View

MRI soon reaches its limits for comprehensive angiographic depiction of vessels with its limited FOV of approximately 400–500 mm. A comprehensive examination of the peripheral arteries, however, typically requires an FOV that covers the abdominal aorta, including the renal arteries down to the pedal arteries – a distance that can be covered with an FOV of about 140 cm. One possibility of extending the effective FOV for such an examination is to divide the examination into several discrete partial examinations, whereby the patient table, together with the patient, is moved relative to the imaging volume in between the partial measurements [26–30]. These are known as so-called multi-station techniques. They exploit the fact that different body regions lie sequentially in the imaging region defined and limited by magnet homogeneity, gradient linearity, and RF signal excitation and reception (■ Fig. 2.1). These limitations remain applicable for each partial imaging FOV with this method; however, in this way the effective FOV may be expanded stepwise over several stations.

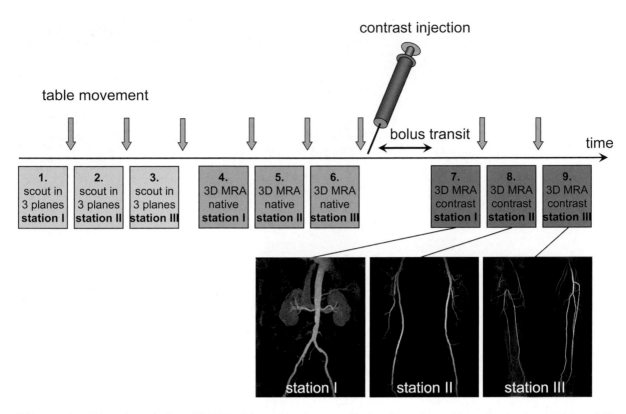

Fig. 2.10. Acquisition scheme for large-FOV MRA of the peripheral vasculature using multi-station moving table techniques. First overview images or »scouts« are acquired at multiple stations covering the region of interest. One table movement takes place between the stations each time to reposition the respective anatomic region to the isocenter of the scanner. Following acquisition of the localizer images, the coronal 3D MRA examination is planned and positioned on each individual station. Prior to the injection of contrast agent, native 3D data sets are acquired consecutively in all stations. The table is then moved back to the starting position and contrast agent is injected. 3D contrast-enhanced acquisition of the first station is started according to the previously determined individual bolus transit time. The 3D acquisitions of the second and third stations follow, after table movement in each case. For additional acquisition of steady state MRA data following this first pass multi-station angiogram, the patient table can simply be stepped back through the isocenter of the magnet in reversed order

2.5.1 Multi-station Peripheral MRA

The basic requirement for the implementation of multi-station techniques is the technical capability to move the patient table relative to the imaging field of the MR scanner. Here, the maximum range of movement of the table directly determines the effective maximum FOV, which can be covered stepwise with an examination of this type. Older-generation MR systems typically have a range of movement limited to less than 150 cm. To examine a patient from head to toe it is therefore unavoidable to reposition the patient at least once during the examination. For example, in the first phase the patient is positioned head-first, in the second phase feet-first. The latest generation of MRI scanners now provide the option to move the table along a distance of about 200 cm, enough distance to provide whole-body MRA imaging capabilities.

The complex interaction between contrast agent injection and stepwise data acquisition with multiple table movement requires careful planning of first pass bolus-chase multi-station MRA examinations. ☐ Figure 2.10 illustrates planning and acquisition of a three-station peripheral MRA examination (☐ Fig. 2.10). First, all three stations are consecutively positioned and overview images (»localizers« or »scouts«) are produced. After the overview images for a station have been acquired, the table moves on to the next station and the next »localizers« are acquired. This is repeated until all anatomic regions of interest have been covered stationwise with overview images (☐ Fig. 2.10). The overview images serve for further planning of the 3D MRA imaging volumes, for example in coronal slab orientation. After carefully planning the 3D MRA imaging volumes at all stations, the examination begins without contrast agent administration starting at the abdomen and moving towards the feet (☐ Fig. 2.10). Following data

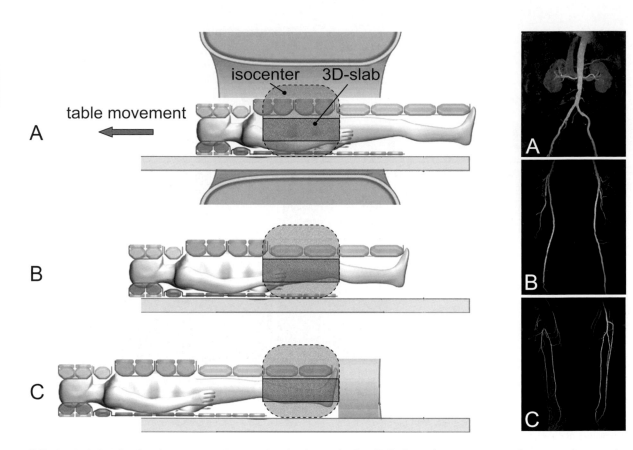

⬛ Fig. 2.11A–C. Peripheral multi-station 3D CE-MRA. The sketches show a longitudinal cross-section of a scanner. The patient with RF surface coils on top is first positioned with the thorax in the isocenter of the scanner (**A**). The coronal 3D acquisition volume (3D slab) is positioned within the isocenter. During the course of the examination, the patient table, together with the patient, is advanced stepwise towards the feet (**B-C**). Given the appropriate synchronization between the contrast agent bolus and the imaging time per station, the contrast agent bolus is followed along its path from the aorta via the pelvis-leg vessels to the feet. This also allows vessels to be depicted whose dimensions exceed the size of a conventional FOV (MRA in **A-C**)

acquisition and reconstruction, unenhanced »native« 3D data sets are available from all three stations, which can later be subtracted from the 3D MRA contrast agent data sets to improve image quality.

Taking into account the contrast agent bolus transit time previously determined, MRA data acquisition is started with the appropriate delay after contrast agent injection so that the data acquisition correlates with the arrival of the first pass contrast agent bolus in the vascular region to be imaged.

On completion of data acquisition at the first station, the table is moved and acquisition follows at the second and the third station (⬛ Figs. 2.10, 2.11). In this way, the first pass contrast agent bolus is followed in its transit from the aorta, through the pelvis-leg arteries, towards the feet. 3D MRA data sets of the individual stations are available at the end of a successful multi-station examination (⬛ Fig. 2.11A–C). Multi-station MRA examinations are widespread in routine clinical CE-MRA of the peripheral arteries nowadays [31–35]. Extending the multi-

station MRA imaging protocol by another one or two stations even allows for whole-body MRA coverage [36-39]. Combining whole-body MRA with parallel imaging [40] now can be considered state-of-the-art on modern MRI systems [41].

2.5.2 Continuously Moving Table Peripheral MRA

The multi-station bolus-chase MRA techniques previously described help to overcome the constraints of conventional FOVs when larger vascular territories are imaged. The stationwise examination of comprehensive vascular anatomy with a limited FOV, however, has other inherent technical limitations: Data acquisition has to be interrupted for typically 3–4 s while the table is moving between successive stations; the partial FOVs for each station typically overlap slightly by several centimeters, requiring additional time for redundant data acquisition;

time is necessary at each station for the re-establishment of the equilibrium magnetization for the image sequence; signal attenuation often arises on the margins of the FOVs, which can lead to inhomogeneities in the resulting combined overview images; and non-linearities in the gradient system lead to geometric distortions on the margins of the partial FOVs, which in turn can cause artifacts on the boundaries between adjacent stations. These limitations inherently reduce the time efficiency of multi-station techniques and/or hamper the evaluation of the images, especially on the boundaries of the partial FOVs [42, 43]. The ideal situation would be a continuous large-FOV 3D MRA data set with uninterrupted and unchanging quality, which can be processed as a whole during image viewing and assessment.

Various techniques have been investigated recently as alternatives to the multi-station techniques [42–47]. These techniques for continuous table movement during data acquisition, also termed »move during scan« techniques, place special requirements on data acquisition, hardware, and image reconstruction: Inhomogeneity of the main magnetic field and non-linearity of the gradients generate image distortions at the margins of the FOV, which are now a function of time, because the table is moved through the scanner during acquisition [48]. In addition, a number of adjustment parameters, which previously were modified once per station for the stationwise examination of the patient, must now be automatically adapted during table movement. These parameters include the tuning of the RF transmitter coil, the transmission and receiver frequency, the RF transmission power, the RF receiver gain, the »shimming« of the magnet, the activation of the RF surface coil elements located in the imaging region and other parameters, all of which are needed to ensure optimal, homogeneous image quality and the safety of the patient. Otherwise, the excitation flip angle can, for instance, have a different value in the pelvic region than in the thoracic region and the image contrast varies unpredictably.

Initial clinical studies of continuously moving table MRA in direct comparison with multi-station MRA with volunteers and patients show promising results [49, 50] (◘ Fig. 2.12). Parallel imaging techniques can also be applied here through the use of surface coils combined with independent RF receivers [49–51] and the potential for faster imaging, larger anatomic coverage in the same time, and/or improved spatial resolution can be exploited. The application of such continuously moving table MRA techniques is rewarded by the depiction of extended anatomic structures in large seamless images and has the potential of achieving a paradigm shift in MRA data acquisition, reconstruction, post-processing and evaluation [49, 50].

Further technical developments will feature increased spatial resolution of the large FOV 3D MRA data sets as

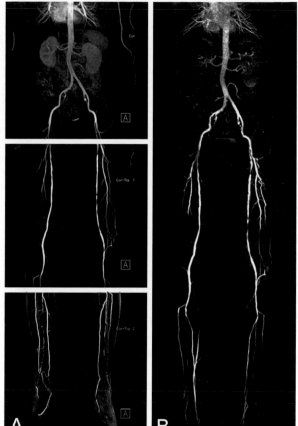

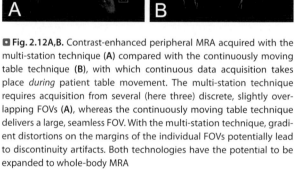

◘ **Fig. 2.12A,B.** Contrast-enhanced peripheral MRA acquired with the multi-station technique (**A**) compared with the continuously moving table technique (**B**), with which continuous data acquisition takes place *during* patient table movement. The multi-station technique requires acquisition from several (here three) discrete, slightly overlapping FOVs (**A**), whereas the continuously moving table technique delivers a large, seamless FOV. With the multi-station technique, gradient distortions on the margins of the individual FOVs potentially lead to discontinuity artifacts. Both technologies have the potential to be expanded to whole-body MRA

well as adaptation of the continuously moving table speed to the individual travel velocity of the contrast bolus [52]. These steps will further increase the efficient use of the contrast bolus. Intravascular contrast agents will fundamentally support the use of continuously moving table techniques by increasing the flexibility of the potential data acquisition schemes. Beyond combining moving table techniques with conventional first pass bolus chase, the addition of steady state imaging opens up a whole new time window for significantly increased data acquisition times. Consequently, the data acquisition schemes – proposed above and illustrated in ◘ Fig. 2.9 – that make use of the steady state to increase spatial resolution, can be combined with the continuously moving table techniques and thus provide significantly increased spatial resolution in large-FOV MRA. Initial experiments combining these data acquisition schemes with multi-station MRA and Vasovist have shown promising results [53]. The combination of such data acquisition and reconstruction techniques with continuously moving tables and blood pool contrast agents is envisaged.

2.6   Conclusion

Magnetic resonance angiography has achieved a high diagnostic status in a short time, not least due to the numerous hardware and software developments, and, as a result, has replaced X-ray-based invasive catheter angiography for many diagnostic investigations. In the process, MRA itself has initiated numerous technical developments in imaging from which modern MRI as a whole has profited enormously. The clinical advance of new intravascular contrast agents such as Gadofosveset allows both for first pass and steady state imaging, thus offering an additional window for high-resolution MRA imaging. This impact of intravascular contrast agents is set to bring attractive applications and to further expand the diagnostic spectrum of MRA.

Take home messages

- The three basic hardware components of an MRI system are: 1) The main magnet providing high magnetic field strength [B0] for magnetization of the spins in the tissue; 2) the gradient system providing spatial and time varying magnetic fields in three dimensions [Gx, Gy, Gz] for spatial encoding of the MRI signal; 3) The radiofrequency (RF) system that excites the spins by sending RF energy [B1] with the built-in body RF coil and that receives weak RF signals being emitted from the tissue.
- MR signals are collected and stored as »raw data« in a two-dimensional (2D) or three-dimensional (3D) matrix also termed »k-space«. Following a mathematical operation called fast Fourier-transformation (FFT), these raw data are transformed into 2D or 3D MR images.
- Parallel imaging strategies (e.g. SMASH, SENSE) in MRI are a technique to increase the speed of the MRI acquisition by skipping a number of phase-encoding lines in k-space during data acquisition – an otherwise time-consuming process. In MR angiography (MRA) parallel imaging techniques can be used to reduce data acquisition time, to increase the spatial resolution per unit acquisition time or even to combine both effects.

- When injecting blood pool contrast agents for MRA, the arterial »first pass« contrast phase known from conventional extracellular contrast agents is followed by an additional prolonged »steady state« of signal enhancement in the arteries and veins. This provides enhanced flexibility for MRA data acquisition, e.g. for increasing spatial resolution.
- Multi-station techniques can be used for extending the limited field-of-view (FOV) of an MRI system in order to perform MRA of the peripheral arteries or even whole-body MRA. For MRA data acquisition with multi-station techniques the patient table is moved through the isocenter of the magnet in multiple successive stations while the »first pass« of contrast agent is traveling towards the patient's feet.
- Continuously moving table techniques are currently being developed to replace multi-station MRA examinations. Continuous techniques instead of multi-station techniques provide one seamless large-FOV MRA data set that is virtually free of discontinuity artifacts. In combination with continuous moving table techniques blood pool contrast agents provide enhanced flexibility and efficiency for large-FOV MRA data acquisition.

References

1. Prince MR (1994) Gadolinium-enhanced MR aortography. Radiology 191:155–164
2. Yucel EK, Anderson CM, Edelman RR, Grist TM, Baum RA, Manning WJ, Culebras A, Pearce W (1999) AHA scientific statement. Magnetic resonance angiography: update on applications for extracranial arteries. Circulation 100:2284–2301
3. Lauffer RB (1991) Targeted relaxation enhancement agents for MRI. Magn Reson Med 22:339–342
4. Lauffer RB, Parmelee DJ, Dunham SU, Ouellet HS, Dolan RP, Witte S, McMurry TJ, Walovitch RC (1998) MS-325: albumin-targeted contrast agent for MR angiography. Radiology 207:529–538

5. Caravan P, Cloutier NJ, Greenfield MT, McDermid SA, Dunham SU, Bulte JW, Amedio JC Jr, Looby RJ, Supkowski RM, Horrocks WD Jr, McMurry TJ, Lauffer RB (2002) The interaction of MS-325 with human serum albumin and its effect on proton relaxation rates. J Am Chem Soc 124:3152–3162
6. Hartmann M, Wiethoff AJ, Hentrich HR, Rohrer M (2006) Initial imaging recommendations for Vasovist angiography. Eur Radiol 16 [Suppl] 2:B15–23
7. Laub G (1999) Principles of contrast-enhanced MR angiography. Basic and clinical applications. Magn Reson Imaging Clin N Am 7:783–795
8. Sodickson DK, Manning WJ (1997) Simultaneous acquisition of spatial harmonics (SMASH): fast imaging with radiofrequency coil arrays. Magn Reson Med. 38:591–603

9. Pruessmann KP, Weiger M, Scheidegger MB, Boesiger P (1999) SENSE: sensitivity encoding for fast MRI. Magn Reson Med 42:952–962

10. Griswold MA, Jakob PM, Heidemann RM, Nittka M, Jellus V, Wang J, Kiefer B, Haase A (2002) Generalized autocalibrating partially parallel acquisitions (GRAPPA). Magn Reson Med 47:1202–1210

11. Blaimer M, Breuer F, Mueller M, Heidemann RM, Griswold MA, Jakob PM (2004) SMASH, SENSE, PILS, GRAPPA: how to choose the optimal method. Top Magn Reson Imaging.15:223–236

12. Weiger M, Pruessmann KP, Kassner A, Roditi G, Lawton T, Reid A, Boesiger P (2000): Contrast-enhanced 3D MRA using SENSE. J Magn Reson Imaging 12:671–677

13. Sodickson DK, McKenzie CA, Li W, Wolff S, Manning WJ, Edelman RR (2000): Contrast-enhanced 3D MR angiography with simultaneous acquisition of spatial harmonics: A pilot study. Radiology 217:284–289

14. Wilson GJ, Hoogeveen RM, Willinek WA, Muthupillai R, Maki JH (2004) Parallel imaging in MR angiography. Top Magn Reson Imaging 15:169–185

15. Glockner JF, Hu HH, Stanley DW, Angelos L, King K (2005) Parallel MR imaging: a user's guide. Radiographics 25:1279–1297

16. Rohrer M, Geerts-Ossevoort L, Laub G (2007) Technical requirements, biophysical considerations and protocol optimization with magnetic resonance angiography using blood-pool agents. Eur Radiol 17 [Suppl 2]:B7–B12

17. Prince M, Grist TM, Debatin JF (2003) 3-D contrast MR angiography, 3rd edn. Springer, Berlin, Heidelberg, New York

18. Nikolaou K, Kramer H, Grosse C, Clevert D, Dietrich O, Hartmann M, Chamberlin P, Assmann S, Reiser MF, Schoenberg SO (2006) High-spatial-resolution multistation MR angiography with parallel imaging and blood pool contrast agent: initial experience. Radiology 241:861–872

19. Wang MS, Haynor DR, Wilson GJ, Leiner T, Maki JH (2007) Maximizing contrast-to-noise ratio in ultra-high resolution peripheral MR angiography using a blood pool agent and parallel imaging. J Magn Reson Imaging 26:580–588

20. Huston J 3rd, Fain SB, Riederer SJ, Wilman AH, Bernstein MA, Busse RF (1999) Carotid arteries: maximizing arterial to venous contrast in fluoroscopically triggered contrast-enhanced MR angiography with elliptic centric view ordering. Radiology 211:265–273

21. Huston J 3rd, Fain SB, Wald JT, Luetmer PH, Rydberg CH, Covarrubias DJ, Riederer SJ, Bernstein MA, Brown RD, Meyer FB, Bower TC, Schleck CD (2001) Carotid artery: elliptic centric contrast-enhanced MR angiography compared with conventional angiography. Radiology 218:138–143

22. Willinek WA, Gieseke J, Conrad R, Strunk H, Hoogeveen R, von Falkenhausen M, Keller E, Urbach H, Kuhl CK, Schild HH (2002) Randomly segmented central k-space ordering in high-spatial-resolution contrast-enhanced MR angiography of the supraaortic arteries: initial experience. Radiology 225:583–588

23. Foo TK, Ho VB, Hood MN, Hess SL, Choyke PL (2001) High-spatial-resolution multistation MR imaging of lower-extremity peripheral vasculature with segmented volume acquisition: feasibility study. Radiology 219:835–841

24. van Bemmel CM, Spreeuwers LJ, Viergever MA, Niessen WJ (2003) Level-set-based artery-vein separation in blood pool agent CE-MR angiograms. IEEE Trans Med Imaging 22:1224–1234

25. Lei T, Udupa JK, Odhner D, Nyúl LG, Saha PK (2003) 3DVIEWNIX-AVS: a software package for the separate visualization of arteries and veins in CE-MRA images. Comput Med Imaging Graph 27:351–362

26. Ho KY, Leiner T, de Haan MW, Kessels AG, Kitslaar PJ, van Engelshoven JM (1998) Peripheral vascular tree stenoses: evaluation with moving-bed infusion-tracking MR angiography. Radiology 206:683–692

27. Wang Y, Lee HM, Khilnani NM, Jaqust MR, Winchester PA, Bush HL, Sos TA, Sostman HD (1998) Bolus-chase MR digital subtraction angiography in the lower extremity. Radiology 207: 263–269

28. Meaney JF, Ridgway JP, Chakraverty S, Robertson I, Kessel D, Radjenovic A, Kouwenhoven M, Kassner A, Smith MA (1998) Stepping-table gadolinium-enhanced digital subtraction MR angiography of the aorta and lower extremity arteries: preliminary experience. Radiology 211:59–67

29. Ruehm SG, Hany TF, Pfammatter T, Schneider E, Ladd ME, Debatin JF (2000) Pelvic and lower extremity arterial imaging: diagnostic performance of three-dimensional contrast-enhanced MR angiography. AJR Am J Roentgenol 174:1127–1135

30. Leiner T, Ho KY, Nelemans PJ, de Haan MW, van Engelshoven JM (2000) Three-dimensional contrast-enhanced moving-bed infusion-tracking (MoBI-track) peripheral MR angiography with flexible choice of imaging parameters for each field of view. J Magn Reson Imaging 11:368–377

31. Goyen M, Ruehm SG, Barkhausen J, Kroger K, Ladd ME, Truemmler KH, Bosk S, Requardt M, Reykowski A, Debatin JF (2001) Improved multi-station peripheral MR angiography with a dedicated vascular coil. J Magn Reson Imaging 13:475–480

32. Ho KY, Leiner T, de Haan MW, van Engelshoven JM (1999) Peripheral MR angiography. Eur Radiol 9:1765–1774

33. Busch HP, Hoffmann HG, Rock J, Schneider C (2001) MR angiography of pelvic and leg vessels with automatic table movement technique (»MobiTrak«): Clinical experience with 450 studies. RoFo Fortschr Röntgenstr 173:405–409

34. Huber A, Scheidler J, Wintersperger B, Baur A, Schmidt M, Requardt M, Holzknecht N, Helmberger T, Billing A, Reiser M (2003) Moving-table MR angiography of the peripheral runoff vessels: comparison of body coil and dedicated phased array coil systems. AJR Am J Roentgenol 180:1365–1373

35. Leiner T, Nijenhuis RJ, Maki JH, Lemaire E, Hoogeveen R, van Engelshoven JM (2004) Use of a three-station phased array coil to improve peripheral contrast-enhanced magnetic resonance angiography. J Magn Reson Imaging 20:417–425

36. Ruehm SG, Goyen M, Barkhausen J, Kroger K, Bosk S, Ladd ME, Debatin JF (2001) Rapid magnetic resonance angiography for detection of atherosclerosis. Lancet 357:1086–1089

37. Ruehm SG, Goyen M, Quick HH, Schleputz M, Schleputz H, Bosk S, Barkhausen J, Ladd ME, Debatin JF (2000) [Whole-body MRA on a rolling table platform (AngioSURF)] Rofo Fortschr Röntgenstr 172:670–674

38. Goyen M, Quick HH, Debatin JF, Ladd ME, Barkhausen J, Herborn CU, Bosk S, Kuehl H, Schleputz M, Ruehm SG (2002) Whole-body three-dimensional MR angiography with a rolling table platform: initial clinical experience. Radiology 224:270–277

39. Herborn CU, Goyen M, Quick HH, Bosk S, Massing S, Kroeger K, Stoesser D, Ruehm SG, Debatin JF (2004). Whole-body 3D MR angiography of patients with peripheral arterial occlusive disease. AJR Am J Roentgenol 182:1427–1434

40. Quick HH, Vogt FM, Maderwald S, Herborn CU, Bosk S, Gohde S, Debatin JF, Ladd ME (2004) High spatial resolution whole-body MR angiography featuring parallel imaging: initial experience. RoFo Fortschr Röntgenstr 176:163–169

41. Kramer H, Schoenberg SO, Nikolaou K, Huber A, Struwe A, Winnik E, Wintersperger BJ, Dietrich O, Kiefer B, Reiser MF (2005) Cardiovascular screening with parallel imaging techniques and a whole-body MR imager. Radiology 236:300–310

42. Dietrich O, Hajnal JV (1999) Extending the coverage of true volume scans by continuous movement of the subject. ISMRM, 7th Scientific Meeting and Exhibition, Philadelphia, p 1653

43. Kruger DG, Riederer SJ, Grimm RC, Rossman PJ (2002) Continuously moving table data acquisition method for long FOV con-

trast-enhanced MRA and whole-body MRI. Magn Reson Med 47:224–231

44. Zhu Y, Dumoulin CL (2003) Extended field-of-view imaging with table translation and frequency sweeping. Magn Reson Med 49:1106–1112

45. Fain SB, Browning FJ, Polzin JA, Du J, Zhou Y, Block WF, Grist TM, Mistretta CA (2004) Floating table isotropic projection (FLIPR) acquisition: a time-resolved 3D method for extended field-of-view MRI during continuous table motion. Magn Reson Med 52:1093–1102

46. Madhuranthakam AJ, Kruger DG, Riederer SJ, Glockner JF, Hu HH (2004) Time-resolved 3D contrast-enhanced MRA of an extended FOV using continuous table motion. Magn Reson Med 51:568–576

47. Zenge MO, Ladd ME, Vogt FM, Brauck K, Barkhausen J, Quick HH (2005) Whole-body magnetic resonance imaging featuring moving table continuous data acquisition with high-precision position feedback. Magn Reson Med 54:707–711

48. Polzin JA, Kruger DG, Gurr DH, Brittain JH, Riederer SJ (2004) Correction for gradient nonlinearity in continuously moving table MR imaging. Magn Reson Med 52:181–187

49. Zenge MO, Vogt FM, Brauck K, Jökel M, Barkhausen J, Kannengiesser S, Ladd ME, Quick HH (2006) High-resolution continuously acquired peripheral MR angiography featuring partial parallel imaging GRAPPA. Magn Reson Med 2006 56:859–865

50. Vogt FM, Zenge MO, Ladd ME, Herborn CU, Brauck K, Luboldt W, Barkhausen J, Quick HH (2007) Peripheral vascular disease: comparison of continuous MR angiography and conventional MR angiography--pilot study. Radiology 243:229–238

51. Keupp J, Aldefeld B, Bornert P (2005) Continuously moving table SENSE imaging. Magn Reson Med 53:217–220

52. Kruger DG, Riederer SJ, Polzin JA, Madhuranthakam AJ, Hu HH, Glockner JF (2005) Dual-velocity continuously moving table acquisition for contrast-enhanced peripheral magnetic resonance angiography. Magn Reson Med 53:110–117

53. Kinner S, Zenge MO, Vogt FM, Ucan B, Ladd ME, Barkhausen J, Quick HH (2007) Ultra-high resolution peripheral MRA with k-space segmentation featuring a blood-pool contrast agent and venous suppression. Proc ISMRM 19-25 May, Berlin

Part II   Safety and Efficacy

tra- and intracellular fluid [15]. This has two important consequences: First, the cell membrane tends to shield the interior of cells very effectively from current flow, which is thus restricted to the extracellular fluid. Second, voltages are induced across the membrane of cells. When the electric voltages are above a tissue-specific threshold level, they can stimulate nerve and muscle cells.

The primary concern with regard to time-varying magnetic fields is cardiac fibrillation, because it is a life-threatening condition. In contrast, peripheral nerve stimulation is of practical concern because uncomfortable or intolerable stimulations would interfere with the examination (e.g., due to patient movements) or even result in a termination of the examination. As determined in animal experiments, excitation thresholds for the heart are substantially greater than those for nerves as long as the pulse duration is sufficiently less than about 3 ms [16]. Therefore, the avoidance of peripheral sensations in a patient provides a conservative safety margin with respect to cardiac stimulation.

Peripheral nerve stimulation has been investigated in various volunteer studies. A systematic evaluation of the available data was presented by Schaefer, Bourland and Nyenhuis in 2000 [17]. They recalculated published threshold levels - often reported for different gradient coils and shapes in different terms - to the maximum dB/dt occurring during the maximum switch rate of the gradient coil at a radius of 20 cm from the central axis of the MR system, i.e., at the border of the volume normally accessible to patients. Bourland et al. also analyzed their stimulation data in the form of cumulative frequency distributions that relate a dB/dt level to the number of subjects that had already reported on perceptible, uncomfortable, or even intolerable sensations [18]. The results indicate that the lowest percentile for intolerable stimulation is approximately 20% above the median threshold for the perception of peripheral nerve stimulation, which can be parameterized by the following empirical relation:

$$\frac{dB}{dt} = 20 \cdot \left(1 + \frac{0.36}{\tau}\right) \quad \text{(in T/s)}. \qquad \text{Eq. (3)}$$

In this equation, t_{eff} is the effective stimulus duration (in ms) defined as the duration of the period of monotonic increasing or decreasing gradient.

In the current safety recommendations issued by the IEC and ICNRIP, the maximum recommended exposure level for time-varying magnetic fields is set equal to a dB/dt of 80% of the median perception threshold given by Eq. (3) for normal operation and 100% of the median for controlled operation. As shown in ☐ Fig. 3.1, the threshold for cardiac stimulation [16] is well above the median perception threshold for peripheral nerve stimulation, except at very long pulse durations, which are, however, not

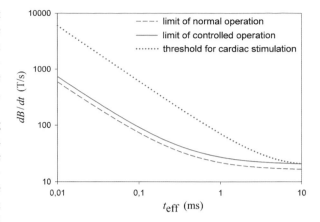

☐ **Fig. 3.1.** Threshold for cardiac stimulation [16] and limits for normal and controlled operation of an MR device. Data are expressed as dB/dt as a function of the effective stimulus duration t_{eff}. The limit for the controlled operation mode is given by the median threshold for the perception of peripheral nerve stimulation

relevant for MR procedures. Instead of using the parameterization given by Eq. (1), mean perception threshold levels can be determined by the manufacturers for a given type of gradient system by means of experimental studies on human volunteers.

3.3.4 Radiofrequency Electromagnetic Fields

Time-varying magnetic fields used for the excitation and preparation of the spin system in MRI typically have frequencies above 10 MHz. In this RF range, the conductivity of cell membranes is comparable to that of the extra- and intracellular fluid, which means that no substantial voltages are induced across the membranes [15]. For this reason, stimulation of nerve and muscle cells is no longer a matter of concern. Instead, thermal effects due to tissue heating by the induced electric tissue currents are of importance. The parameter relevant for the evaluation of biological effects of RF fields is the increase in tissue temperature, which is dependent not only on localized power absorption and the duration of RF exposure, but also on heat transfer and the activation of thermoregulatory mechanisms leading to thermal equalization within the body.

Absorption of energy in the human body strongly depends on the size and orientation of the body with respect to the RF field as well as on the frequency of the field. Theoretical and experimental considerations reveal that RF absorption in the body approaches a maximum when the wavelength of the field is on the order of the body size. Unfortunately, the wavelength of the RF fields used in MRI falls into this »resonance range«.

◻ Table 3.1. Basic restrictions for body temperature rise and partial-body temperatures for patients undergoing MRI procedures [9, 10]

Operating mode	Rise of body-core temperature (°C)	Spatially localized temperature limits		
		Head (°C)	Trunk (°C)	Extremities (°C)
Normal	0.5	38	39	40
Controlled	1	38	39	40
Experimental	> 1	> 38	> 39	> 40

◻ Table 3.2. SAR limits (in W/kg) for patients when a volume coil is used to excite a greater field-of-view [9, 10]. The values hold at environmental temperatures below 24°C

Body region → Operating mode ↓	Averaging time 6 min		
	Whole-body	Partial-body	
		any region, except head	head[b]
Normal	2	2–10[a]	3.2
Controlled	4	4–10[a]	3.2
Experimental	> 4	> (4–10)[a]	> 3.2

Short-term SAR: The SAR limit over any 10-s period shall not exceed three times the corresponding average SAR limit.

[a] Partial-body SARs scale dynamically with the ratio r between the patient mass exposed and the total patient mass:
 – normal operating mode: $SAR = (10 - 8 \cdot r)$ W/kg
 – controlled operating mode: $SAR = (10 - 6 \cdot r)$ W/kg
[b] Partial-volume SARs given by IEC; ICNIRP limits SAR exposure to the head to 3 W/kg.

The time rate of electromagnetic energy absorption by a unit of tissue mass is defined as specific absorption rate (SAR in W/kg). In good approximation, the time-averaged SAR of an RF pulse is proportional (a) to the square of the static magnetic field, B_0, which means that energy absorption is markedly higher with high-field than with low-field MR systems, and (b) to the square of the pulse angle, so that MRA sequences with large-angle pulses will result in relatively high SAR levels. From the point of view of safety, CE-MRA at 3 T is thus much more challenging than at 1.5 T and makes it necessary to use optimized coil designs as well as sophisticated pulse sequences utilizing SAR reduction techniques such as parallel imaging or hyperechos.

According to published studies, no adverse health effects are expected if the RF-induced increase in body-core temperature does not exceed 1°C. In case of infants, pregnant women, or persons with cardiocirculatory impairment, it is desirable to limit body-core temperature increases to 0.5°C [10]. As indicated in ◻ Table 3.1, these values have been laid down in the current safety recommendations to limit the body-core temperature for the normal and controlled operating mode. Additionally, lo-

cal temperatures under exposure to the head, trunk, and extremities are limited for each of the two operating modes to the values given in ◻ Table 3.1.

However, temperature changes in the different parts of the body are difficult to control during an MR procedure in clinical routine. Therefore, SAR limits have been derived on the basis of experimental and theoretical studies which should not be exceeded, in order to limit the temperature rise to the values given in ◻ Table 3.1. As only parts of the body – at least in the case of adult patients – are exposed simultaneously during an MR procedure, not only the whole-body SAR but also partial-body SAR values for the head, the trunk, and the extremities have to be estimated by means of suitable patient models [19] and limited to the values given in ◻ Table 3.2 for the normal and controlled operating mode. With respect to the application of the SAR limits defined in ◻ Table 3.2, it has to be taken into account that they do not relate to an individual MR sequence, but rather to running SAR averages computed over each 6-min period, which is assumed to be a typical thermal equilibration time of smaller masses of tissue [20].

4.2.2 Recommended clinical dose (0.03 mmol Gd/kg)

Patients from this subgroup received a dose of 0.03 mmol/kg Vasovist® across all clinical studies using Vasovist® and part of the overall assessment of all dose ranges (0.01–0.15 mmol Gd/kg) as described above. For the recommended dose of 0.03 mmol Gd/kg, safety results in phase II and III studies have been described in detail for a pooled collective of 767 patients [64]. In summary, the incidence rates and the profile of adverse events in patients who had received Vasovist® at the clinically recommended dose were comparable with those in patients who had received placebo, and in fact the proportion of patients with adverse events was lower in the Vasovist® group than in the placebo group. Most (~82%) of the adverse events in the Vasovist® group were assessed as mild in intensity. Seventeen severe adverse events were reported for 15 patients (2%) in the Vasovist® group. Six events were considered to be at least possibly related to the treatment with Vasovist® and included burning sensation, dysgeusia, headache, pruritus, rash, and pain. Individual adverse events are shown in ▫ Table 4.3 including the subgroup for the clinically recommended dose of 0.03 mmol Gd/kg. The most common adverse events (▫ Table 4.2) following treatment with Vasovist® (possibly or probably related to treatment) were pruritus (4%), nausea (4%), paresthesia (3%), and vasodilatation (3%). Onset was generally (70% of all treatment-related events) within 2 h of dosing, and symptoms usually resolved in most cases (75% of treatment-related events) within 2 h after onset. Four of

the 767 patients (0.5%) experienced five serious adverse events, which included aggravated coronary artery disease, hypoglycemia (both of these reported by one patient), gangrene, chest pain, and anaphylactoid reaction. The instances of gangrene and chest pain were deemed unlikely to be related to the study drug. Overall, no clinically significant changes in any laboratory parameters were seen after injection of Vasovist®. Hematology, coagulation, and urine values were normal, with sporadic deviations only. Specifically, there was no evidence of a depletion of zinc, calcium, or iron from serum following administration of Vasovist®. Individual changes in immunological variables (complement C3, complement C4 plasma histamine, IgE, tryptase-CAPS), ECG parameters and the results of physical examination all raised no safety concerns.

One prospectively planned phase IIIb study was conducted between 2006 and 2007 [77] for which a total of 264 patients with aortoiliac disease Fontaine stage IIb–IV were enrolled; 261 patients received Vasovist®. The age of the patients ranged from 32 to 86 years (mean 65 years); 171 patients (65.5%) were male and 90 (34.5%) were female, and they received a dose of 0.03 mmol Gd/kg Vasovist®. A total of 39 patients (14.9%) experienced 51 adverse events; 33 adverse events were assessed as being (probably: 16, possibly: 17) related to the study drug. The most common events were grouped to gastrointestinal disorders (nausea), followed by nervous system disorders (burning sensations) and reproductive system/breast disorders (genital burning). The intensities of all drug-related adverse events were mild or moderate. No serious adverse drug reactions were reported.

▫ **Table 4.2.** Number and percentage of patients who experienced the most common Gadofosveset-related adverse events [30]

	Placebo		Dose (mmol Gd/kg)								All doses combined	
			<0.03		0.03		0.05		>0.05			
	n=49		n=95		n=767		n=348		n=111		n=1321	
	n	%	n	%	n	%	n	%	n	%	n	%
Any Gadofosveset-related AE	16	33	14	15	176	23	150	43	75	67	415	31
Pruritus *	1	2	1	1	34	4	39	11	20	18	94	7
Paresthesia	1	2	–	–	20	3	39	11	19	17	78	6
Headache *	2	4	1	1	17	2	13	4	3	3	34	3
Nausea	–	–	1	1	29	4	25	7	5	5	60	5
Vasodilatation	–	–	1	1	22	3	19	5	22	20	64	5
Burning sensation*	–	–	–	–	15	2	28	8	17	15	60	5
Dysgeusia	6	12	2	2	17	2	20	6	5	5	44	3
Feeling cold	–	–	2	2	5	1	10	3	–	–	17	1

*Not otherwise specified
Cut-off: 1% of all patients. n is the total number of patients in the dose group; % is based on n

Summary

Adverse events which were recorded as related to the intravenous injection of Vasovist in all company-sponsored clinical studies to date are available for a total of 1821 subjects. They are grouped in ◘ Table 4.3 according to MedDRA [35] system organ classes and adapted to the current version of MedDRA terminology, as well as to applicable frequency conventions. A total of five serious adverse events were experienced by patients who received 0.03 mmol/kg Vasovist® across all clinical studies using Vasovist®. These events were coronary artery disease, hyperglycemia, gangrene, chest pain, and anaphylactoid reaction. Only the anaphylactoid reaction was considered to be probably related to Vasovist® and was resolved within 5 min.

◘ **Table 4.3.** Frequency of adverse reactions from clinical trial data. Based on experience of more than 1800 patients, the following undesirable effects have been observed and classified by investigators as drug-related (possibly, probably, or definitely). The Table below reports adverse reactions by MedDRA system organ classes (MedDRA SOCs)

System Organ Class (MedDra)	Common (≥1:100)	Uncommon (≥1:1000, <1:100)	Rare (<1:1000)
Infections and infestations		nasopharyngitis	cellulites
Immune system disorders		hypersensitivity	
Metabolism and nutrition disorders		hyperglycemia, electrolyte imbalance (incl. hypocalcemia)	
Psychiatric disorders		anxiety, confusion	
Nervous system disorders	headache, paresthesia, dysgeusia, burning sensation	ageusia, dizziness (excl. vertigo), tremor, hypoesthesia, parosmia, muscle contractions involuntary	
Eye disorders		lacrimation increased, vision abnormal	
Ear and labyrinth disorders			ear pain
Cardiac disorders		atrioventricular block first degree, tachycardia	cardiac flutter, bradycardia, palpitations
Vascular disorders	vasodilatation (incl. flushing)	hypertension, phlebitis, peripheral coldness	hypotension, anaphylactoid reaction
Respiratory, thoracic and mediastinal disorders		dyspnea, cough	
Gastrointestinal disorders	nausea	Vomiting, diarrhea, abdominal discomfort, abdominal pain, dry mouth, flatulence, hypoesthesia lips, salivary hypersecretion, dyspepsia, pharyngolaryngeal pain, pruritus ani	
Skin and subcutaneous tissue disorders	pruritus	urticaria, erythema, rash, sweating increased	swelling face
Musculoskeletal, connective tissue and bone disorders		muscle cramps, muscle spasms, neck pain, pain in limb	
Renal and urinary disorders		hematuria, microalbuminuria, glycosuria	micturition urgency
Reproductive system and breast disorders		genital burning sensation, genital pruritus	pelvic pain
General disorders and administration site conditions	feeling cold	pain, chest pain, fatigue, feeling abnormal, groin pain, feeling hot, injection site reaction	pyrexia, rigors
Investigations		electrocardiogram QT prolonged , electrocardiogram abnormal	electrocardiogram ST segment depression, electrocardiogram T-wave amplitude decreased, eosinophil count increased

ample, the average specificity across the precontrast TOF sequence was only around 31% and could be increased after Gadofosveset application to between 59.4 and 66.4%. Sensitivity was also increased by Vasovist® application (◘ Table 5.3). However, clinically this value is of only minor significance, since for patients with an indication for foot artery angiography the question of the possibility of extremity-saving bypass surgery, and therefore primarily a high degree of accuracy with unequivocal exclusion (true negatives, which are factored into the calculation of specificity, ◘ Table 5.2) of significant vascular stenosis is the primary focus. Only vessels appearing non-stenosed in angiography, with findings reflecting reality, are suitable as connecting vessels for bypass.

Contrary to the other phase III trials, the study performed on 156 patients with suspected stenosis/occlusion of the foot arteries showed for both non-contrast-enhanced TOF MRA and Gadofosveset-enhanced MRA unusually high sensitivity values in the detection of vascular stenosis. A statistically significant sensitivity increase due to Vasovist® administration was shown for only one reader. However, for all three blinded readers, the specificity was statistically significantly superior after Vasovist® administration. The diagnostic accuracy increased with the administration of Vasovist® for all three readers and was statistically significant for two of the three (◘ Table 5.3).

5.3.5 Stenosis Quantification

All four phase III trials not only examined the accuracy of detection of significant vascular stenosis compared with DSA, but also included quantification (in % stenosis) by measurement. These studies revealed that Gadofosveset-enhanced MRA not only far surpasses the accuracy of TOF angiography but also delivers results comparable to those of DSA.

5.4 Efficacy of Vasovist® at Low Albumin Levels

The contrast behavior of Vasovist® is critically dependent on its interaction with albumin. Thus, an analysis across several studies examined whether the diagnostic accuracy of MRA after administration of Vasovist® decreases in patients with low serum albumin levels. The unchanged values show that even in patients with pathologically low albumin levels a sufficient number of albumin molecules are still available for ensuring satisfactory efficacy of Vasovist®.

Take home messages

- Data from all the phase III studies showed an excellent overall efficacy compared with DSA as a clinical standard.
- Due to significantly higher relaxivity compared with extracellular agents, Vasovist® provides much stronger (brighter) signal, thereby improving the signal to-noise and contrast-to-noise ratios.
- Individual MRA readers had a mean accuracy for Gadofosveset-enhanced MRA of 88%, while the mean accuracy for non-contrast MRA was 75%.
- In addition, it was shown that the proportion of non-diagnostic angiographies after Vasovist® administration falls to below 1%; this is clearly lower than in TOF MRA (~14%) and even below DSA (~8%).

References

1. Grist TM, Korosec FR, Peters DC, Witte S, Walovitch RC, Dolan RP, Bridson WE, Yucel EK, Mistretta CA (1998) Steady state and dynamic MR angiography with MS-325: initial experience in humans. Radiology 207:539–544
2. Bluemke DA, Stillman AE, Bis KG, Grist TM, Baum RA, D'Agostino R, Malden ES, Pierro JA, Yucel EK (2001) Carotid MR angiography: phase II study of safety and efficacy for MS-325. Radiology 219:114–122
3. Perreault P, Edelman MA, Baum RA, Yucel EK, Weisskoff RM, Shamsi K, Mohler ER 3rd (2003) MR angiography with gadofosveset trisodium for peripheral vascular disease: phase II trial. Radiology 229:811–820
4. Rapp JH, Wolff SD, Quinn SF, Soto JA, Meranze SG, Muluk S, Blebea J, Johnson SP, Rofsky NM, Duerinckx A, Foster GS, Kent KC, Moneta G, Middlebrook MR, Narra VR, Toombs BD, Pollak J, Yucel EK, Shamsi K, Weisskoff RM (2005) Aortoiliac occlusive disease in patients with known or suspected peripheral vascular disease: safety and efficacy of gadofosveset-enhanced MR angiography – multicenter comparative phase III study. Radiology 236:71–78
5. Goyen M, Edelman M, Perreault P, O'Riordan E, Bertoni H, Taylor J, Siragusa D, Sharafuddin M, Mohler ER 3rd, Breger R, Yucel EK, Shamsi K, Weisskoff RM (2005) MR angiography of aortoiliac occlusive disease: a phase III study of the safety and effectiveness of the blood-pool contrast agent MS-325. Radiology 236:825–833
6. Pipe J (2001) Limits of time-of-flight magnetic resonance angiography. Top Magn Reson Imaging 2:163–174

Part III Blood Pool Agents in MRA: Indications, Clinical Applications and Benefits

of the carotid bifurcation, CE-MRA also yields useful supplemental information about such conditions as coexistent infarction, ischemia, intracranial aneurysms [32], and arteriovenous malformations [33], as well as arteriovenous fistulae. Crucially, and in addition, although CE-MRA depicts only the lumen accurately, non-enhanced, mainly fat-suppressed T1- and T2-weighted imaging proved to be effective for detection of vessel dissection, vascular wall and parenchymal hematoma, and subarachnoid bleeding. These diagnoses are not achievable with other imaging modalities [34].

6.6   Protocols for Supra-aortic Vessel Visualization

MRA provides the opportunity for both morphological and functional imaging. If multiple 3D data sets are acquired during the passage of the contrast agent bolus, the dynamics of blood flow can be monitored, providing a functional dimension to the technique that allows detection of blood-flow abnormalities. With extracellular gadolinium-based contrast agents and a 1.5-T scanner, a series of MRA data sets can be obtained with a 3D fast low-angle shot (FLASH) pulse sequence [35]. However, for most extracellular contrast agents, a conflict arises between the spatial resolution required for diagnostic accuracy of stenosis and the temporal resolution required for functional imaging. Therefore, for a combination of morphological and functional imaging, two separate injections are usually necessary when an extracellular contrast agent is used.

Technical innovations, including the introduction of parallel imaging allow reduction in acquisition time or increase the spatial resolution, or both [36]. The result is that, by virtue of improved sub-millimeter resolution, increased accuracy of contrast-enhanced MRA may be anticipated, thus meeting the requirements for detection and accurate grading of clinically significant carotid stenosis, notwithstanding the fact that comparison with catheter angiography (DSA) is unlikely now that it is no longer a widely employed diagnostic tool.

Another robust technique, the time-resolved echo-shared angiography technique (TREAT), provides additional functional information in areas or lesions with rapid blood flow. TREAT MRA combines morphological and functional information of the cerebral vasculature and addresses the specific physiological demands of some vascular lesions, e.g., short arteriovenous transit time. The advantage of using TREAT in dynamic MRA is that it provides images with reasonable resolution (voxel size $1.5 \times 1.3 \times 3$ mm) that approach the accuracy of DSA.

6.7   Benefits of the Blood pool MR Contrast Agent Vasovist®

Vasovist® is the first intravascular contrast agent approved for use with MRA in the European Union, Switzerland, Turkey, Canada, and Australia. The agent reversibly binds to albumin, providing extended intravascular enhancement [37], which should overcome the limitations of conventional contrast agents in MRA. The long intravascular residence time, combined with the highest available T1 relaxivity of all approved agents, enables high-resolution imaging of the carotid vessel walls and yields morphological and functional information with a single injection.

The optimum dose, clinical efficacy, and safety of Vasovist® have been evaluated in two phase II and four multicentre, phase III clinical trials. The optimum dose was found to be 0.03 mmol/kg and an injection time of 2–3 ml/s is recommended for first pass imaging [38, 39]. The phase III trials showed that the overall accuracy of Vasovist®-enhanced MRA was similar to that of catheter-based DSA, as determined by blinded readings [39]. In the four studies, nine of 12 readers reported statistically significant improvement in sensitivity, 12 of 12 readers greater specificity, and 11 of 12 readers greater accuracy in both vascular beds representative of areas of turbulent blood flow and of slow flow.

The excellent performance of the agent in MRA is based on two mechanisms: First, the agent binds reversibly and non-covalently to albumin, allowing an elimination half-life of approximately 15 h. The protein binding also reduces the tumbling rate of the molecule, resulting in a significantly higher relaxivity and an extended imaging time compared with other contrast agents [40]. The relaxivity (at 20 mHz) of Vasovist® measured in human plasma and ex vivo samples from rabbits and monkeys is approximately six to ten times greater that that of gadolinium diethylenetriaminepentaacetic acid (Magnevist®, Gd-DTPA, BayerSchering Pharma AG, Berlin, Germany) [41]. Because Vasovist® remains in the blood vessels in the steady state longer than extravascular agents, an imaging window of at least 30–60 min is provided which makes it possible to obtain not only a first pass MRA (◘ Fig. 6.1), but also high-resolution steady state imaging with no time restrictions from the contrast media side [42–44] (◘ Fig. 6.2). Compared with first pass imaging, steady state imaging sequences yield more morphological information than conventional MRA type sequences. This makes it possible to get additional information about parenchymal structures such as the vessel wall or adjacent pathologies (◘ Fig. 6.3). Thus, there is the potential to integrate the different diagnostic requirements of morphological and functional imaging in one comprehensive scan, with only one injection of contrast agent [39] (◘ Fig. 6.3).

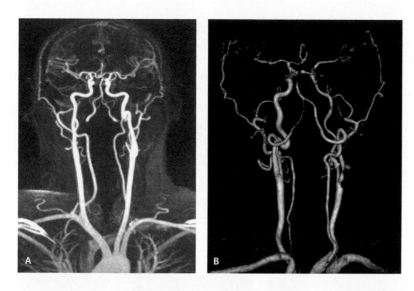

■ **Fig. 6.1A,B.** Supra-aortic 1.5-Tesla (Magnetom Avanto, Siemens Medical Solutions, Erlangen, Germany) first pass MRA with 0.03 mmol/kg of Vasovist® in a healthy volunteer (**A**) and in a patient with cerebrovascular disease (**B**). The contrast media allows a homogeneous enhancement of all displayed vessel segments including the intracerebral vasculature. MIP projection (**A**) and volume-rendered display (**B**) both allow a high-quality diagnosis of the complete supra-aortic vasculature with visualization of even the small peripheral branches. In the patient study (**B**) the pathology, a tandem stenosis of the left carotid artery, was clearly visualized using a standard dose. Due to the high vessel contrast and the possibility to achieve high-resolution data even a subtotal stenosis can be diagnosed with high accuracy

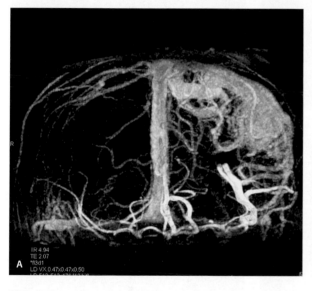

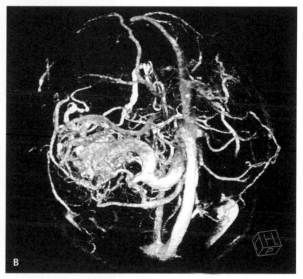

■ **Fig. 6.2A,B.** High-resolution 1.5-T (Magnetom Avanto, Siemens Medical Solutions, Erlangen, Germany) steady state MRA in a patient with a large cerebral arteriovenous malformation. The spatial resolution was 0.5 x 0.5 x 0.5 mm using a fast GRE sequence 5 min after injection of 0.03 mmol/kg of Vasovist®. Both the MIP projection (**A**) and the volume-rendered display (**B**) enable a detailed visualization of the complex angioarchitecture, including the venous drainage patterns. This information is very important for treatment decision and planning

The reversible binding of Vasovist® to albumin enhances its efficiency and, for diagnostic purposes, allows the administration of a smaller dose compared with existing extracellular contrast agents. The result is a reduced injection volume and flow rate, which avoids the need to change sequence parameters, as in conventional MRA [45].

Correct bolus timing for the first pass imaging is along routine lines with either a test bolus of Vasovist® of 1 ml injected at 1 ml/s followed by a 20-ml saline bolus injected at the same rate or, preferably, using MR fluoroscopy [44].

With exact timing, first pass imaging shows excellent image quality, which is comparable to that obtained with extracellular contrast agents. Processing of the images using thin maximum intensity projection or volume rendering techniques reduced venous overlay in the reconstructed image.

After reaching the equilibrium phase, Vasovist® enables repeated imaging at a high or ultra high spatial resolution. Even using low-level systems, steady state acquisition of isotropic voxels of <1 mm³ is possible, with acquisition times ≤1 min. As well as determining high resolution, this allows for reformatting of the data into any projection without compromising image quality. A recent study found that, for steady state imaging of the carotid arteries, an isotropic voxel dimension of 0.80 mm appeared to be the ideal compromise between resolution and acquisition time (40 s) to avoid movement-based artifacts and allowed the differentiation of the venous structures from the carotid arteries [44].

When Vasovist® is used for steady state imaging of the carotid arteries, it provides a high diagnostic image quality without the need for special post-processing. Steady state imaging provides all diagnostic information in contrast to first pass data. Vasovist®-enhanced MRA

resulted in high sensitivity and specificity (100% and 96%, respectively) for detection of significant stenosis [44]. In cases with suboptimal bolus timing during first pass imaging, steady state imaging enables several repeated acquisitions.

Because of the intravascular persistence and the possibility to achieve high-resolution steady state imaging, Vasovist® has the potential to be used for an improved diagnosis of intracranial vascular disease, such as aneurysms and vascular malformations (◘ Fig. 6.4), and can also demonstrate tumor vascular supply (◘ Fig. 6.5).

The protein binding increases both the T1 and the T2 relaxivity. The improved T1 relaxivity is responsible for

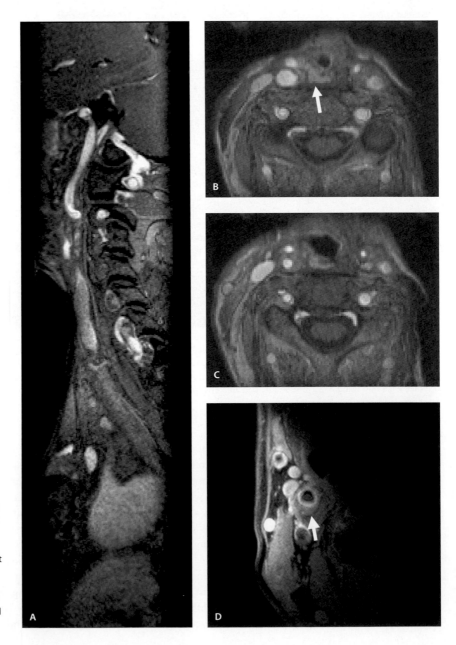

◘ **Fig. 6.3A–D.** High-resolution 3T (Magnetom Trio, Siemens Medical Solutions, Erlangen, Germany) steady state Vasovist® (0.03 mmol/kg)-enhanced MRA in a patient with squamous cell carcinoma. The GRE VIBE sequence used allows for ultra high spatial resolution imaging while still obtaining anatomical information (**A–C**). This enables a clear description of the relation of the tumor (*arrow* in **B**) to the right carotid artery. As an additional finding a stenosis of the left carotid artery was diagnosed. Steady state imaging also allows for better depiction of the vessel wall, as can be seen in a different patient with carotid artery disease panel **D** (*arrow*)

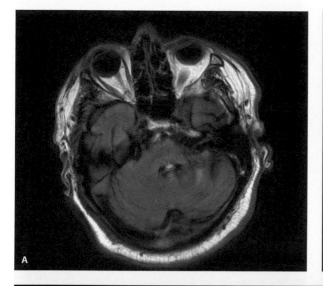

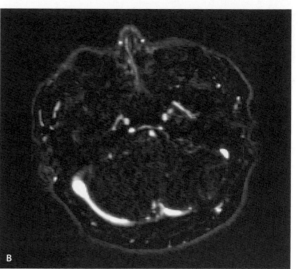

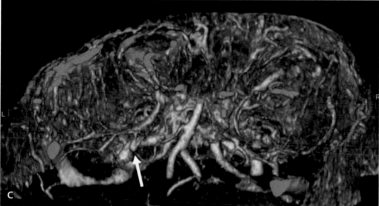

Fig. 6.4A–C. Vasovist®-enhanced MRA (0.03 mmol/kg) in a patient with small residual arteriovenous malformation after bleeding who was referred for treatment decision (**A**) While TOF-MRA was not able to diagnose residual AVM components, the contrast-enhanced 3-T MRA (Magnetom Trio®, Siemens Medical Solutions, Erlangen, Germany) using TRICKS (**B**) showed a small residual AVM nidus at the lateral border of the cerebellum, fed by an early-appearing branch from the left PICA. The high-resolution steady state MRA that followed (**C**) allowed a detailed 3D view of the nidus in relation to the feeding arteries and draining vein. Based on the MRA, the patient was identified as a candidate for high-precision radiosurgical treatment

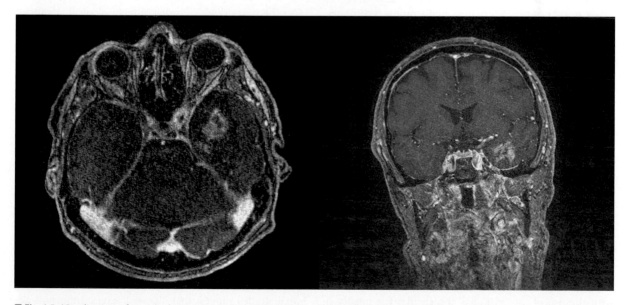

Fig. 6.5. Visualization of a radiotherapeutic induced blood-brain barrier breakdown in a patient with arteriovenous malformation. Following injection of a standard dose of Vasovist® both first pass multiphase TRICKS MRA and high-resolution steady state were not able to illustrate residual components. However, the enhancement in the AVM bed was well-displayed due to an extravasation of Vasovist® via the disrupted blood-brain barrier

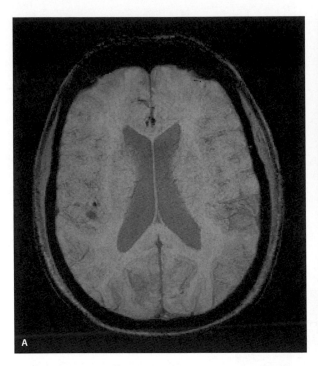
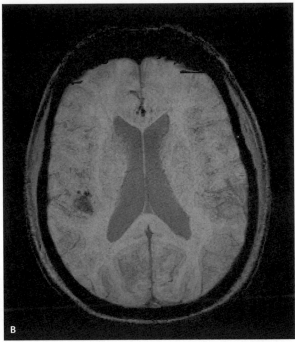

Fig. 6.6A,B. 3-Tesla (Magnetom Trio, Siemens Medical Solutions, Erlangen, Germany) susceptibility-weighted MRI prior to (**A**) and after (**B**) injection of 0.03 mmol/kg of Gadofosveset in a cavernoma patient. Following contrast medium injection the quality of the SWI MRI substantially increased, with enhanced display of small venous vascular structures. On the displayed identical slices the venous vascular malformation appears to be larger due to the stronger susceptibility effect, induced by the higher relaxivity of the agent

the substantially better MRA performance, and because of the improved T2 relaxivity it is possible to enhance the image quality of new alternative angiographic techniques, e.g., susceptibility-weighted MR imaging.

High-resolution susceptibility-weighted imaging (SWI) (initially called high-resolution magnetic resonance blood oxygenation level-dependent venography) is a three-dimensional MRA method that has been developed within the past few years [46, 47].

The BOLD (blood oxygenation level-dependent) sensitive method combines magnitude and phase image information from a high-resolution 3D T2*-weighted gradient echo sequence to visualize small cerebral vessels, mainly veins, in high spatial resolution and detail. The technique has so far been applied for imaging vascular malformations [48], brain tumors [49], trauma, stroke, microhemorrhages, and as a functional imaging method [49].

Methods to improve this interesting new angiographic technique are the use of 3T and the use of a T1-shortening paramagnetic contrast agent [50]. First experience with the use of Vasovist® has shown that the quality of susceptibility-weighted MRA is superior with respect to vessel visualization and description of extent of disease (■ Fig. 6.6).

6.8 Conclusions

Over the past decade, a series of technological advances, such as fast gradient echo imaging and better understanding of the contrast dynamics of extravascular contrast agents, has resulted in the development of highly accurate, safe imaging of the head and neck arteries. The development of Vasovist® – the first approved blood pool contrast agent – combined with advances in acquisition strategies and more advanced post-processing techniques has resulted in sub-millimeter resolution of carotid stenosis. This degree of resolution and accuracy of CE-MRA has already resulted in MRA replacing DSA as the gold standard for assessing carotid artery disease and identifying patients who are likely to benefit most from surgical intervention. Future studies will have to address the optimization of imaging time, reconstruction time, and interpretation strategies – as well as the further optimization of image quality – for steady state imaging data. Although it has yet to be evaluated extensively in the clinical setting, initial studies suggest that Vasovist® gives important additional information in the evaluation of both carotid and intracranial disease, not only at the structural but also the functional level.

References

1. Feigin VL, Lawes CM, Bennett DA, Anderson CS (2003) Stroke epidemiology: a review of population-based studies of incidence, prevalence, and case-fatality in the late 20th century. Lancet Neurol 2:43–53

2. Beers MHH, Porter RS (2003) The Merck manual of diagnosis and therapy, 18th edn. Merck Research Laboratories, Whitehouse Station

3. World Health Organization (2003) Cardiovascular disease fact file. World Health Organization, Geneva

4. Chang HS (2006) Simulation of the natural history of cerebral aneurysms based on data from the International Study of Unruptured Intracranial Aneurysms. J Neurosurg 104:188–194

5. Bots ML, Hoes AW, Hofman A, Witteman JCM, Grobbee DE (1999) Cross-sectionally assessed carotid intima-media thickness relates to long-term risk of stroke, coronary heart disease and death as estimated by available risk functions. J Intern Med 245:269–276

6. Hademenos GJ, Massoud TF (1997) Biophysical mechanisms of stroke. Stroke 28:2067–2077

7. European Carotid Surgery Trialists' Collaborative Group (1998) Randomised trial of endarterectomy for recently symptomatic carotid stenosis: final results of the MRC European Carotid Surgery Trial (ECST). Lancet 351:1379–1387

8. Barnett HJ, Taylor DW, Eliasziw M, Fox AJ, Ferguson GG, Haynes RB, Rankin RN, Clagett GP, Hachinski VC, Sackett DL, Thorpe KE, Meldrum HE, Spence JD (1998) Benefit of carotid endarterectomy in patients with symptomatic moderate or severe stenosis. North American Symptomatic Carotid Endarterectomy Trial Collaborators. N Engl J Med 339:1415–1425

9. Mayberg MR, Wilson SE, Yatsu F, Weiss DG, Messina L, Hershey LA, Colling C, Eskridge J, Deykin D, Winn HR (1991) Carotid endarterectomy and prevention of cerebral ischemia in symptomatic carotid stenosis. JAMA 266:3289–3294

10. Barth A, Arnold M, Mattle HP, Schroth G, Remonda L (2006) Contrast-enhanced 3-D MRA in decision making for carotid endarterectomy: a 6-year experience. Cerebrovasc Dis 21:393–400

11. Kaufmann TJ, Kallmes DF (2005) Utility of MRA and CTA in the evaluation of carotid occlusive disease. Semin Vasc Surg 18:75–82

12. U-Kim-Im JM, Trivedi Ra, Graves MJ et al (2004) Contrast-enhanced MR angiography for carotid disease: diagnostic and potential clinical impact. Neurology 27:1282–1290

13. Jewells V, Castillo M (2003) MR angiography of the extracranial circulation. Magn Reson Imaging Clin N Am 11:585–597

14. Beltramello A, Piovan E, Rosta L (1994) Double blind comparison of safety and efficaxo of iomeprol and iopamidol in carotid digital subtraction angiography. Eur J Radiol 18:S67–72

15. Barth A, Arnold M, Mattle HP, Schroth G, Remonda L (2006) Contrast-enhance 3-D MRA in decision making for carotid endarterectomy: a 6-year experience. Cerebrovasc Dis 21:393–400

16. Nieman K, van der Lugt A, Pattynama PM, de Feyter PJ (2003) Noninvasive visualization of atherosclerotic plaque with electron beam and multislice spial computed tomography. J Interv Cardiol 16:123–128

17. Adams WM, Laitt RD, Thorne J, Jackson A (1999) MRA visualization of cerebral aneurysms. Medica Mundi 43:2–9

18. Ozsarlak O, Van Goethem JW, Maes M, Parizel PM (2004) MR angiography of the intracranial vessels: technical aspects and clinical applications. Neuroradiology 46:955–972

19. Wilkerson DK, Keller I, Mezrich R, Schroder WB, Sebok D, Gronlund-Jacobs J, Conway R, Zatina MA (1991) The comparative evaluation of three-dimensional magnetic resonance for carotid artery disease. J Vasc Surg 14:803–809

20. Chiesa R, Melissano G, Castellano R, Triulzi F, Anzalone N, Veglia F, Scotti G, Grossi A (1993) Three dimensional time of flight magnetic resonance angiography in carotid artery surgery: a comparison with digital subtraction angiography. Eur J Vasc Surg 7:171–176

21. DeMarco JK, Huston J, 3rd, Bernstein MA (2004) Evaluation of classic 2D time-of-flight MR angiography in the depiction of severe carotid stenosis. AJR Am J Roentgenol 183:787–793

22. Carr JC, Shaibani A, Russell E, Finn JP (2001) Contrast-enhanced magnetic resonance angiography of the carotid circulation. Top Magn Reson Imaging 12:349–357

23. U-King-Im JM, Trivedi RA, Graves MJ, Higgins NJ, Cross JJ, Tom BD, Hollingworth W, Eales H, Warburton EA, Kirkpatrick PJ, Antoun NM, Gillard JH (2004) Contrast-enhanced MR angiography for carotid disease: diagnostic and potential clinical impact. Neurology 62:1282–1290

24. Nael K, Ruehm SG, Michaely HJ, Pope W, Laub G, Finn JP, Villablanca JP (2006) High spatial-resolution CE-MRA of the carotid circulation with parallel imaging: comparison of image quality between 2 different acceleration factors at 3.0 Tesla. Invest Radiol 41:391–399

25. Naganawa S, Koshikawa T, Fukatsu H, Sakurai Y, Ichinose N, Ishiguchi T, Ishigaki T (2001) Contrast-enhanced MR angiography of the carotid artery using 3D time-resolved imaging of contrast kinetics: comparison with real-time fluoroscopic triggered 3D-elliptical centric view ordering. Radiat Med 19:185–192

26. Earls JP, Rofsky NM, DeCorato DR, Krinsky GA, Weinreb JC (1996) Breath-hold single-dose gadolinium-enhanced three-dimensional MR aortography: usefulness of a timing examination and MR power injector. Radiology 201:705–710

27. Foo TK, Saranathan M, Prince MR, Chenevert TL (1997) Automated detection of bolus arrival and initiation of data acquisition in fast, three-dimensional, gadolinium-enhanced MR angiography. Radiology 203:275–280

28. Wilman AH, Riederer SJ, King BF, Debbins JP, Rossman PJ, Ehman RL (1997) Fluoroscopically triggered contrast-enhanced three-dimensional MR angiography with elliptical centric view order: application to the renal arteries. Radiology 205:137–146

6

29. Blakeley DD, Oddone EZ, Hasselblad V, Simel DL, Matchar DB (1995) Noninvasive carotid artery testing. A meta-analytic review. Ann Intern Med 122:360–367

30. Nederkoorn PJ, van der Graaf Y, Hunink MG (2003) Duplex ultrasound and magnetic resonance angiography compared with digital subtraction angiography in carotid artery stenosis: a systematic review. Stroke 34:1324–1332

31. Atlas SW, Sheppard L, Goldberg HI, Hurst RW, Listerud J, Flamm E (1997) Intracranial aneurysms: detection and characterization with MR angiography with use of an advanced postprocessing technique in a blinded-reader study. Radiology 203:807–814

32. Duran M, Schoenberg SO, Yuh WT, Knopp MV, van Kaick G, Essig M (2002) Cerebral arteriovenous malformations: morphologic evaluation by ultrashort 3D gadolinium-enhanced MR angiography. Eur Radiol 12:2957–2964

33. Essig M, Reichenbach JR, Schad LR, Schoenberg SO, Debus J, Kaiser WA (1999) High-resolution MR venography of cerebral arteriovenous malformations. Magn Reson Imaging 17:1417–1425

34. Schellinger PD, Fiebach JB (2004) Intracranial hemorrhage: the role of magnetic resonance imaging. Neurocrit Care 1:31-45

35. Fellner C, Strotzer M, Fraunhofer S, Held P, Spies V, Seitz J, Fellner F (1997) MR angiography of the supra-aortic arteries using a dedicated head and neck coil: image quality and assessment of stenoses. Neuroradiology 39:763–771

36. Weiger M, Pruessmann KP, Kassner A, Roditi G, Lawton T, Reid A, Boesiger P (2000) Contrast-enhanced 3D MRA using SENSE. J Magn Reson Imaging 12:671–677

37. Caravan P, Cloutier NJ, Greenfield MT, McDermid SA, Dunham SU, Bulte JW, Amedio JC Jr, Looby RJ, Supkowski RM, Horrocks WD Jr, McMurry TJ, Lauffer RB (2002) The interaction of MS-325 with human serum albumin and its effect on proton relaxation rates. J Am Chem Soc 124:3152–3162

38. Bluemke DA, Stillman AE, Bis KG, Grist TM, Baum RA, D'Agostino R, Malden ES, Pierro JA, Yucel EK (2001) Carotid MR angiography: phase II study of safety and efficacy for MS-325. Radiology 219:114–122

39. Perreault P, Edelman MA, Baum RA, Yucel EK, Weisskoff RM, Shamsi K, Mohler ER 3rd (2003) MR angiography with gadofosveset trisodium for peripheral vascular disease: phase II trial. Radiology 229:811–820

40. Goyen M, Shamsi K, Schoenberg SO (2006) Vasovist-enhanced MR angiography. Eur Radiol 16 [Suppl 2]:B9–B14

41. Lauffer RB, Parmelee DJ, Dunham SU, Ouellet HS, Dolan RP, Witte S, McMurry TJ, Walovitch RC (1998) MS-325: albumin-targeted contrast agent for MR angiography. Radiology 207:529–538

42. Rohrer M, Bauer H, Mintorovitch J, Requardt M, Weinmann HJ (2005) Comparison of magnetic properties of MRI contrast media solutions at different magnetic field strengths. Invest Radiol 40:715–724

43. Grist TM, Korosec FR, Peters DC, Witte S, Walovitch RC, Dolan RP, Bridson WE, Yucel EK, Mistretta CA (1998) Steady state and dynamic MR angiography with MS-325: initial experience in humans. Radiology 207:539–544

44. Nikolaou K, Kramer H, Grosse C, Clevert D, Dietrich O, Hartmann M, Chamberlin P, Assmann S, Reiser MF, Schoenberg SO (2006) High-spatial-resolution multistation MR angiography with parallel imaging and blood pool contrast agent: initial experience. Radiology 241:861–872

45. Hartmann M, Wiethoff AJ, Hentrich HR, Rohrer M (2006) Initial imaging recommendations for Vasovist angiography. Eur Radiol 16 [Suppl 2]:B15–B23

46. Haacke EM, Xu Y, Cheng YC, Reichenbach JR (2004) Susceptibility weighted imaging (SWI). Magn Reson Med 52:612–618

47. Reichenbach JR, Venkatesan R, Schillinger et al (1997) Small vessels in the human brain: MR venography with deoxyhemoglobin as an intrinsic contrast agent. Radiology 204:272–277

48. Essig M, Reichenbach JR, Schad LR, et al (1999) High-resolution MR venography of cerebral arteriovenous malformations. Mag Res Imaging 17:1417–1425

49. Sehal V, Delproposto Z, Haacke EM, et al (2005) Clinical applications of neuroimaging with susceptibility-weighted imaging. J Magn Reson Imaging 22:439–450

50. Barth M, Noebauer-Huhmann I-M, Reichenbach JR, et al (2003) High resolution, three dimensional contrast-enhanced blood oxygenation level-dependent magnetic resonance venography of brain tumors at 3 Tesla: first experience and comparison with 1.5 Tesla. Invest Radiol 38:409–414

Pulmonary MRA

Christian Fink, Ulrike Attenberger, and Konstantin Nikolaou

7.1 Introduction

Computed tomography angiography (CTA) of the lung is nowadays considered the clinical gold standard for the assessment of pulmonary vascular disease [1, 2]. Different to other vascular territories (e.g., the peripheral arteries, renal arteries), contrast-enhanced magnetic resonance angiography (MRA) is usually not considered a first-line imaging tool for the assessment of the pulmonary circulation. When compared with CT, the inferior spatial resolution and long breath-hold times of pulmonary MRA are regarded as major drawbacks.

On the other hand, there are potential advantages of MRA for the evaluation of lung disease. Above all, this includes the lack of ionizing radiation, which is of major importance in congenital disease and chronic diseases requiring frequent follow-up examinations. Moreover, MRI is considered the standard of reference for the assessment of cardiac function; thus MRI can provide a comprehensive assessment of pulmonary vascular disease, including measurement of the right heart function pulmonary artery pressure [3, 4]. Ongoing technical developments, such as parallel imaging techniques, have further improved the feasibility of pulmonary MRA and moved the application from a pure research tool to a clinical practice. The recent introduction of the blood pool MR contrast agent Vasovist® (Gadofosveset, Bayer Schering Pharma AG, Berlin, Germany) has further increased the options of pulmonary MRA [5]. The albumin-binding characteristic of the contrast agent extends the vascular lifetime and thus allows for longer vascular imaging time, potentially higher spatial resolution, and greater anatomic coverage. During the first pass of the contrast agent, pulmonary perfusion can be assessed. During the equilibrium or »steady state« phase of the contrast, the pulmonary vasculature – as well as other parts of the body vasculature such as the veins of the abdomen and lower extremities – can be scanned at high spatial resolution, without additional injections of contrast agent required. With the introduction of such contrast agents, limitations of today's thoracic MRA might be overcome, and imaging strategies could further be developed and improved [6].

7.2 Technical Considerations

7.2.1 General Considerations

Three-dimensional gradient echo MRA after injection of an extracellular MR contrast agent (ECCM) has been established as the method of choice for pulmonary MRA. In general, there are two different approaches to first pass contrast-enhanced pulmonary MRA. In addition to a single high-resolution 3D MRA, time-resolved multiphase MRA

of the pulmonary vasculature may be performed. Along with improved arteriovenous separation, time-resolved pulmonary MRA is less sensitive for incorrect bolus timing and less sensitive for motion artifacts. The latter may be relevant in dyspneic patients. Also, and probably most important, time-resolved MRA also makes it possible to obtain functional information of the pulmonary circulation, such as the characterization of shunts or the assessment of capillary perfusion of the lung parenchyma. Several studies have shown the feasibility of pulmonary perfusion MRI using a time-resolved MRA technique [7–11].

The anatomy of the pulmonary circulation has some specific implications for pulmonary MR imaging. The multiple air-tissue interfaces of the lungs result in a very high susceptibility. This substantially affects the achievable signal intensity of small peripheral lung vessels in MRI. On the other hand, the low signal of the lung parenchyma usually results in a high vessel-to-background contrast of pulmonary MRA. In general, short echo times, i.e., potentially lower than 2–3 ms, should be used to eliminate susceptibility effects [12]. Moreover, the lungs have a very short transit time, i.e., in the range of 3–5 s [13]. As a consequence, first pass pulmonary MRA often has substantial venous contamination, potentially affecting the diagnostic accuracy. To reduce venous contamination, the aim should be a very compact bolus profile. Using ECCM, this can be achieved by using a low contrast agent volume and high injection rates (e.g. 5 ml/s).

7.2.2 Introduction of Intravascular Contrast Agents

Compared with standard ECCM, the intravascular contrast agent Vasovist® provides a much smaller and therefore very compact injection volume of approximately 7–10 ml for a standard dose (0.12 ml/kg body weight). Similar to standard ECCM, Vasovist® can also be used for first pass high-resolution MRA or first pass perfusion imaging [14]. Because the relaxivity of Vasovist® is five to seven times higher than that of conventional 0.5 mol/l extracellular contrast agents (used at 1.5 T), the injection of Vasovist® at 1 ml/s translates into a conventional contrast agent injection rate of about 5–7 ml/s, resulting in a high vascular signal intensity (SI) and high image quality of the Vasovist®-enhanced first pass imaging data. This benefit of high signal-to-noise ratio during the first pass of Vasovist® might be of particular advantage for time-resolved imaging. For first pass MRA, regardless of using ECCM or Vasovist®, the shortest achievable TE and TR should be used. However, in contrast to ECCM, Vasovist® can also be used for an additional high-resolution MRA during steady state distribution of the contrast agent (◘ Fig. 7.1). If possible, the sequence parameters for steady state MRA with Vasovist® should be adapted using longer TR (7–20 ms) and lower flip angles (15–25°) [15]. However, using a longer TR might increase the scan time, so that a breath-hold exam is no longer feasible. Also, cardiac motion artifacts can pose considerable problems in acquisition optimization. One solution to maintain a high spatial resolution of the steady state MRA datasets could be the acquisition of two separate sagittal slabs covering the pulmonary arteries and both lungs in two subsequent breath-holds [16]. In addition, refined acquisition techniques involving free-breathing navigator approaches – possibly combined with electrocardiographic gating – could be effective to optimize image quality. Navigator-gated MRA has already been evaluated for free-breathing pulmonary MRA in various animal and volunteer studies [17–20]. A potential drawback of navigator-gated MRA is the increased scan time, which might limit the value of this imaging technique in clinical practice.

Several studies have already evaluated the use of various blood pool MR contrast agents for pulmonary MRA. In a study by Nolte-Ernsting et al., pulmonary MRA was performed in pigs using a superparamagnetic iron oxide blood pool agent. In correlation to conventional X-ray angiography, the pulmonary vasculature was visualized down to the first order sub-segmental branches, including vessel diameters of approximately 1.5 mm [21]. A subsequent feasibility study by Weishaupt et al. evaluated ultra-small superparamagnetic iron oxide-enhanced pulmonary MRA in two volunteers and a pig model of pulmonary hemorrhage [22]. The use of the blood pool agent allowed excellent delineation of central, segmental, and sub-segmental pulmonary arteries in the volunteer studies. In the pig model, pulmonary hemorrhage was visualized. In a volunteer study by Ahlstrom et al., pulmonary MRA was performed with a superparamagnetic iron oxide using navigator respiratory gating. With increasing doses of the contrast agent, higher signal intensities and vessel branch order visualization were achieved. A subsequent animal study by Abolmaali et al. demonstrated the feasibility of navigator-gated pulmonary MRA using the gadolinium-based blood pool contrast agent Gadomer-17 [20]. Zheng et al. evaluated the protein-binding blood pool contrast agent B-22956/1 for the assessment of pulmonary embolism by perfusion MRI and high-resolution MRA in a pig model [23]. They found that whole-lung-coverage perfusion MRI and high-resolution target MRA could be performed after a single contrast bolus injection. Motivated by these studies, we assessed the feasibility of contrast-enhanced 3D perfusion MRI and MRA of pulmonary embolism using a single injection of Gadomer-17. Perfusion MRI allowed the visualization of typical wedge-shaped perfusion defects. Compared with a standard ECCM, the blood pool contrast agent achieved a higher SNR [24].

7.2.3 Perfusion MRI of the Lungs: Qualitative and Quantitative Approach

For a number of clinical indications, knowledge of the regional pulmonary microcirculation is essential, such as in patients suffering from acute or chronic pulmonary embolism or various other forms of pulmonary hypertension. Presurgical information on the most poorly perfused lung area before lung reduction is as important as postoperative quantification of lung perfusion after lung transplantation or in postoperative complications, such as obliterative bronchiolitis. The desire for both qualitative and quantitative information on pulmonary microcirculation in a single study without exposure to ionizing radiation drives the investigation of magnetic MRI techniques for the assessment of pulmonary perfusion.

More than 10 years ago it was reported that qualitative assessment of pulmonary microcirculation in human subjects was feasible using a contrast-enhanced inversion recovery fast gradient-echo technique with ultra-short echo times [25]. Subsequent clinical studies have shown the clinical utility of dynamic MRI for the evaluation of lung diseases such as pulmonary embolism by detecting the first pass of a paramagnetic contrast medium (CM) through lung tissue [26, 27]. The clinical introduction of parallel imaging techniques has brought along significant advantages, primarily in terms of acquisition time and/ or an increase of spatial resolution [10, 28]. These advantages are particularly attractive for time-resolved, contrast-enhanced MRI of tissue microcirculation, because a high temporal resolution is necessary for acquisition of sufficient data points during the first passage of a contrast bolus. With the application of these techniques, MRI has been shown to be sensitive to gravity-dependent differences of pulmonary perfusion and to agree well with conventional radionuclide perfusion scintigraphy in healthy volunteers and in patients with lung cancer [7].

In addition to qualitative imaging of lung perfusion, the quantitative assessment of the pulmonary microcirculation would be desirable for several reasons: It would enable interindividual comparison of patients with various pathologies, and an intraindividual assessment after surgical or other medical treatment, e.g., longitudinal assessment of drug treatment of pulmonary hypertension using prostaglandin derivates [29]. However, several technical difficulties in absolute quantification of lung perfusion have to be overcome: susceptibility artifacts reducing the obtainable signal, necessary optimization of the dosage of contrast agent to avoid systematic errors in perfusion quantification, and choosing the correct theoretical or mathematical model to calculate lung perfusion. Difficulties in obtaining MR signal from lung parenchyma can be decreased by using an ultra-short echo time (TE) of <1 ms, which reduces the effect of local magnetic field

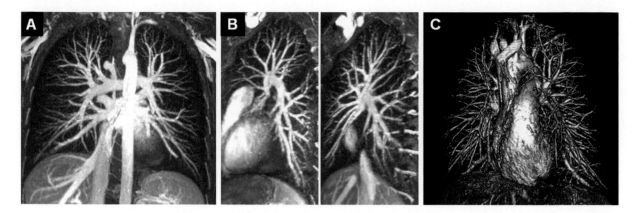

◻ **Fig. 7.1A–C.** High-resolution steady state MRA of the lung acquired with Vasovist® in a healthy volunteer. After first pass imaging (during which either perfusion imaging or first pass high-resolution MR angiography can be performed), a long acquisition window of up to 60 min can be used for high-resolution imaging of various vascular beds. Using parallel imaging for high-resolution steady state MRA, isotropic spatial resolution of about 1.0–1.5 mm³ can be achieved in a scan time of approximately 20 s. The nearly isotropic spatial resolution allows for a true 3D volumetric assessment of the pulmonary arterial tree [**A** coronal maximum intensity projection (MIP); **B** sagittal MIPs of the right lung; **C** 3D volume rendering of the complete MRA dataset]. (Modified from [50], with permission)

inhomogeneities caused by the multiple air/soft tissue interfaces of pulmonary alveolar architecture. Promising results concerning quantification of pulmonary perfusion in an animal model using a time-resolved inversion recovery technique with ultra-short echo times have been published [30]. Initial studies have presented data on absolute quantification of pulmonary perfusion in human subjects, including a limited number of patients and reporting a broad interindividual variation of results [1, 10, 32]. Also – as mentioned above - the effect of the CM dosage and CM type on the correctness of quantification of pulmonary microcirculation in human subjects has been brought up and seems to be crucial for the reliability of quantitative results [10, 33]. CM dosages appropriate for absolute quantification are small, resulting in only small signal increases. So far, only a few studies have systematically investigated the effect of the amount and type of the paramagnetic contrast agent applied in time-resolved pulmonary MRA [10]. It has been reported that administration of a CM with a higher concentration of gadolinium chelates (e.g., 1.0 M Gadobutrol, Gadovist®) but maintaining the absolute amount of chelates does not offer significant advantages over standard 0.5 M Gd-DTPA for contrast-enhanced 3D MRI of the lung [33]. It seems reasonable that the use of a higher total CM dose tended to provide a higher degree of visual parenchymal enhancement [34, 35]. However, using these high CM concentrations, absolute quantification of microcirculatory parameters is not practicable because of saturation effects affecting the shape of the arterial input function. An approximately linear correlation between signal intensity and CM concentration is an indispensable requirement for reliable assessment of the arterial input function. For this reason, the CM dose administered for quantification of pulmonary blood flow and volume must be markedly lower than the dose typically used for qualitative, visual assessment of pulmonary perfusion. Furthermore, for a quantitative estimation of pulmonary blood flow and volume, typically simplified models such as an open one-compartment model are being used. However, this simple model reflects the presumption that CM extravasation is negligible during first pass through the lungs (or, least probable, that CM exchange between the capillaries and the interstitial space is extremely fast). The use of blood pool agents such as Vasovist® may resolve this dilemma because their prolonged retention time circumvents the possibility of extravasation during the first pass [36]. Several initial studies have employed a blood pool contrast agent for qualitative evaluation of pulmonary perfusion, with promising results (◻ Fig. 7.1 and 7.2) [23, 24, 37]. One study has also demonstrated the successful quantification of perfusion indices on a 3T system, using an intravascular contrast agent [38]. The prolonged intravascular time of an intravascular contrast agent ensures the linearity of the signal response to tracer concentration, which is necessary for application of the indicator dilution theory [39]. This results in an improved fitting, and accurate quantification of perfusion indices such as time-to-peak (TTP), mean-transit-time (MTT), maximal-signal-intensity (MSI) and others becomes feasible. Overall, in terms of qualitative and quantitative assessment of pulmonary perfusion, intravascular contrast agents such as Vasovist® have two major advantages: First, after perfusion imaging during first pass of the contrast, it is still possible to obtain high-resolution steady state MRA data. Second, due to the lack of contrast extravasation during first pass, absolute quantification should be more reliable and reproducible.

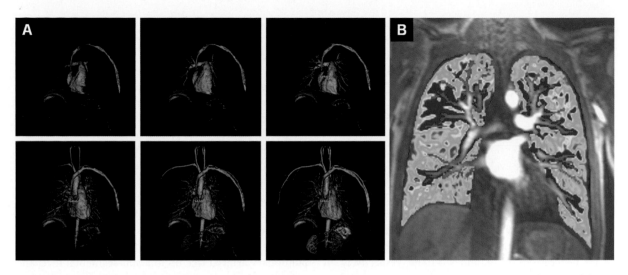

Fig. 7.2A,B. Time-resolved MRA (**A**, **B**) of the lung acquired with Vasovist® in a healthy volunteer. **A**: Selected frames from a time-resolved MRA acquired during the first pass of the contrast agent bolus showing a homogeneous lung perfusion **B**: Color-coded perfusion map computed from the time-resolved MRA data (pulmonary perfusion MRI). Using parallel imaging techniques and a state-of-the-art MR scanner with strong gradients, single 3D slabs can be acquired in about 1.0–1.2 s, acquiring a dynamic dataset of 20 slabs in an acceptable breath-hold time of less than 25 s during the first pass of Vasovist®. (Modified from [50], with permission)

7.2.4 Imaging the Pulmonary Vasculature at 3 Tesla

The implementation of parallel acquisition techniques generally results in a reduction of the minimum scan time, which then can be used to increase the speed and/or the spatial resolution. However, the signal-to-noise ratio (SNR) penalty of parallel imaging can be limiting in clinical practice, depending on several factors, such as the degree of K-space undersampling [40]. Strategies to preserve SNR while maximizing the efficiency of parallel acquisition include raising the baseline signal by increasing field strength [41, 42], minimizing noise amplification by using new array coils [43], and using contrast agents with higher concentration or T1 relaxivity [44, 45]. In a recently published study, Nael et al. evaluated the feasibility of contrast-enhanced pulmonary perfusion MRI at 3 T using Gadomer-17 in a pig model [38]. The high T1 relaxivity of the blood pool contrast agent facilitated the acquisition of perfusion data sets with high image quality and allowed for the calculation of quantitative perfusion parameters.

In general, the introduction of multichannel 3 T MR systems into clinical practice has the potential to significantly improve the performance of pulmonary MR perfusion and high-resolution MRA in terms of spatial and temporal resolution [41]. However, in the lungs the higher magnetic susceptibility gradients associated with high magnetic field can be limiting, resulting in signal loss and relatively lower parenchymal enhancement in comparison

to 1.5 T [46]. Dielectric resonances and radiofrequency (RF) eddy currents can also be potentially troublesome at 3 T [47]. The use of an intravascular contrast agent with shorter T1 may be advantageous to trade off the signal loss associated with magnetic susceptibility effects and further support highly accelerated parallel acquisition. Also, since the longitudinal relaxation time (T1) of unenhanced blood increases with field strength, the sensitivity to injected gadolinium (Gd) agents is heightened, and thus less contrast material is required [48]. However, initial studies have shown a relatively lower parenchymal enhancement at 3 T in comparison to 1.5 T. One possible explanation is that signal loss occurs due to magnetic susceptibility gradients of the lungs resulting from multiple air/soft-tissue interfaces. Since the susceptibility effect increases with magnetic field [32], the T2* of the lung is expected to be smaller at 3.0 T than at 1.5 T [49]. This signal loss has constrained the application of parallel acquisition to an acceleration factor of 2 for pulmonary imaging at both 1.5 T and 3.0 T. An intravascular contrast agent with shorter T1, such as Vasovist®, may be used to enhance the performance of pulmonary perfusion protocols at 3.0 T and support parallel acquisition with a higher acceleration factor.

7.3 Clinical Applications

Pulmonary MRA has been proposed for several pulmonary vascular disorders. The imaging technique can be tailored to the clinical problem, ranging from detailed morphological evaluation using high spatial resolution MRA to functional time-resolved MRA studies characterizing shunts or lung perfusion. In the following, the most important applications are reviewed in detail.

7.3.1 Pulmonary MRA in Acute Pulmonary Embolism

Several studies have evaluated the performance of pulmonary contrast-enhanced MRA for the diagnosis of pulmonary embolism (PE) [50]. In a pivotal study, Meaney et al. examined 30 patients with suspected PE using contrast-enhanced pulmonary MRA and DSA. Contrast-enhanced MRA yielded a sensitivity and specificity for the detection of PE between 75–100% and 95–100%, respectively. In addition, a good interobserver agreement (kappa values of 0.57–0.83) was demonstrated [51]. A subsequent study by Gupta et al. evaluated the accuracy of pulmonary contrast-enhanced MRA in 36 patients with intermediate or low probability lung scintigraphy. In this study as well, all patients underwent pulmonary DSA, which demonstrated PE in 13 patients. Pulmonary contrast-enhanced MRA diagnosed 12 patients as having PE but missed two cases. This resulted in a sensitivity of 85% and specificity of 96%. Both missed pulmonary emboli were isolated and sub-segmental in location [52]. In the largest study so far, Oudkerk et al. assessed the accuracy of pulmonary contrast-enhanced MRA in 141 patients with an abnormal perfusion lung scintigraphy and compared the findings with those of pulmonary DSA. Contrast-enhanced MRA detected 27 of 35 cases with confirmed PE, resulting in an overall sensitivity of 77%. The sensitivity for isolated sub-segmental, segmental, and central/lobar PE was 40%, 84%, and 100%, respectively. Contrast-enhanced MRA demonstrated emboli in two patients with a normal angiogram, i.e., the specificity was 98% [53]. In a more recent study, Blum et al. examined 89 patients with suspected PE using coronal, axial, and sagittal-orientated contrast-enhanced MRA. The images were interpreted independently by two teams of radiologists. Different to the previous studies, a heterogeneous combination of clinical probability, D-dimer testing, spiral CT, compression venous ultrasound, and pulmonary DSA served as the gold standard in this study [54]. In addition, the study cohort had a much higher prevalence of PE (i.e. 71%). Depending on the team of readers, the sensitivity and specificity of contrast-enhanced MRA ranged between 31–71% and 85–92%. In a study of 48 patients with suspected PE, Pleszewski reported a sensitivity and specificity of 82% and 100%, respectively [55]; similar to the study by Blum et al., a combination of different imaging methods served as the gold standard in this study. In a study by Kluge et al., pulmonary contrast-enhanced MRA was performed in 62 patients with suspected PE. Using parallel imaging their MRA technique achieved a substantially higher spatial resolution ($0.7 \times 1.2 \times 1.5$ mm) than the previous studies in a short acquisition time of 15 s. With this technique pulmonary contrast-enhanced MRA achieved a sensitivity of 81% and a specificity of 100% in comparison to 16-slice CTA [56].

In addition to these results of high-resolution MRA of the pulmonary vasculature, time-resolved contrast-enhanced MRA has been evaluated for the assessment of patients with suspected PE. In a feasibility study, Goyen et al. examined eight dyspneic patients with known or suspected PE using a time-resolved contrast-enhanced MRA with a scan time of less than 4 s. Pulmonary contrast-enhanced MRA allowed the assessment of the pulmonary arterial tree up to a sub-segmental level and identified PE in all four subsequently confirmed cases. All patients were able to hold their breath for at least 8 s, during which a dataset with an angiogram of the pulmonary arteries was obtained [57]. In a more recent study Ohno et al. compared the diagnostic accuracy of time-resolved contrast-enhanced MRA with parallel imaging (SENSE) versus CTA and ventilation-perfusion scintigraphy (VQ scan) in 48 patients with suspected PE. Conventional pulmonary DSA served as the gold standard. In this study time-resolved MRA had a higher sensitivity [92% vs. 83% (CTA) and 67% (VQ scan)] and specificity [94% vs. 94% (CTA) and 78% (VQ scan)] for the detection of PE than CTA and VQ scan [58].

7.3.2 Venous Imaging

It has been estimated that in the United States alone, as many as 5 million episodes of pulmonary embolism, a dreaded complication of deep venous thrombosis, occur every year. Radiographic venography or venous ultrasonography is still considered the gold standard for the diagnosis of deep venous thrombosis; however, venography is an invasive X-ray based procedure requiring iodinated contrast agent, and ultrasonography suffers from diagnostic limitations, e.g., of the pelvic veins. Recently, MR venography has also been proposed for the assessment of the venous system as a potential source of PE. Non-enhanced as well as direct and indirect contrast-enhanced MR venography techniques have been described. According to a recently published meta-analysis [59], the sensitivity of MR venography ranges between 0% and 100%, while the specificity ranges between 43% and 100%. The pooled estimate of the sensitivity and specificity of the included studies was 91.5% and 94.8%, respectively. In a recent study, 207 patients underwent a comprehensive MR protocol of non-enhanced and contrast-enhanced pulmonary MRA, pulmonary perfusion MRI and contrast-enhanced MR venography. The imaging time for the entire protocol (including the patient positioning) was less than 20 min. However, agreement with venous ultrasound was overall only moderate [60]. Also, for contrast-enhanced MR venous angiography, timing of the contrast material injection is crucial, and contrast administration has to be repeated to image more than one anatomic level. Intravascular contrast agents such as Vasovist® have several advantages. For example, the bolus transit time does not need to be determined, which simplifies the injection technique and avoids timing errors. Furthermore, insufficient spatial resolution is one of the major problems with contrast-enhanced MR angiography using extracellular contrast agents. Intravascular contrast agents allow for longer scanning times than extracellular contrast agents, thus potentially improving the spatial resolution. A third advantage of contrast-enhanced MR angiography using intravascular contrast agents is the possibility of scanning as many vascular regions as needed after administration of a single contrast bolus. An obvious gain is the visualization of the pelvic and abdominal vessels and the deep femoral vein, compared with what can be depicted on radiographic venography. Furthermore, scanning for deep venous thrombosis and pulmonary embolism can be performed during a single MRA session [61]. A potential drawback of contrast-enhanced MR venography using intravascular contrast agents is the need for postprocessing, because the contrast agent is present in arteries as well as in veins. In some anatomic regions, such as below the knee, this limitation could constitute a problem. Here, multiplanar reconstructions and maximum intensity projections are crucial to differentiate venous from arterial structures. Improvements of these tools (e.g., in vessel separation) are being developed and will most certainly speed up the postprocessing phase. To date no clinical studies on Vasovist®-enhanced pulmonary MRA of patients with PE have been published. However, based on our own experience from an ongoing study, Vasovist® can be used for a comprehensive evaluation of PE and deep venous thrombosis using first pass pulmonary perfusion MRI, high-resolution steady state pulmonary MRA, and steady state whole-body MR venography (Fig. 7.3, 7.4).

7.3.3 Imaging of Patients with Pulmonary Arterial Hypertension

Pulmonary arterial hypertension (PAH) is a progressive disease that leads to substantial mortality and eventually death. Elevated pulmonary arterial pressure and pulmonary vascular resistance with right ventricular failure of varying degree are the main hemodynamic features of this disease. Many different disorders have been identified as causing pulmonary hypertension, and medical management of hypertension is based on these underlying conditions [62]. Recurrent pulmonary thromboembolism is one of the causes of PAH. Hypertension that is caused by recurrent pulmonary thromboembolism is classified as chronic thromboembolic pulmonary arterial hypertension (CTEPH) and may be treated with surgery [63]; other forms of pulmonary hypertension can be treated with vasodilating drugs. Comprehensive workup to differentiate the various causes of pulmonary hypertension, especially CTEPH, typically requires a series of clinical examinations and imaging procedures. Because treatment of CTEPH differs considerably from that of other causes of pulmonary hypertension, an accurate diagnosis is essential. A prerequisite for the correct and reliable

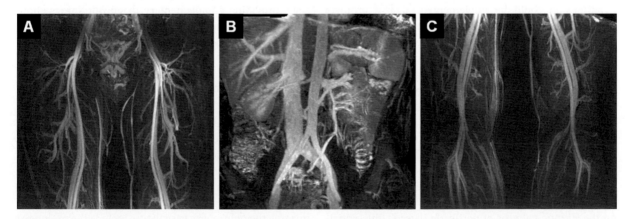

 Fig. 7.3A–C. Contrast-enhanced MR venography using the intravascular contrast agent Vasovist® in a healthy volunteer. After injection of the contrast agent, an acquisition window of up to 60 min can be used not only for high resolution of the thoracic vasculature, but also for imaging the complete venous anatomy of the abdomen and the lower extremities. Coronal maximum-intensity-projection images of abdomen and pelvis (A), the upper leg vasculature (B), and the knee/proximal lower leg (C) show normal anatomy of arterial and venous structures with no evidence of venous thrombosis

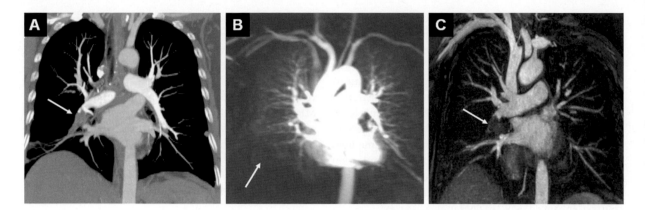

Fig. 7.4A–C. Images of a 53-year-old man with dyspnea. **A** 64-slice CT angiography demonstrates a large thrombus in the right lower lobe pulmonary artery (*arrow*). **B** The maximum-intensity-projection (MIP) image of a single perfusion phase obtained during contrast-enhanced, first pass MR perfusion imaging with Vasovist® clearly shows a segmen-tal perfusion defect in the right lower lobe owing to the thromboem-bolic occlusion (*arrow*). **C** The high-resolution MR angiogram of same patient obtained during the steady state window after injection of Vasovist® demonstrates the dark thromboembolic material in the pulmonary artery of the lower right lobe (*arrow*), similar to the CTA image

diagnosis of CTEPH is the depiction of occluding thrombotic material and concomitant perfusion defects. As discussed above, pulmonary magnetic resonance perfusion imaging and high-resolution angiography are rather new and promising non-invasive imaging techniques for assessing the pulmonary circulation. Detection of chronic occlusive and non-occlusive changes in the pulmonary arteries at the segmental or sub-segmental level requires high spatial resolution, which is limited by the imaging time of a single breath hold. Recently, parallel imaging techniques have become widely available. With these techniques, the temporal and spatial resolution can be improved substantially [9, 10]. In combination with intravascular contrast agents such as Vasovist®, an optimized, fully comprehensive protocol for the assessment and differential diagnosis of patients with pulmonary hypertension could be implemented. Such a protocol could include first pass perfusion imaging (potentially with quantification of results – see above), steady state high-resolution MRA, assessment of venous structures as a potential source of recurrent emboli, and an examination of the right heart to look for changes caused by the increased pulmonary arterial pressure. This comprehensive protocol would be feasible after a single injection of intravascular contrast.

MR perfusion imaging adds valuable information in patients with PAH; it can demonstrate the exact extent of perfusion defects and has increased diagnostic accuracy in the differentiation of various causes of PAH, depending on the specific patterns of perfusion defects, differentiating occlusive (segmental) from non-occlusive (patchy) forms of defects.

To maintain a sufficient SNR during first pass perfusion imaging – which is a crucial prerequisite when searching for sometimes subtle perfusion defects in PAH patients – typically high injection rate of about 5 ml/s have to be used when applying extracellular MR contrast agents. Here, contrast agents with a higher relaxivity (such as Vasovist® provides) could be beneficial. In a recent study, a combined approach for the correct differentiation of CTEPH from other forms of PAH was applied by performing time-resolved dynamic MR perfusion imaging and MRA with parallel imaging acquisition techniques at the same time [11]. The combination of first pass and high-resolution MRA data significantly enhanced diagnostic accuracy, which reached 90%. Thus, the application of an intravascular contrast agent could enable a comprehensive protocol in patients with PAH, combining MR first pass perfusion imaging with high-resolution pulmonary MR angiography and MR venography in steady state, providing complementary diagnostic information, and increasing the diagnostic value of pulmonary MR imaging in these patients.

7.4   Conclusions

Recent technical developments in the field of MR hardware and pulse sequence design have substantially improved the potential of MRI for the assessment of the pulmonary circulation. With the clinical introduction of the first intravascular MR contrast agent Vasovist®, new options arise. The main advantages of this contrast agent for imaging the pulmonary vasculature include the prolonged acquisition time during the equilibrium phase of the contrast agent and its higher relaxivity as compared with most extracellular contrast agents. This enables the setup of a comprehensive MR protocol for various vascular diseases of the thorax, including first pass perfusion imaging, high-resolution steady state MRA, and MR venography. Due to its intravascular character, Vasovist® could also be ultimately implemented for the calculation of true quantitative parameter maps of parenchymal perfusion. The higher available SNR at 3 T and the high T1 relaxivity of Vasovist could efficiently support highly accelerated parallel acquisition and generate an optimized combination of temporal and spatial resolution. In certain patient groups, such as subjects with contraindications to iodinated contrast media, or younger women with a low clinical probability for PE or during pregnancy, Vasovist-MRA might soon be considered as a radiation-free first-line imaging test for acute PE. Furthermore, Vasovist MRA of the pulmonary vasculature could be complemented by

additional functional measurements, such as assessments of cardiac function in the right side of the heart and MR venography to detect the potential source of emboli. A similar protocol would be ideally suited for patients with pulmonary arterial hypertension, reliably differentiating chronic thrombembolic forms of the disease from other causes of PAH or including an assessment of the treatment effects of vasodilative drug therapy in such patients. Acquisition techniques will have to be further adapted in future studies. Perhaps the use of electrocardiographic or respiratory gating techniques can further improve the image quality that is achievable during steady state MRA of the thorax. Future studies will also have to address the optimization of reconstruction times and interpretation strategies.

Take home messages

- Recent technical developments in the field of MR hardware and pulse sequence design have substantially improved the potential of MRI for the assessment of the pulmonary circulation.
- The introduction of an intravascular contrast agent such as Vasovist® brings along a number of potential advantages for imaging the pulmonary vasculature, including the prolonged acquisition time during the equilibrium phase of the contrast agent and its higher relaxivity as compared with most extracellular contrast agents, enabling the setup of a comprehensive MR protocol for various vascular diseases of the thorax, including first pass perfusion imaging, high-resolution steady state MRA, and MR venography.
- Due to its intravascular character, Vasovist® could also be ultimately implemented for the calculation

of true quantitative parameter maps of parenchymal pulmonary perfusion.
- The higher available SNR at 3 T and the high T1 relaxivity of Vasovist® could efficiently support highly accelerated parallel acquisition and generate an optimized combination of temporal and spatial resolution.
- In certain patient groups, such as subjects with contraindications to iodinated contrast media, or younger women with a low clinical probability for pulmonary embolism or during pregnancy, Vasovist-MRA might soon be considered as a radiation-free first-line imaging test for acute pulmonary embolism.
- In patients with pulmonary embolism, Vasovist® MR venography could be routinely implemented during steady state to detect the potential source of emboli.

References

1. Schoepf UJ, Costello P (2004) CT angiography for diagnosis of pulmonary embolism: state of the art. Radiology 230:329–337
2. Remy-Jardin M, Pistolesi M, Goodman LR, Gefter WB, Gottschalk A, Mayo JR et al (2007) Management of suspected acute pulmonary embolism in the era of CT angiography: a statement from the Fleischner Society. Radiology 245:315–329
3. Kreitner KF, Ley S, Kauczor HU, Mayer E, Kramm T, Pitton MB et al (2004) Chronic thromboembolic pulmonary hypertension: pre- and postoperative assessment with breath-hold MR imaging techniques. Radiology 232:535–543
4. Sanz J, Kuschnir P, Rius T, Salguero R, Sulica R, Einstein AJ et al (2007) Pulmonary arterial hypertension: noninvasive detection with phase-contrast MR imaging. Radiology 243:70–79
5. Fink C, Goyen M, Lotz J (2007) Magnetic resonance angiography with blood-pool contrast agents: future applications. Eur Radiol 17 [Suppl 2]:B38–44.:B38–B44
6. Perrault LP, Edelman RR, Baum RA, Yucel EK, Weisskoff RM, Shamsi K et al (2003) MR angiography with gadofosveset trisodium for peripheral vascular disease: phase II trial. Radiology 229:811–820
7. Fink C, Puderbach M, Bock M, Lodemann KP, Zuna I, Schmahl A et al (2004) Regional lung perfusion: assessment with partially parallel three-dimensional MR imaging. Radiology 231:175–184
8. Fink C, Bock M, Puderbach M, Schmahl A, Delorme S (2003) Partially parallel three-dimensional magnetic resonance imaging for the assessment of lung perfusion – initial results. Invest Radiol 38:482–488
9. Ohno Y, Kawamitsu H, Higashino T, Takenaka D, Watanabe H, Van Cauteren M et al (2003) Time-resolved contrast-enhanced pulmonary MR angiography using sensitivity encoding (SENSE). J Magn Reson Imaging 17:330–336
10. Nikolaou K, Schoenberg SO, Brix G, Goldman JP, Attenberger U, Kuehn B et al (2004) Quantification of pulmonary blood flow and volume in healthy volunteers by dynamic contrast-enhanced magnetic resonance imaging using a parallel imaging technique. Invest Radiol 39:537–545

11. Nikolaou K, Schoenberg SO, Attenberger U, Scheidler J, Dietrich O, Kuehn B et al (2005) Pulmonary arterial hypertension: diagnosis with fast perfusion MR imaging and high-spatial-resolution MR angiography – preliminary experience. Radiology 236:694–703

12. Prince MR, Grist TM, Debatin JF (2003) 3D Contrast MR angiography, 3rd edn. Springer Verlag, Berlin Heidelberg New York

13. Fishman AP (1963) Dynamic of the pulmonary circulation. In: Hamilton WF, editor. Handbook of physiology, Sect 2: Circulation. Washington, DC: American Physiological Society, p 1708

14. Rohrer M, Geerts-Ossevoort L, Laub G (2007) Technical requirements, biophysical considerations and protocol optimization with magnetic resonance angiography using blood-pool agents. Eur Radiol 17 [Suppl 2]:B7–12.:B7–12

15. Hartmann M, Wiethoff AJ, Hentrich HR, Rohrer M (2006) Initial imaging recommendations for Vasovist angiography. Eur Radiol 16 [Suppl 2]:B15–23.:B15–B23

16. Nikolaou K, Kramer H, Grosse C, Clevert D, Dietrich O, Hartmann M et al (2006) High-spatial-resolution multistation MR angiography with parallel imaging and blood pool contrast agent: initial experience. Radiology 241:861–872

17. Hui BK, Noga ML, Gan KD, Wilman AH (2005) Navigator-gated three-dimensional MR angiography of the pulmonary arteries using steady state free precession. J Magn Reson Imaging 21:831–835

18. Wang Y, Rossman PJ, Grimm RC, Riederer SJ, Ehman RL (1996) Navigator-echo-based real-time respiratory gating and triggering for reduction of respiration effects in three-dimensional coronary MR angiography. Radiology 198:55–60

19. Ahlstrom KH, Johansson LO, Rodenburg JB, Ragnarsson AS, Akeson P, Borseth A (1999) Pulmonary MR angiography with ultrasmall superparamagnetic iron oxide particles as a blood pool agent and a navigator echo for respiratory gating: pilot study. Radiology 211:865–869

20. Abolmaali ND, Hietschold V, Appold S, Ebert W, Vogl TJ (2002) Gadomer-17-enhanced 3D navigator-echo MR angiography of the pulmonary arteries in pigs. Eur Radiol 12:692–697

21. Nolte-Ernsting C, Adam G, Bucker A, Berges S, Bjornerud A, Gunther RW (1998) Experimental evaluation of superparamagnetic iron oxide particles in pulmonary MR angiography (in German). Rofo Fortschr Geb Rontgenstr Neuen Bildgeb Verfahr 168:508–513

22. Weishaupt D, Hilfiker PR, Schmidt M, Debatin JF (1999) Pulmonary hemorrhage: imaging with a new magnetic resonance blood pool agent in conjunction with breath-held three-dimensional magnetic resonance angiography. Cardiovasc Intervent Radiol 22:321–325

23. Zheng J, Carr J, Harris K, Saker MB, Cavagna FM, Maggioni F et al (2001) Three-dimensional MR pulmonary perfusion imaging and angiography with an injection of a new blood pool contrast agent B-22956/1. J Magn Reson Imaging 14:425–432

24. Fink C, Ley S, Puderbach M, Plathow C, Bock M, Kauczor HU (2004) 3D pulmonary perfusion MRI and MR angiography of pulmonary embolism in pigs after a single injection of a blood pool MR contrast agent. Eur Radiol 14:1291-1296

25. Hatabu H, Gaa J, Kim D, Li W, Prasad PV, Edelman RR (1996) Pulmonary perfusion and angiography: evaluation with breath-hold enhanced three-dimensional fast imaging steady state precession MR imaging with short TR and TE. AJR Am J Roentgenol 167:653–655

26. Berthezene Y, Croisille P, Wiart M, Howarth N, Houzard C, Faure O et al (1999) Prospective comparison of MR lung perfusion and lung scintigraphy. J Magn Reson Imaging 9:61–68

27. Amundsen T, Torheim G, Kvistad KA, Waage A, Bjermer L, Nordlid KK et al (2002) Perfusion abnormalities in pulmonary embolism studied with perfusion MRI and ventilation-perfusion scintigraphy: an intra-modality and inter-modality agreement study. J Magn Reson Imaging 15:386–394

28. Sodickson DK, McKenzie CA (2001) A generalized approach to parallel magnetic resonance imaging. Med Phys 28:1629–1643

29. Sitbon O, Humbert M, Simonneau G (2002) Primary pulmonary hypertension: Current therapy. Prog Cardiovasc Dis 45:115–128

30. Rizi RR, Saha PK, Wang B, Ferrante MA, Lipson D, Baumgardner J et al (2003) Co-registration of acquired MR ventilation and perfusion images – validation in a porcine model. Magn Reson Med 49:13–18

31. Fink C, Risse F, Buhmann R, Ley S, Meyer FJ, Plathow C et al (2004) Quantitative analysis of pulmonary perfusion using time-resolved parallel 3D MRI – initial results. Rofo Fortschr Geb Rontgenstr Neuen Bildgeb Verfahr 176:170–174

32. Ley S, Fink C, Puderbach M, Plathow C, Risse F, Kreitner KF et al (2004) [Contrast-enhanced 3D MR perfusion of the lung: application of parallel imaging technique in healthy subjects]. Rofo Fortschr Geb Rontgenstr Neuen Bildgeb Verfahr 176:330–334

33. Fink C, Puderbach M, Ley S, Plathow C, Bock M, Zuna I et al (2004) Contrast-enhanced three-dimensional pulmonary perfusion magnetic resonance imaging: intraindividual comparison of 1.0 M gadobutrol and 0.5 M Gd-DTPA at three dose levels. Invest Radiol 39:143–148

34. Halliburton SS, Paschal CB, Rothpletz JD, Loyd JE (2001) Estimation and visualization of regional and global pulmonary perfusion with 3D magnetic resonance angiography. J Magn Reson Imaging 14:734–740

35. Hatabu H, Gaa J, Kim D, Li W, Prasad PV, Edelman RR (1996) Pulmonary perfusion: qualitative assessment with dynamic contrast-enhanced MRI using ultra-short TE and inversion recovery turbo FLASH. Magn Reson Med 36:503–508

36. Dong Q, Hurst DR, Weinmann HJ, Chenevert TL, Londy FJ, Prince MR (1998) Magnetic resonance angiography with gadomer-17. An animal study original investigation. Invest Radiol 33:699–708

37. Berthezene Y, Vexler V, Price DC, Wisner-Dupon J, Moseley ME, Aicher KP et al (1992) Magnetic resonance imaging detection of an experimental pulmonary perfusion deficit using a macromolecular contrast agent. Polylysine-gadolinium-DTPA40 [published erratum appears in Invest Radiol (1992) 27:582]. Invest Radiol 27:346–351

38. Nael K, Saleh R, Nyborg GK, Fonseca CG, Weinmann HJ, Laub G et al (2007) Pulmonary MR perfusion at 3.0 Tesla using a blood pool contrast agent: Initial results in a swine model. J Magn Reson Imaging 25:66–72

39. Atkinson DJ, Burstein D, Edelman RR (1990) First pass cardiac perfusion: evaluation with ultrafast MR imaging. Radiology 174 (3 Pt 1):757–762

40. Pruessmann KP, Weiger M, Scheidegger MB, Boesiger P (1999) SENSE: sensitivity encoding for fast MRI. Magn Reson Med 42:952–962

41. Nael K, Michaely HJ, Kramer U, Lee MH, Goldin J, Laub G et al (2006) Pulmonary circulation: contrast-enhanced 3.0-T MR angiography–initial results. Radiology 240:858–868

42. Michaely HJ, Kramer H, Dietrich O, Nael K, Lodemann KP, Reiser MF et al (2007) Intraindividual comparison of high-spatial-resolution abdominal MR angiography at 1.5 T and 3.0 T: initial experience. Radiology 244:907–913

43. Weiger M, Pruessmann KP, Leussler C, Roschmann P, Boesiger P (2001) Specific coil design for SENSE: a six-element cardiac array. Magn Reson Med 45:495–504

44. Meaney JF, Goyen M (2007) Recent advances in contrast-enhanced magnetic resonance angiography. Eur Radiol 17 [Suppl 2]:B2–B6

45. Rohrer M, Geerts-Ossevoort L, Laub G (2007) Technical requirements, biophysical considerations and protocol optimization with magnetic resonance angiography using blood-pool agents. Eur Radiol 17 [Suppl 2]:B7–B12

46. Nael K, Michaely HJ, Lee M, Goldin J, Laub G, Finn JP (2006) Dynamic pulmonary perfusion and flow quantification with MR imaging, 3.0T vs. 1.5T: initial results. J Magn Reson Imaging 24:333-339

47. Kangarlu A, Baertlein BA, Lee R, Ibrahim T, Yang L, Abduljalil AM et al (1999) Dielectric resonance phenomena in ultra high field MRI. J Comput Assist Tomogr 23:821-831

48. Rinck PA, Muller RN (1999) Field strength and dose dependence of contrast enhancement by gadolinium-based MR contrast agents. Eur Radiol 9:998-1004

49. Marzola P, Osculati F, Sbarbati A (2003) High field MRI in preclinical research. Eur J Radiol 48:165-170

50. Fink C, Ley S, Schoenberg SO, Reiser MF, Kauczor HU (2007) Magnetic resonance imaging of acute pulmonary embolism. Eur Radiol 17:2546-2553

51. Meaney JF, Weg JG, Chenevert TL, Stafford-Johnson D, Hamilton BH, Prince MR (1997) Diagnosis of pulmonary embolism with magnetic resonance angiography. N Engl J Med 336:1422-1427

52. Gupta A, Frazer CK, Ferguson JM, Kumar AB, Davis SJ, Fallon MJ et al (1999) Acute pulmonary embolism: diagnosis with MR angiography. Radiology 210:353-359

53. Oudkerk M, van Beek EJ, Wielopolski P, van Ooijen PM, Brouwers-Kuyper EM, Bongaerts AH et al (2002) Comparison of contrast-enhanced magnetic resonance angiography and conventional pulmonary angiography for the diagnosis of pulmonary embolism: a prospective study. Lancet 359:1643-1647

54. Blum A, Bellou A, Guillemin F, Douek P, Laprevote-Heully MC, Wahl D (2005) Performance of magnetic resonance angiography in suspected acute pulmonary embolism. Thromb Haemost 93:503-511

55. Pleszewski B, Chartrand-Lefebvre C, Qanadli SD, Dery R, Perreault P, Oliva VL et al (2006) Gadolinium-enhanced pulmonary magnetic resonance angiography in the diagnosis of acute pulmonary embolism: a prospective study on 48 patients. Clin Imaging 30:166-172

56. Kluge A, Luboldt W, Bachmann G (2006) Acute pulmonary embolism to the subsegmental level: diagnostic accuracy of three MRI techniques compared with 16-MDCT. AJR Am J Roentgenol 187:W7-14

57. Goyen M, Laub G, Ladd ME, Debatin JF, Barkhausen J, Truemmler KH et al (2001) Dynamic 3D MR angiography of the pulmonary arteries in under four seconds. J Magn Reson Imaging 13:372-377

58. Ohno Y, Higashino T, Takenaka D, Sugimoto K, Yoshikawa T, Kawai H et al (2004) MR angiography with sensitivity encoding (SENSE) for suspected pulmonary embolism: comparison with MDCT and ventilation-perfusion scintigraphy. AJR Am J Roentgenol 183:91-98

59. Sampson FC, Goodacre SW, Thomas SM, van Beek EJ (2007) The accuracy of MRI in diagnosis of suspected deep vein thrombosis: systematic review and meta-analysis. Eur Radiol 17:175-181

60. Kluge A, Mueller C, Strunk J, Lange U, Bachmann G (2006) Experience in 207 combined MRI examinations for acute pulmonary embolism and deep vein thrombosis. AJR Am J Roentgenol 186:1686-1696

61. Sandstede JJ, Krause U, Pabst T, Hoffmann V, Braun H, Kenn W et al (2000) Deep venous thrombosis and consecutive pulmonary embolism as the first sign of an ovarian cancer: MR angiography using an intravascular contrast agent (CLARISCAN). J Magn Reson Imaging 12:497-500

62. Rich S (2000) Primary pulmonary hypertension. Curr Treat Options Cardiovasc Med 2:135-140

63. Fedullo PF, Auger WR, Kerr KM, Rubin LJ (2001) Chronic thromboembolic pulmonary hypertension. N Engl J Med 345:1465-1472

9.1   Introduction

Since the first description of moving-bed contrast-enhanced magnetic resonance angiography (CE-MRA) in 1998 [1], the technique has seen numerous refinements and is now widely applied in clinical practice throughout the world. The most widely used technique is to obtain a luminogram during first arterial passage of an extracellular MR contrast agent, often in combination with background subtraction to improve vessel-to-background contrast.

There are several important boundary considerations when performing peripheral MRA. Because of the inherently slow MR image acquisition process it is very important to carefully synchronize first arterial passage of the contrast medium with acquisition of the center K-space lines. Also, one always has to make a trade-off between acquisition duration, spatial resolution, and the capability of the patient to remain motionless and to sustain a breath hold. Furthermore, manual table movement was needed in the earliest iterations of the technique, whereas today all major MR vendors market hard- and software that allows for easy and near full-automated workflow once the 3D volumes are in the desired position in relation to the vasculature.

A major improvement that challenges these traditional conceptions about CE-MRA is the recent clinical introduction of the first blood pool agent, Vasovist® (Gadofosveset, Bayer Schering Pharma AG, Berlin, Germany). First described in 1998 [2], Vasovist® came on the market in the European Union in 2005 and has since expanded the diagnostic armamentarium of the radiologist, not only by providing superior first pass imaging, but also by enabling ultra-high spatial resolution equilibrium-phase imaging of both arteries and veins at previously unseen spatial resolutions that come very close to that of the gold standard in vascular imaging, conventional intra-arterial X-ray-based digital subtraction angiography (IA-DSA).

This chapter discusses some of the theoretical considerations and provides practical advice about and examples of how Vasovist® can be used to improve imaging of the peripheral vasculature.

9.2   Technical Considerations and Imaging Protocols

9.2.1   Vasovist® Versus Conventional Contrast Media

Vasovist® can be used exactly the same way as extracellular agents with regard to first pass imaging, as has been demonstrated by Klessen et al. [3]. The advantage of using this agent for first pass imaging lies in its much higher relaxivity (see also the chapter by Rohrer). This means that a higher signal-to-noise ratio can be obtained when parameters are kept identical or, conversely, that spatial resolution can be increased while the same signal-to-noise ratio is maintained. The truly interesting property of blood pool agents in general, however, is the much longer intravascular residence time. Equilibrium phase imaging is possible because, despite the fact that dilution of the injected contrast medium after first arterial passage leads to a T1 increase of the blood pool compared with the first pass, the value is still much lower than that of fat. Hartmann et al. estimated that T1 of blood in the equilibrium phase, 3–5 min after injection of 0.03 mmol/kg Vasovist® is about 130 ms, increasing to about 150 ms after 10–15 min [4]. This prolonged T1 reduction offers the opportunity to obtain images of the peripheral vascular tree up to about 45–60 min after injection. The extended imaging window can be used to acquire images with much higher spatial resolution without a significant loss of vessel-to-background contrast (◘ Fig. 9.1). In clinical practice this means that scan duration is no longer determined by the transient T1 shortening, but by the capacity of the patient to sustain a breath hold or to remain motionless. An exciting work-in-progress that is likely to further improve image quality

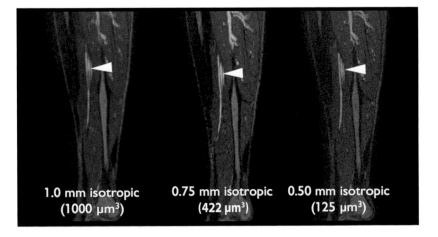

◘ Fig. 9.1. Source images of equilibrium-phase acquisitions at three different isotropic spatial resolutions demonstrating progressively improving visualization of the right anterior tibial artery surrounded by accompanying veins (*arrowheads*). Left panel: 1.0 x 1.0 x 1.0 mm³ (1000 µm³); middle panel: 0.75 x 0.75 x 0.75 mm³ (422 µm³); right panel: 0.5 x 0.5 x 0.5 mm³ (125 µm³) resolution. Note relative preservation of vessel-to-background enhancement despite the eightfold decrease in voxel size

is the combination of navigator gating with equilibrium-phase imaging of the abdominal aorta and its branches. By synchronizing the acquisition to end-expiration by means of tracking diaphragmatic motion it will be possible to extend imaging to several minutes as well (◨ Fig. 9.2).

The apparent drawback of using a blood pool agent is the simultaneous enhancement of venous structures close to arteries. This phenomenon is a well-known problem at first pass imaging, often resulting in images that cannot be used for clinical decision-making. However, because equilibrium phase images can be acquired at much higher spatial resolution, often with a 5- to 15-fold decrease in voxel size compared with first pass protocols, arteries can be readily separated from accompanying veins. Empirically, the authors recommend that the acquisition for the iliac arteries last no longer than 20 s, because usually a breath hold is desired. When imaging the vascular system in the pelvis only, no breath hold is needed and the acquisition can be extended to a few minutes. For the upper and lower legs we recommend that acquisitions last no longer than 5 min.

9.2.2 Considerations with Regard to Vasovist®-enhanced Peripheral MRA Imaging Protocols

The MR sequence parameters used in conventional first pass CE-MRA are not suitable for equilibrium phase imaging, as short repetition (TR) and echo times (TE), high bandwidths, high flip angles, and relatively low spatial resolutions are used to achieve short scan times aimed at obtaining a selective arterial phase within a breath hold.

Imaging in the equilibrium-phase places other demands on the imaging protocol. For instance, much higher spatial resolution is needed in order to reliably separate arteries from veins. However, higher resolution comes at the expense of signal-to-noise ratio (SNR), which must remain sufficient to provide adequate vessel-to-background contrast. Since there is no requirement to complete the acquisition in the period of first arterial passage of contrast material, significantly longer acquisition times can be used in the equilibrium phase to compensate

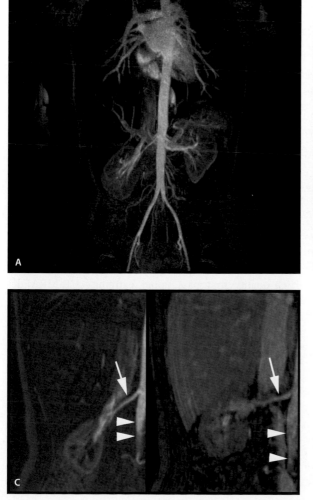

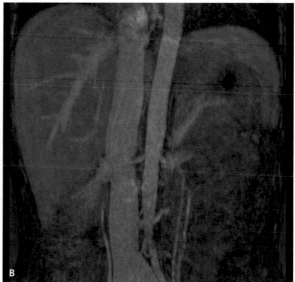

◨ **Fig. 9.2A–C.** Whole-volume MIP of first pass acquisition (**A**) in a 35-year-old patient suspected of having renovascular hypertension. There is slight venous enhancement of the left renal vein and inferior vena cava (resolution was 1.2 x 1.0 x 2.2 mm³). Cardiac-triggered and respiratory navigator-gated equilibrium-phase acquisition (**B**) demonstrates improved sharpness of the vessel borders compared with the first pass images. Resolution was 1.0 x 1.0 x 1.0 mm³. Zoomed detail of the right renal artery confirms high-fidelity depiction of the renal artery in the equilibrium-phase (**C**, *right panel*) compared with first pass (**c**, *left panel*). Again, note sharper delineation of the right renal artery (*arrow*) and aorta (*arrowheads*)

for the loss in SNR due to increased spatial resolution. Both in vitro and in vivo work by our groups with regard to equilibrium-phase sequence parameter optimization has demonstrated that optimal image quality demands an increase of TR from to 2–4 to about 10–12 ms, a TE below 5 ms, and a decrease in flip angle from about 35–40 to 20–29 degrees, depending on the type of coil and parallel imaging factor used [5]. These parameters are optimized for an equilibrium-phase voxel size of 0.5 x 0.5 x 0.5 mm^3 (125 µm), which provides sufficiently high spatial resolution to clearly distinguish arteries from veins at still reasonable imaging times.

Practically, we recommend an imaging protocol that consists of time-of-flight localizer images, followed by non-enhanced mask images. Subsequently, we use real-time bolus tracking of the injected contrast material, which is immediately followed by high-resolution first pass imaging of the pelvic, upper leg, and lower leg stations using moving-table software. After the first pass acquisitions are completed, equilibrium-phase images can be obtained using the relatively minor modifications in imaging parameters as described above, yielding high-quality ultra-high spatial resolution equilibrium-phase images of the entire peripheral vascular tree. We recommend limiting the 125-µm equilibrium-phase acquisition to the upper and lower leg stations. For the aortoiliac station we use the same imaging parameters as in the first pass acquisition in order to combine the acquisition with breath holding.

When imaging the upper extremity a very similar imaging protocol in terms of sequences and spatial resolution can be used. Voxel sizes down to 0.4 x 0.4 x 0.4 mm^3 are feasible.

9.2.3 Vasovist® Injection Protocol

The approved clinical dose of Vasovist® is 0.03 mmol/kg body weight. Considering that the drug comes in 10-ml vials at a concentration of 0.25 mol/l, the typical 75-kg adult would receive a dose of 9 ml. Conversely, a single vial can be used for patients up to 83.3 kg. Considering the rather small volume of the contrast injection compared with regular extracellular chelates, we recommend an injection rate of 1.0 ml/s at the highest in order to avoid having too short a bolus. This is especially pertinent when imaging the lower extremity vasculature in a multiple station imaging protocol because of the desire to achieve uniform vascular opacification over the entire duration of the first pass acquisition. The contrast injection should be followed by at least 25–30 ml of saline chaser injected at the same rate, in order to avoid pooling of the contrast medium in upper extremity veins.

9.3 Clinical Indications

9.3.1 Upper Extremities

Anatomical and Physiological Considerations

With the elbow extended, the upper extremity of a 170-cm-tall adult is about 75 cm long. This implies that at least two fields-of-view (FOV) of about 40 cm in the craniocaudal direction are needed to depict all the relevant arteries. A FOV of 20–25 cm suffices if the main area of interest is the distal forearm and hand. The diameter of the subclavian artery is about 1.0–1.3 cm, and the diameter of the axillary artery is about 6–8 mm. Distally, the arteries progressively taper to a diameter of about 1–2 mm at the level of the palmar arch in the hand. It is of paramount importance that depiction of the arteries in the distal forearm and hand requires higher spatial resolution compared with more proximal vessels. The preferred voxel size is on the order of 1 mm^3 or even smaller. While this is not easily achieved in combination with first pass imaging, acquisition in the equilibrium-phase facilitates ultra-high spatial resolution images.

The mean time of selective arterial opacification in the upper extremity is relatively short. Winterer et al. found a mean bolus arrival time of 27 s measured at the level of the terminal radial and ulnar arteries and a mean time window of selective arterial enhancement of 11–14 s [6]. However, large interindividual differences in contrast medium circulation times were found. The period between arterial and venous enhancement can be substantially lengthened by applying supra- or sub-systolic compression (>200 mmHg) just proximal to the wrist with an MR-compatible blood pressure cuff. This effectively increases the period of selective arterial enhancement and hence the imaging window needed to achieve the ultra-high spatial resolution required for optimal evaluation of arterial occlusive disease in the small hand vessels [7, 8].

Imaging Protocol and Parameters

High-quality first pass upper extremity CE-MRA demands large FOV imaging with high spatial resolution, short imaging times, and dedicated multi-element parallel imaging capable surface coils. In combination with a multiphase acquisition a timing bolus is not needed. This is advantageous because of the small volume of contrast agent that is available.

A multiphase acquisition ensures adequate synchronization of peak arterial contrast enhancement with acquisition of the center of K-space. Alternatively, real-time bolus visualization software (e.g. BolusTrak [Philips Medical Systems]; SmartPrep [GE Health] or CareBolus [Siemens Medical Solutions]) can be used [9–11]. In ◻ Tables 9.1 and 9.2, recommended sequence parameters are listed for

◾ **Table 9.1.** Recommended MR sequence parameters for first pass and equilibrium-phase MRA of the aortic arch and proximal upper extremity

Sequence	Orientation	Coverage	TR/TE (ms)	FA (degrees)	FOV (mm)	Matrix	Slice thickness* (mm)	No. of partitions	Duration (s)	Comments
bSSFP	Coronal	Aortic arch to distal brachial artery	6.0 / 3.0	90	430 x 430	400 x 256	5–10	30–60	30–60	
2D PCA	Transverse	Neck / carotid and vertebral arteries	20 / 5	15	260 x 260	256 x 256	10	1	30–60	To detect subclavian steal set VENC to 120 cm/s
3D GRE (first pass)	Coronal	Aortic arch to distal brachial artery	<4.0 / <2.0	30–40	430 x 300	430 x 300	1.0–2.0	Tailor to anatomy	40–50 (≥2 dyn)	Use parallel imaging
3D GRE (equilibrium-phase)	Sagittal	Upper extremity with suspected abnormality. Include aortic arch	<12.0 / <3.0	20	385 x 270	550 x 386	0.7	Tailor to anatomy	Several min	Use parallel imaging

bSSFP balanced steady state free precession; TR repetition time; TE echo time; FA flip angle; FOV field-of-view (frequency x phase); BW band width; NSA number of signals averaged (number below 1 indicates partial or fractional echo); dyn dynamic scans; * non-interpolated, truly acquired slice thickness

◾ **Table 9.2.** Recommended MR sequence parameters for first pass and equilibrium-phase MRA of the forearm and hand

Sequence	Orientation	Coverage	TR/TE (ms)	FA (degrees)	FOV (mm)	Matrix	Slice thickness* (mm)	No. of partitions	Duration (s)	Comments
bSSFP	Coronal	Distal brachial artery to digits	6.0 / 3.0	90	430 x 430	400 x 256	5–10	30–60	30–60	
3D GRE (first pass)	Coronal	Distal brachial artery to digits	<4.0 / <2.0	30–40	430 x 300	430 x 300	1.0	Tailor to anatomy	40–50 (≥2 dyn)	Use parallel imaging
3D GRE (equilibrium-phase)	Sagittal	Upper extremity with suspected abnormality. Include aortic arch	<12.0 / <3.0	20	385 x 270	770 x 540	0.5	Tailor to anatomy	Several min	Use parallel imaging

bSSFP balanced steady state free precession; TR repetition time; TE echo time; FA flip angle; FOV field-of-view (frequency x phase); BW band width; NSA number of signals averaged (number below 1 indicates partial or fractional echo); dyn dynamic scans; * non-interpolated, truly acquired slice thickness

localizer and timing scans as well as high spatial resolution 3D CE-MRA and equilibrium-phase imaging of the upper extremity arteries.

When information is needed about both the proximal and distal upper extremity arteries, two FOVs need to be imaged. This can be done either with a single injection of contrast medium in combination with table movement in between acquisitions, or by performing two separate acquisitions with separate injections of half the total amount of contrast medium each. Owing to the short circulation times in the upper extremity, the latter approach is recommended because it usually leads to better results, especially when the forearm and hand are imaged first. Another important caveat of upper extremity CE-MRA is to inject contrast medium on the asymptomatic side in order to avoid susceptibility-induced intra-arterial signal loss [12.]. When both upper extremities need to be imaged it is advisable to inject contrast medium on the right because of the greater distance of the right brachiocephalic vein and the superior vena cava to the large arteries.

Clinical Applications of Upper Extremity MRA

CE-MRA is a powerful technique for the diagnosis of, pre-interventional treatment planning and post-interventional follow-up of a broad spectrum of congenital and acquired upper extremity occlusive disease (■ Table 9.3). It is important to keep in mind that sub-millimeter isotropic resolutions are necessary to reliably depict distal upper extremity arterial disease. The use of Vasovist® facilitates both high-quality first pass imaging as well as exquisitely detailed images of the small vessels in the hand in the equilibrium phase.

Atherosclerotic occlusive disease

Although atherosclerosis is the most common cause of upper extremity arterial stenosis in the large arteries down to the wrist, its incidence is much lower compared with that of the lower extremities. The most frequent site of occlusion is the brachiocephalic trunk or the proximal subclavian artery. In case of occlusion collateral blood supply is established via the side branches of the subclavian artery and the axillary artery. Subclavian artery stenosis or occlusion is not infrequently accompanied by retrograde collateral blood flow in the ipsilateral vertebral artery. This is also known as *subclavian steal*. Retrograde flow can be depicted on the 2D time-resolved test-bolus scan or with non-enhanced time-of-flight or phase-contrast MRA acquisitions [13–15]. Although in general equilibrium-phase acquisitions are not needed to establish the diagnosis in the proximal *arterial* tree, they are very useful for the depiction of abnormalities in the *venous* system (■ Fig. 9.3).

Vasculitis

The vasculitides regularly affect upper extremity arteries. Wall thickening and enhancement on post-contrast T_1-weighted imaging as well as central aneurysms without a history of trauma or infection suggest a vasculitis [16, 17]. Vasculitides affecting the subclavian artery are Takayasu's disease and Behçet's syndrome. The axillary artery is involved in giant cell arteritis and systemic lupus erythematosus (SLE). Thromboangiitis obliterans (TAO; Buerger's disease) often specifically affects the forearm arteries in patients with this disease. The angiographic hallmark of TAO is widespread arterial occlusion with numerous corkscrew collaterals [18, 19]. Arteries of the hand are discussed below.

Aneurysmal disease

Aneurysms of upper extremity arteries are frequently secondary to iatrogenic arterial trauma (e.g., arterial catheterizations or dialysis access fistula creation) or as the result of blunt or penetrating trauma to the chest. Less frequent causes include vasculitis and hematogenous infection (mycotic aneurysm). Because the first pass contrast-enhanced portion of the exam provides only a lu-

■ **Table 9.3.** Indications for Vasovist®-enhanced MRA of the upper extremity

Indication	Advantages of using Vasovist®
Atherosclerotic occlusive disease of aortic arch and branches	High relaxivity in F/P; Ultra-high spatial resolution in E/P
Aneurysmal disease	High relaxivity in F/P; Definition of mural thrombus in E/P
Vasculitis	High relaxivity in F/P; Ability to depict vessel wall in E/P
Suspected thoracic outlet syndrome	Ability to depict both arteries and veins
Hand imaging	High relaxivity in F/P; Ultra-high spatial resolution and definition of thrombus in E/P

F/P first pass; *E/P* equilibrium phase

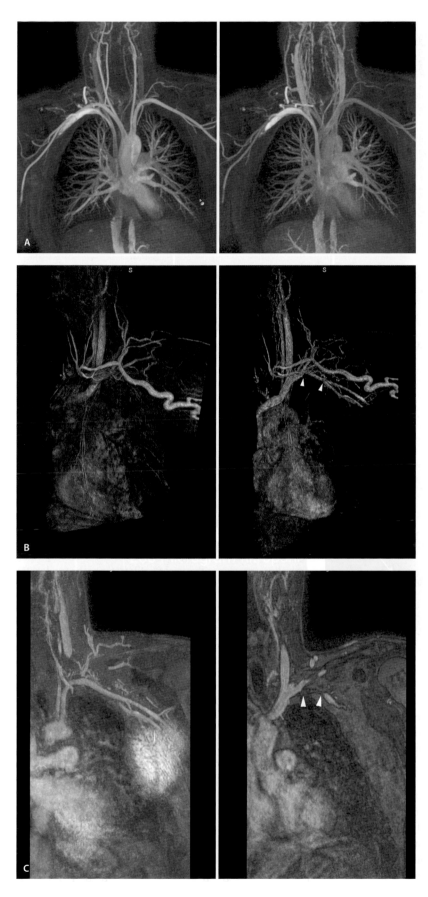

Fig. 9.3A–C. Whole-volume MIPs of dynamic acquisition in the arterial (**A**, *left panel*) and early venous phases (**A**, *right panel*) in a 54-year-old patient suspected of having thoracic outlet syndrome. The subclavian artery shows no abnormalities. Color volume renderings (cVR) at different thresholds of equilibrium-phase acquisitions (0.7 x 0.7 x 0.7 mm³) demonstrate a large superficial venous collateral in the left anterior oblique view (**B**, *left panel*). When the cVR threshold is increased, an interruption is suggested in the subclavian vein (demarcated by *arrowheads* in **B**, *right panel*). Review of equilibrium-phase source images confirms normal subclavian artery (**C**, *left panel*) and near occlusion of the subclavian vein (demarcated by *arrowheads* in **C**, *right panel*)

The arterial part of the AVF is visualized according to the method of Staple, using a proximal cuff to interrupt flow in order to achieve retrograde filling of the arterial part of the AVF [22]. Analysis of DSA images acquired with this method can be difficult due to vessel overlap, especially at the level of the anastomoses. Owing to the temporary flow interruption, the hemodynamic situation is altered, which potentially limits the value of DSA. Furthermore, because of incomplete retrograde filling, the feeding artery and arterial part of the AVF are not always depicted in their entirety [23, 24].

Because of the reasons outlined above, the pre-interventional workup in patients with hemodialysis access failure requires imaging from the aortic valve and superior vena cava down to the distal arteriovenous anastomosis in the elbow or forearm region. The demands of a large FOV combined with the extremely high flow rates in these shunts make parallel imaging particularly useful for imaging dialysis access fistulae and supplying arteries and draining veins. Furthermore, 3D CE-MRA provides unlimited viewing angles that are very helpful in planning the proper intervention. For instance, Planken et al. demonstrated that multiphase 3D CE-MRA detected flow-limiting stenoses in two patients (13%) with failing hemodialysis access fistulae that were not seen with conventional DSA. Only after these stenoses were removed did flow improve [25].

Despite these obvious advantages of MRA, patients on dialysis are not good candidates to receive gadolinium-based contrast agents because of the probability of developing nephrogenic systemic fibrosis (NSF). Although NSF has been described mainly in relation to administration of Gadodiamide (Omniscan®, GE Health, Chalfont St-Giles, United Kingdom), this is certainly not the only compound that has been associated with the disease [26].

9.3.2   Lower Extremity CE-MRA

Anatomical and Physiological Considerations

The lower extremity peripheral arterial tree extends from the infrarenal aorta down to the feet and has a total length of about 90–120 cm. To depict all relevant arteries, at least three separate acquisitions are needed: one acquisition to cover the aortoiliac arteries, one to cover the superficial femoral and proximal popliteal arteries, and an additional acquisition to cover the distal popliteal, lower leg, and pedal arteries. As outlined in the section on upper extremity CE-MRA above, best results are obtained when the acquisition is tailored to the arterial dimensions in the specific FOV [27]. The diameter of the infrarenal aorta is usually around 2.0–2.5 cm, the diameter of the superficial femoral artery is about 7–10 mm, and the arteries at the level of the ankle and foot have diameters of

around 1.0–2.0 mm. In most patients, peripheral arteries are slightly curved in the anteroposterior direction and the coverage needed is usually less than 10 cm. In the presence of an aortic aneurysm, iliac arterial elongation, collaterals bridging iliac or superficial femoral arterial obstructions, or a femorofemoral crossover bypass graft the AP coverage needed to depict these vessels may be markedly increased (up to 15–20 cm). Review of the transverse localizer images ensures that these structures are not excluded from the 3D CE-MRA imaging volume. This is particularly important if a patient has a femorofemoral crossover bypass graft because these grafts are usually not seen on TOF MIPs due to in-plane saturation artifacts [28, 29]. Other patients who require special attention are those with (thoraco-) abdominal aortic aneurysms where flow may be markedly slower than in patients without aneurysms [30]. If insufficient delay time is observed between injection of contrast and imaging, this will result in incomplete opacification of the aneurysm at the time of imaging. To avoid this problem, either a longer delay between injection and start of acquisition, or a multiphase acquisition should be used [31]. In addition, the use of Vasovist® enables an equilibrium-phase acquisition, which should always be performed when possible.

The mean time of selective arterial opacification at different levels in the lower extremity varies widely. Patients with a history of heart failure usually exhibit slower venous return, while patients with ulcers often have an extremely short arteriovenous window. Prince et al. demonstrated that after arrival in the common femoral artery (CFA), intravenously injected contrast material travels down the peripheral arteries at about 6 s per station. In 87 patients undergoing time-resolved 2D CE-MRA, the mean travel time of contrast material to the CFA was 24 s, with an additional 5 s to reach the popliteal artery and 7 s to reach the ankle arteries. In the same study they found that the mean time window of arterial enhancement was 49 s in the pelvis, 45 s in the thigh, and 35 s in the calf [32].

It was recently found that applying venous compression could substantially lengthen the period between arterial and venous enhancement. Suppression of venous enhancement in the distal lower extremity is already achieved with a blood pressure cuff inflated to 50–60 mmHg either just proximal to or just distal to the knee joint [33–35].

Imaging Protocol and Parameters

Because of the lower injection rate and hence the lower vessel-to-background contrast, non-enhanced 'mask' acquisitions are usually acquired prior to the contrast-enhanced acquisitions in patients undergoing lower extremity MRA. After the acquisition has ended, the non-enhanced images are subtracted from the enhanced images to suppress non-vascular background signal. Mask scans are not needed for equilibrium-phase acquisitions, as MIP is not the preferred mode of evaluation.

Currently, the most commonly used and easiest approach to lower extremity CE-MRA is acquisition of three consecutive anatomically tailored imaging volumes during injection of a fixed dose (0.2–0.3 mmol/kg) or volume (30–45 ml) of 0.5 M gadolinium chelate [1, 36, 37].

Although the injected volume is smaller when using Vasovist®, an identical approach can be used for the first pass acquisition [3]. The first pass technique is well suited for the diagnostic imaging workup of the vast majority of patients with intermittent claudication. However, it is of paramount importance that inferior image quality due to insufficient spatial resolution as well as disturbing venous enhancement becomes clinically relevant in patients with severely diseased lower leg arteries. Specific groups in whom first pass imaging with a 3-consecutive station approach does not work well are patients with diabetes mellitus, especially with concomitant arteriovenous malformations, who are known to primarily have very distal disease [38], patients with cellulitis, and patients with chronic critical ischemia who have severe stenoses and occlusions from the aorta down to the feet ('multilevel' disease).

There are several general acquisition strategies that can be used to decrease the chance for disturbing venous enhancement (◻ Table 9.4). These are: (a) lowering TR and TE; (b) use of a separate acquisition for the lower leg station; (c) use of centric K-space filling; (d) use of a time-resolved acquisition strategy (keyhole or TRICKS); (e) use of infrasystolic venous compression, and (f) use of parallel imaging to amplify the other strategies. The most straightforward way of preventing venous enhancement is by shortening acquisition duration. This should be done,

first of all, by lowering TR and TE to the shortest possible value without excessively increasing bandwidth. In addition, partial or fractional echo should be used. When the 3-consecutive station approach is used it is particularly important to image the first two stations (i.e., aortoiliac and upper legs) as fast as possible. Once the acquisition of the lower legs is started, this will allow a relatively long (and thus high-resolution) scan, given that none or minimal venous enhancement is already present and centric K-space filling is used in this station. With the introduction of multi-element (peripheral) surface coils and parallel imaging acquisition speed can be increased further [39–41]. Another way to obtain venous free images of the lower legs is to switch from a 3D high-resolution acquisition to a 2D projectional acquisition, analogous to IA-DSA [42]. A disadvantage of this latter method is that additional views demand separate injections of contrast medium.

To avoid the limitations of imaging three consecutive stations, an alternative approach is a dual-injection protocol in which the lower legs are imaged first and the aortoiliac arteries and upper legs are imaged afterwards in a separate acquisition. The rationale for this 'hybrid' approach [43] is that it is easier in this way to obtain high-resolution 3D images of the lower leg station free of disturbing venous enhancement. The initial acquisition of the lower legs is typically done using up to 15–20 ml 0.5 M Gd-DTPA and can be either mono- or multiphasic. Because synchronization of central K-space lines is optimized with regards to contrast enhancement in the lower leg arteries, venous enhancement is virtually eliminated. After imaging of the lower legs is completed, a moving-table acquisition is performed to image the aortoiliac and upper leg arteries using the remaining volume of contrast agent. When Vasovist® is used, the entire dose of contrast agent can be used for the multiphase lower leg station

◻ **Table 9.4.** Strategies to reduce venous enhancement in first pass lower extremity MRA

Strategy	Advantages	Drawbacks
Separate acquisition for lower legs	Multiphase DSA-like images	Aortoiliac and upper leg vessels need to be acquired separately
Infrasystolic venous compression	Delays venous filling	Can be perceived as uncomfortable by patients; takes time to apply
Lowering TR/TE	Faster acquisition	Lowers SNR
Centric K-space filling	Suppression of venous enhancement	None, even when contrast present in veins
Time-resolved acquisition	Multiphase DSA-like images	Still requires compromise between spatial and temporal resolution
Parallel imaging	Can substantially speed up acquisition	Lowers SNR; can lead to disturbing artifacts

SNR signal-to-noise ratio

9

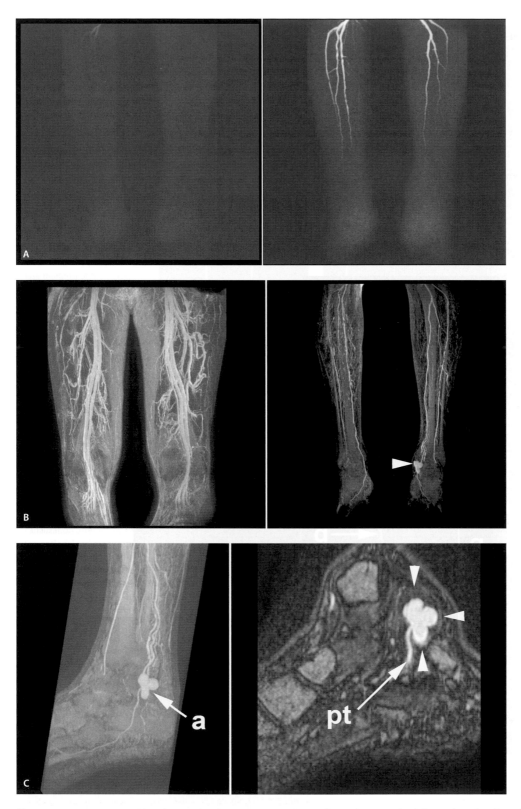

⬛ **Fig. 9.12A–C.** A 70-year-old male patient who presented with a pulsatile mass of the medial aspect of the ankle. First pass imaging (**A**) shows a mistimed acquisition with no filling in the initial phase (**A**, *left panel*) and incomplete filling of the distal lower leg arteries in the second phase (**A**, *right panel*). Subsequent equilibrium-phase acquisitions (0.5 x 0.5 x 0.5 mm³) demonstrate normal superficial femoral arteries (**B**, *left panel*) and a clover-leaf-shaped aneurysm of the posterior tibial artery (**B**, *arrowhead* in *right panel*). A more detailed examination of the aneurysm reveals connections with posterior tibial artery (**C**, *left panel*) and that the aneurysm is partially thrombosed (**C**, *right panel*). *a*, aneurysm; *pt*, posterior tibial artery

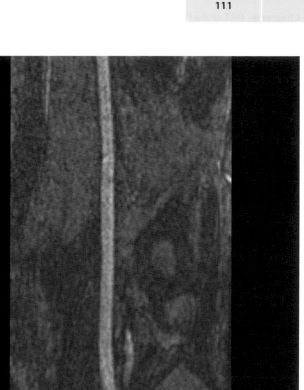

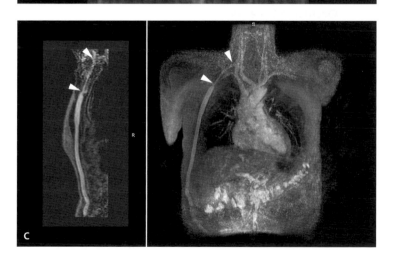

◘ **Fig. 9.13A–C.** Multi-station maximum-intensity projection of first pass CE-MRA in a 55-year-old patient with extra-anatomic bypass suffering from renewed intermittent claudication in the left leg. The right lower leg had been amputed previously. The patient was referred for CE-MRA because routine follow-up of the femoropopliteal bypass with duplex ultrasonography in the left leg showed slow flow and questionable stenosis of the distal anastomosis. First pass imaging after injection of 0.03 mmol/kg Vasovist shows no major stenoses in the distal part of the graft (*boxed area* in **A**). Subsequent higher resolution imaging in the equilibrium phase at 0.6 x 0.6 x 0.6 mm³ (216 µm³) corroborates first pass findings and shows normal caliber of distal bypass and runoff into the distal popliteal artery (*arrow* in **B**). Because of the extended intravascular retention of Vasovist it is possible to image additional arterial territories as well as the venous compartment. **C** Curved multiplanar reformation (*left panel*) and subvolume maximum-intensity projection (*right panel*) of the origin and proximal part of the extra-anatomic bypass. Despite the fact that vessel-to-background is lower compared with first pass imaging, a flow-limiting, significant stenosis can clearly be appreciated (*arrowheads*)

In the management and diagnosis of KTWS it is particularly important, prior to considering surgical intervention or sclerotherapy, to eliminate the possibility of DVT and check the integrity of the deep veins, which are often aberrant with enlarged lateral thigh veins or persistent sciatic veins [14].

The assessment of arteriovenous malformations (AVM) is a further example of the utility of blood pool contrast agents. They give excellent first pass arterial imaging to delineate inflow anatomy, and also provide exquisite detail of the AVM nidus and any muscular or skeletal involvement as well as the venous drainage pathways (■ Fig. 10.12).

In the assessment of lower limb superficial veins as potential conduits for bypass grafting, CE-MRV again provides a rapidly interpretable visual map, and modern workstation

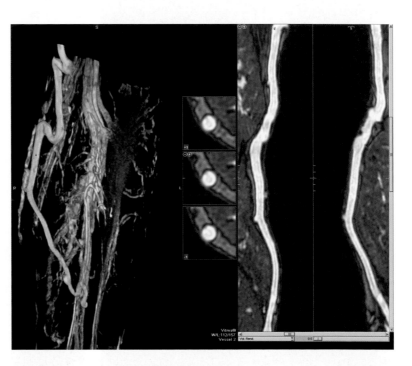

■ **Fig. 10.11.** Steady state phase of contrast-enhanced MRV of thigh veins. Volume-rendered slab reconstruction (*left*) with accompanying automated CPR unfolded vessel view (*right*) and orthogonal reconstructions axial to vein (*middle*). Patient with extensive varicose veins of left leg and particularly dilated and tortuous long saphenous vein

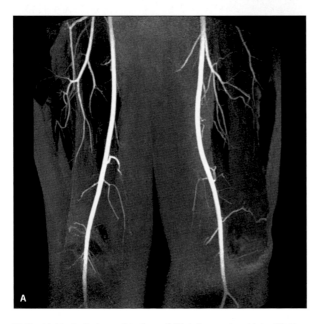

■ **Fig. 10.12a,b.** Patient with deep AVM, left anterior thigh. (**A**) First pass coronal MRA shows normal vasculature of thighs apart from small lateral superior geniculate artery branch feeding deep AVM on the left. (**B**) Steady state phase shows deep nidus of AVM in vastus intermedius anterior to distal left femur, including small phleboliths manifest as tiny foci of susceptibility artifact. There is no bony involvement, and no large draining veins are demonstrated

analysis software with automated center-line definition for curved MPR allows accurate quantification of vessel caliber throughout the length of the vein. Clearly, this is a major advantage of using a blood pool contrast agent such as Vasovist® when performing CE-MRA for peripheral arterial occlusive disease, since the simple addition of steady state high-resolution sequences at the end of the standard first pass scan will provide all the venous information required to plan any potential surgical intervention, obviating the scheduling of additional studies (☐ Figs. 10.13, 10.14).

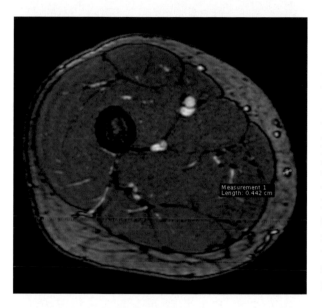

☐ **Fig. 10.13.** Thin-slab MIPs of normal (4-mm caliber) long saphenous veins suitable for use as bypass conduits

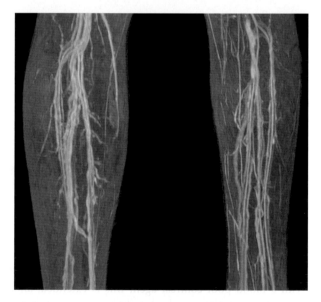

☐ **Fig. 10.14.** Coronal overview MIP of calves in patient with critical lower limb ischemia showing poor-quality long saphenous veins with nothing suitable for bypass conduit

10.6   Abdominal and Pelvic Veins

10.6.1   Inferior Vena Cava and Pelvic Veins

The inferior vena cava (IVC) is most commonly evaluated along with the pelvic veins when lower limb venous thrombosis is assessed, since extension of DVT to the large iliac veins and IVC poses an increased potential threat of pulmonary thromboembolism. The use of MRI for IVC evaluation is advantageous as it may be poorly opacified on CT, the interpretation of which can be challenging since the IVC is prone to flow artifacts with complex admixture of unopacified blood. IVC patency and caliber determination are important to determining the safety of potential intervention in terms of caval filter placement; in particular, the size of the IVC will determine the type of caval filter to be used, as in cases of megacava a 'bird's-nest' type filter is required. Determining the position of the main renal veins and any accessory/aberrant renal veins can alter the position of deployment, as these may necessitate suprarenal placement, a priori knowledge of which is helpful prior to obtaining the patient's consent and planning the intervention. Variants of the IVC itself such as duplicated infrarenal IVC (which occurs in up to 3% of subjects; solitary left infrarenal IVC is less common at ~1% [15]) will also affect management. As in other areas- the use of blood pool contrast agent is beneficial and steady state high-resolution imaging is easily achieved for the fixed retroperitoneal IVC- as it is not disturbed by respiratory motion artifacts.

An advantage of simultaneous venous and arterial imaging in the steady state is ready depiction of the relationships of the common iliac vessels for the diagnosis of May-Thurner syndrome, where thrombosis of the left iliac veins is precipitated through compression of the proximal left common iliac vein by the right common iliac artery crossing point. While May-Thurner syndrome as a cause of left iliofemoral DVT is well recognized it has been thought relatively uncommon; however, recent work has suggested a more subtle and hitherto unrecognized role of iliac vein compression in non-thrombotic chronic venous insufficiency [16, 17].

10.6.2   Gonadal Veins

For male patients with simple scrotal varicocele the pre-procedural evaluation of gonadal venous anatomy is seldom required prior to embolotherapy. However, in female patients with vulval varicosities or suspected pelvic congestion syndrome it is helpful to define whether there is abnormality of ovarian veins, particularly as their pelvic connections may be complex. MRV for gonadal veins with blood pool contrast agent can be performed with standard CE-MRA acquisitions or fat-suppressed T1w GRE se-contrast agent is usually performed with standard breath-hold CE-MRA (◘ Fig. 10.18) or fat-suppressed T1w GRE sequences (such as THRIVE, VIBE, and LAVA) to eliminate respiratory artifacts, though the optimized steady state high-resolution non-breath-hold sequences may be surprisingly successful for these retroperitoneal structures even without the addition of navigator techniques which are being researched.

Despite the excellent image quality now afforded by modern multislice CT imaging there is still occasion to use MRI when investigating suspected renal vein thrombosis. MRI is particularly indicated in younger patients without malignant disease and in pregnancy, for example, in nephrotic syndrome and other systemic conditions such as the connective tissue disorders. Although renal vein thrombus is often well-visualized when renal and adrenal carcinomas are staged on multislice CT, the differentiation of bland from malignant thrombus may not be easy, and studies have shown that gadolinium enhancement of the thrombus on delayed-phase MRI, indicating neovascularity, is predictive of malignancy. There are of course concerns about the use of gadolinium-based contrast agents in severe renal failure (i.e., patients with chronic kidney disease stage 5 on dialysis), but in milder degrees of renal impairment (CKD stages 3 and 4) the use of a low dose of a kinetically stable agent may be less risky than administration of iodinated contrast medium, precipitating a worsening of renal function.

10.6.4 Portal Venous Circulation

Portal and mesenteric venous imaging with contrast-enhanced MRA has been very successful but with the use of ECS contrast agents this relies on accurate timing of breath-hold acquisitions, which may be unreliable, and the ideal portal phase can be missed unless time-resolved MRA sequences are available. With a blood pool contrast agent the imaging window is prolonged and hence more easily captured and since there is little extraction to the ECS compared with conventional agents the venous conspicuity in the first pass of the portal phase is increased. Portal MRV with a blood pool contrast agent is currently best performed with standard resolution breath-hold CE-MRA acquisitions or fat-suppressed T1w GRE sequences (such as THRIVE, VIBE and LAVA) since the optimized steady state high-resolution sequences applicable in the limbs are not suitable for the upper abdomen, where respiratory movement artifacts are problematic. This limitation may in future be overcome with the use of navigator techniques.

10.7 Upper Limbs and Thorax

The indications for venous imaging in the upper limbs and thorax are similar to those for the lower limbs, except that nowadays the most common request is to evaluate for iatrogenic upper extremity venous thrombosis and/or central vein stenosis as complications of prior central venous catheterization. Placement of central venous catheters (CVC) via the jugular or subclavian routes and PICC lines are increasingly common procedures in modern medicine to facilitate patient monitoring and administration of therapies and to provide parenteral nutrition.

Unfortunately, the use of CVCs can be complicated by both venous thrombosis and stenosis which may become symptomatic with either unilateral upper limb/neck edema or even a full superior vena caval occlusion syndrome. Furthermore, occult central venous stenosis and/or thrombosis may complicate what was initially thought to be an uncomplicated catheter insertion in up to 65% of patients, particularly where there has been prior intervention [25–34]. Hence visualization of the central thoracic veins prior to attempted CVC placement is playing an increasing role for patients with problematic vascular access, with the aim of optimizing the lifespan, durability, and effectiveness of central venous catheters. Ultrasonography can assess the veins in the arms, however, the more

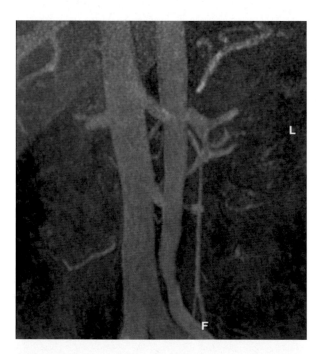

◘ **Fig. 10.18.** Breath-hold coronal contrast-enhanced MRA thin-slab MIP image in equilibrium phase of potential living renal donor after administration of Vasovist®. Image shows circumaortic left renal venous collar; part of the left renal venous drainage is complex, anastomosing to lumbar veins and then passing retro-aortic and caudal to join IVC. Note short length of right renal vein from union of two tributaries prior to cava

central veins are inaccessible to direct ultrasonographic visualization while MRV provides excellent imaging.

Visualization of the central veins of the thorax is also useful in assessment of superior caval obstructing diseases as, while CT will usually define simple SVC obstructions, from lung cancer, for example, more diffuse inflammatory diseases such as fibrosing mediastinitis and granuloma-

tous disorders may benefit from MRI, particularly as it can be used for follow-up in assessment of response to immunosuppressive therapies without concerns regarding excessive radiation exposure. In this context the high relaxivity of a blood pool contrast agent is helpful for assessing venous stent patency, increasing the conspicuity of blood within the stent lumen (◘ Figs. 10.19, 10.20).

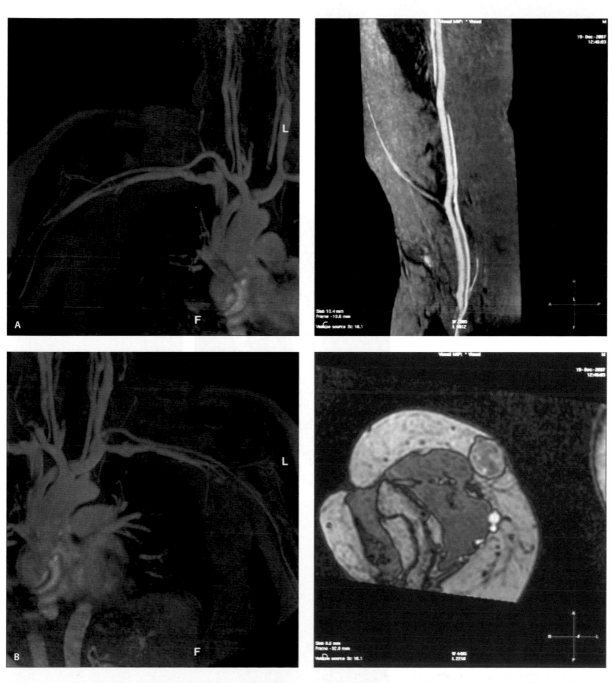

◘ **Fig. 10.19. A,B** Breath-hold coronal contrast-enhanced MRA MIPs in first pass arterial and equilibrium phases of upper thoracic vessels in patient with three previous bilateral failed arteriovenous fistulae. Note occlusive damage to left axillary vein. **C,D** Subsequent steady state high-resolution imaging of right arm shows sites of two of the previous failed arteriovenous fistulae (*arrows* to anastomoses) and small-caliber basilic vein (*asterisk* – smaller than and adjacent to brachial artery) unsuitable for basilic transposition operation

11.1   Introduction

The morbidity and mortality statistics of developed countries still show vascular diseases in a leading position. Probably the most common manifestation of the systemic disease atherosclerosis is peripheral vascular occlusive disease (PAOD), while the most threatening manifestations are carotid, renal, and coronary artery stenoses [1–5]. All of these manifestations have in common that they need adequate imaging for early detection and optimized treatment planning. There are a number of diagnostic tools for each of these vascular territories, but none of them is regarded as the standard of reference for the entire arterial vascular bed. Until a few years ago, magnetic resonance angiography (MRA) was a preferred diagnostic tool for the assessment of single anatomical territories, but it was not possible to perform a whole-body MRA. Today this drawback has been overcome, and by combining parallel imaging strategies with whole-body MR systems, the complete vasculature of the body can be examined at once. However, the last persisting constraint is the somewhat limited spatial resolution compared with other imaging methods such as conventional digital subtraction angiography (DSA), duplex ultrasonography, or computed tomography angiography (CTA) [6–10]. Due to the absence of ionizing radiation and recent developments regarding hard- and software, as well as sequence technology and new contrast agents (CA), magnetic resonance angiography (MRA) should be considered the best candidate and a comprehensive diagnostic tool to image the complete body vasculature.

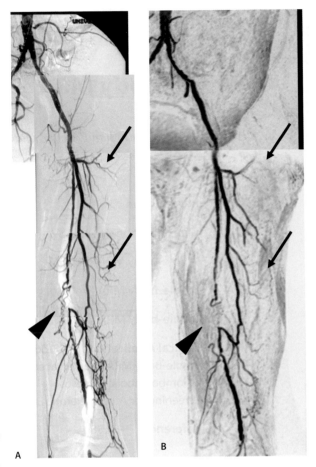

Fig. 11.1A,B. Comparison of a DSA (**A**) and an MRA (**B**, colors inverted) dataset. Due to the higher spatial resolution, small muscle-arterial branches (*arrows*) as well as collateral vessels (*arrowhead*) are better depicted

11.2   Clinical Rationale

With an increasing average age of the population in the industrialized world, the incidence and prevalence of atherosclerotic and other vascular diseases rise steadily. However, treatment options for vascular-related diseases are improving. In this respect, an early diagnosis of vascular disease, if possible in an asymptomatic stage, is of high interest. There are several clinical and laboratory tests such as the ankle-brachial-index (ABI) for the diagnosis of PAOD or prognostically important risk factors for developing atherosclerotic plaques such as the absolute levels and relations of high- and low-density lipoproteins (HDL/LDL), but before a treatment decision is made, detailed imaging of the diseased vascular region is required [11, 12]. As mentioned above, there are several established vascular imaging modalities for different vascular regions. Digital subtraction angiography (DSA) is still regarded as the standard of reference in most vascular territories [13] (◘ Fig. 11.1). However, the combination of ionizing radiation, invasiveness, and potentially nephrotoxic contrast agents (CA) demonstrates

the need for alternative, less harmful, and ideally non-invasive imaging techniques. Imaging of the carotid arteries for example is – among other techniques – a domain of duplex ultrasound [14, 15] (◘ Fig. 11.2). With this method, the superficially localized common carotid arteries as well as the proximal parts of the internal carotid arteries are excellently imaged; it is possible not only to measure the vessel lumen but also to assess the vessel wall. However, this method is very user dependent and cannot be used in every anatomical region. The evaluation of the renal arteries, for example, is often challenging with ultrasound, because of the location of these vessels deep in the body and the surrounding structures such as the bowel, which can impair the accessibility and assessability. Because of its high spatial resolution and easy application, CTA constitutes another promising and non-invasive method for imaging of nearly all vascular regions at a high spatial resolution [8, 16, 17] (◘ Fig. 11.3). On the other hand, ionizing radiation and the need for iodinated CA constitute a definite drawback.

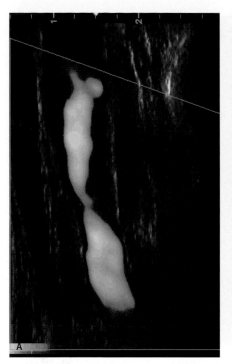
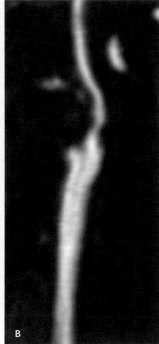

Fig. 11.2A,B. Comparison of a duplex ultrasound image (**A**) and a magnified MRA image (**B**) showing an occlusion of the internal carotid artery

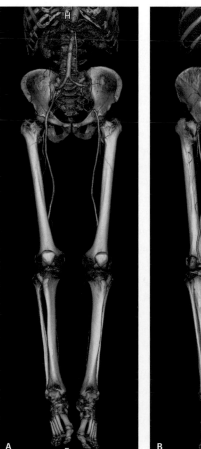
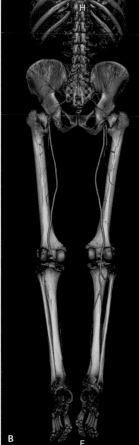
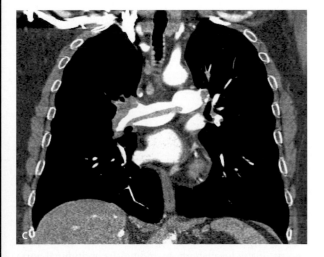

Fig. 11.3A–C. Examples of CTA datasets. (**A**) Anterior and (**B**) posterior VRT view of a peripheral run-off CTA showing occlusion of the arterial vessels of the left calf. **C** Coronal reconstruction of a pulmonary CTA showing major central pulmonary embolism

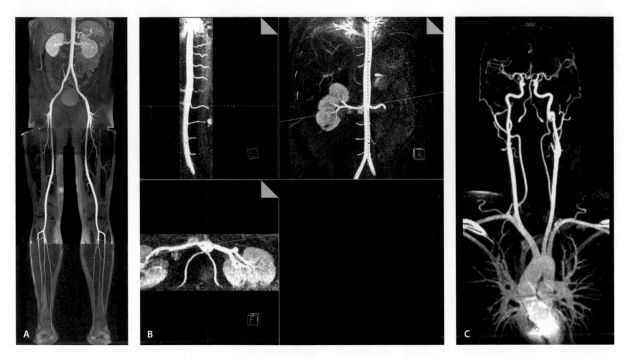

▣ Fig. 11.4A–C. MRA examinations of different anatomical regions. **A** Run-off study acquired in three stations in arterial first pass without venous opacification. **B** The possibility of 3D reformatting due to iso- tropic spatial resolution. **C** First pass carotid MRA with nice display of the carotid arteries

Magnetic resonance angiography is the only non-invasive imaging method which does not entail the disadvantage of ionizing radiation and which provides good image quality at a high spatial resolution throughout the entire body (▣ Fig. 11.4). Even the CA used are very well tolerated if renal function is not impaired [18].

Recent developments in MR system technology can further expand the application of MRA from imaging dedicated anatomical regions to a »real« whole-body MRA [19, 20].

11.3 Whole-body MRA

First attempts to image the entire arterial system from the skull base down to the feet were limited by MR system technology. The majority of MR systems have a restricted range of patient table movement of typically less than 150 cm. This means that whole-body imaging can be performed only with two contrast injections, requiring repositioning of the patient during the examination. This way, in a first step only the thoracic and head and neck vessels can be displayed, and after repositioning of the patient the vessels of the lower body including the abdominal aorta and the iliac and peripheral arteries are imaged in a second step. This second part covers a very large anatomical area which often leads to an impaired image quality in the

most distal vessel station, i.e. the lower leg, due to venous opacification [20] (▣ Fig. 11.5).

To overcome the limited range of table movement and to avoid having to reposition the patient during whole-body MRA, crucial impetus was provided by independent research groups for technical implementations to achieve whole-body MRA. Manually movable table platforms were developed, e.g., »SKIP« (Stepping Kinematic Imaging Platform, Magnetic Moments, Bloomfield, MI, USA) and »AngioSURF« (Angiographic System for Unlimited Rolling Field-of-views, MR-Innovation GmbH, Essen, Germany), which exceeded the range of movement of the motorized patient tables used in MR scanners, thereby extending the achievable FOV to approximately 200 cm and giving rise to »real« whole-body MRA [21, 22] (▣ Fig. 11.6). With these table platforms, a step-by-step whole-body MRA is possible with five to six stations. The inadequate coverage of this examination field with RF surface coils is circumvented by a stationary RF surface coil pair positioned in the isocenter of the magnet. A phased-array coil is system inbuilt in most scanners in the patient table and delivers signals from the posterior region of the patient. On the anterior side of the patient, a second phased-array surface coil is mounted on a coil glider, which is height-adjustable and held in position by two arms at the isocenter of the magnet. The patient is positioned on an MR-compatible table platform mounted on rollers. Using this technique, the patient can be manu-

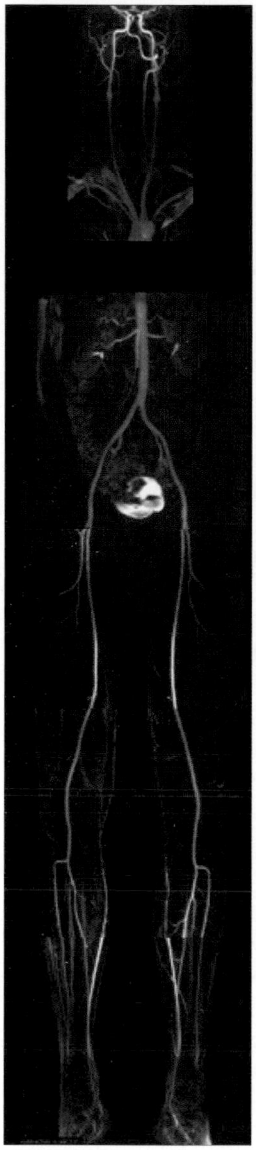

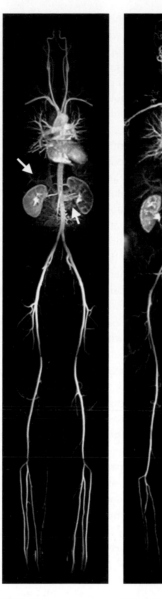

■ Fig. 11.5.   ■ Fig. 11.6. 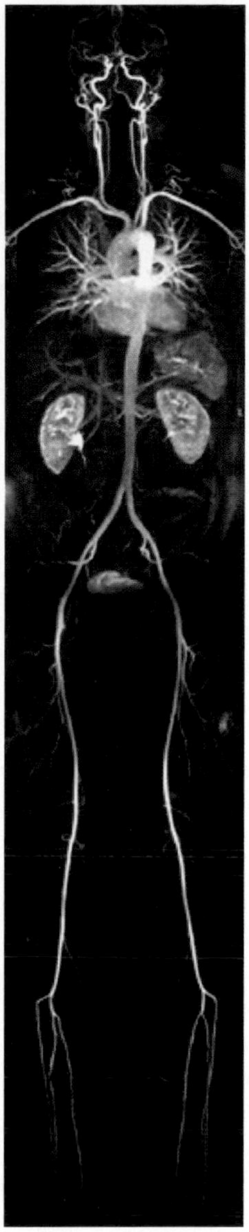   ■ Fig. 11.7.

■ **Fig. 11.5.** Whole-body MRA dataset acquired with a standard MR system. Note the gap between the first MRA station (carotid arteries) and the second part of the whole-body MRA after the patient was repositioned

■ **Fig. 11.6.** Whole-body MRA dataset acquired with a standard MR system in combination with a rolling table platform. Whole-body-MRA is performed in six steps from head to feet. Note the beginning venous enhancement of the renal veins (*shorter arrow*) and the portal vein (*arrow*)

■ **Fig. 11.7.** Whole-body MRA dataset acquired with a dedicated whole-body MR system in four steps from head to feet

ally pulled stepwise through the magnet passing between the two surface coils. The RF surface coils provide the SNR required for high image quality without the need to completely enclose the patient in RF coils from head to toe. First results using this technique have been promising but come along with a somewhat reduced spatial resolution, due to the necessity of fast imaging and coverage of a large FOV.

In 2004, a new MR system generation with an extensive moving table in combination with a dedicated matrix coil system for whole-body imaging was presented. With this type of MR system, the patient does not need to be repositioned, and no dedicated rolling table platform is necessary. The system's patient table allows a movement of more than 200 cm and the patient can be completely cov-

ered with dedicated surface coils before the examination. During the examination, every anatomical region can be moved to the isocenter of the magnet, and the activated coils or respective coil elements can be chosen as needed [19, 20, 23] (■ Fig. 11.7).

11.4   Whole-body MRA Protocols

To achieve the best possible image quality, dedicated imaging and/or optimized CA application protocols are recommended. When using standard extracellular CA, the primary goal is to image every vessel region in a purely arterial phase, without any venous contamination. When imaging various vascular territories, this can be achieved by several techniques such as test-bolus or bolus-chase applications for a precise timing of the CA arrival or, potentially, by additional venous compression to slow down venous enhancement, especially in the lower extremity. In whole-body MRA, these techniques are of major importance, but they are often enough not sufficient to get optimal results. Here, acquisition time, spatial resolution, and table movement have to be compromised [24]. It is certainly possible to image the first vascular region without venous contamination and at high spatial resolution, but in the following vascular regions image quality may decrease. For example, it is not possible to image the renal arteries without venous overlay directly after imaging the carotid arteries. During data acquisition of the carotid arteries, contrast runs down to the lower body part and leads to venous contamination, for example, in the renal veins, and later on in the venous vessels of the lower leg. One solution to restrict the amount of venous enhancement is to shorten the acquisition time of every imaged station, which will automatically result in a reduced spatial resolution and a decreased signal-to-noise ratio (SNR).

The introduction of the aforementioned dedicated whole-body MR systems helped to overcome many of these limitations. The large range of table movement offers the flexibility to move to every vascular region in a very short time, and the combination with dedicated matrix surface coil systems allows for implementing parallel imaging techniques for an enhanced data acquisition. For such a setup of hard- and software (i.e., MR sequences), several different imaging protocols for whole-body MRA exist [20, 25, 26]. The most promising approach seems to be a protocol using two separate contrast injections, to avoid imaging of the entire arterial vasculature with only one contrast bolus. With such a dual-bolus technique, the arteries of the upper thorax, neck, and head are imaged first. Then the table moves the patient down to the calf station and during this table movement, the first contrast bolus is overtaken. This way, the most distal vascular station, i.e., the calves, can be acquired without venous contamination. After a short break, the abdominal arteries are imaged with a second contrast bolus followed by acquisition of the thigh arteries. With this protocol it is possible to perform »real« whole-body MRA without disturbing venous contamination at good arterial contrast.

11.5 Whole-body MRA with Intravascular Contrast Agents

When using intravascular or »blood pool« contrast agents such as Vasovist® (Gadofosveset, Bayer Schering Pharma AG, Berlin, Germany) for whole-body MRA, it is certainly not possible (and also not necessary) to perform the afore-

mentioned dual injection CA application protocol [27]. Before whole-body MRA with blood pool agents is done, some important questions have to be answered:

1. Do I need to image the entire vasculature in an arterial first pass?
2. If not, which vascular regions are most important and should be imaged during arterial first pass?

As mentioned above, it is not possible to image all vascular territories at high spatial resolution without venous overlay with only one CA bolus. On the one hand, when using blood pool agents, spatial resolution can be compromised during first pass of the contrast to get a whole-body MRA dataset without venous overlay, because there is the opportunity to acquire high spatial resolution datasets during the steady state or »equilibrium phase« [28]. On the other hand, a maximum of two vascular regions can be acquired at high spatial resolution in the arterial first pass, and every other region is acquired at high spatial resolution during steady state [29–31] (◨ Fig. 11.8).

In whole-body MRA with intravascular contrast during steady state, there are significant inherent differences when examining various vascular beds. Thigh and calf stations are not vulnerable to movement artifacts from breathing or pulsation. Here, steady state imaging or respective acquisition time is more or less unlimited, and acquisition times of more than 5 min can be tolerated, leading to an unprecedented spatial resolution. However, the upper body, with the aortic arch and neck and head vessels, as well as the abdomen, can be affected by breathing artifacts and potentially by cardiac pulsation artifacts. This is mostly true for the thorax and abdomen, while the internal carotid arteries are typically not affected by this. The most challenging vascular region to be acquired during first pass imaging of the intravascular contrast is the abdominal station. Here, breathing and pulsation artifacts occur in datasets with long acquisition times. Until there are respiratory-triggered acquisition strategies that can be used for imaging this region, steady state imaging will be restricted to the duration of a single breath hold, and the full capacity of spatial resolution cannot be exploited.

11.6 Clinical Applications

Although most patients initially complain about problems in a single vascular territory, vascular diseases typically affect the entire arterial system, from the intracranial down to the pedal vessels. Therefore, whole-body vascular imaging seems to be a fast and attractive diagnostic approach for different clinical scenarios. Here, application of an intravascular contrast agent such as Vasovist® could result in extended imaging time, potentially higher spatial resolution, and larger anatomical coverage.

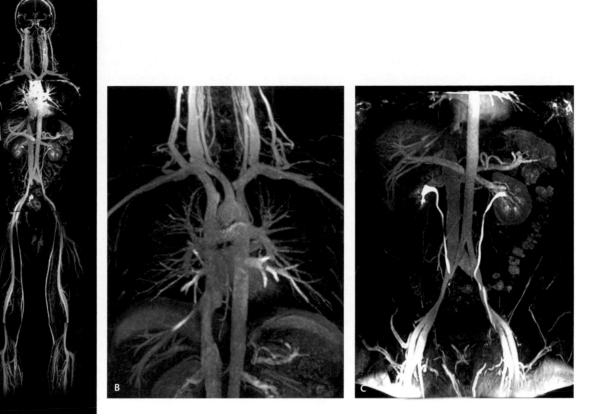

Fig. 11.8A–C. Whole-body MRA dataset acquired in the steady state with Vasovist®. (**A**) Arterial first pass imaging of every anatomical station without any venous enhancement is not possible, but every station can be acquired in the steady state with high spatial resolution, limited only by motion due to breathing (**B** and **C**)

11.6.1 Whole-body MRA as a Replacement for Run-off Studies

Multistation MR angiography covering the abdominal aorta down to the pedal arteries is a well-established technique for the evaluation of peripheral artery disease (PAD). However, using the recent hard- and software developments described above, the examination can easily be extended to whole-body MRA without increasing the dose of contrast. The scan time, the in-room time, and the time required for post-processing and reading of the examination increase to a certain degree; however, the high prevalence of concomitant atherosclerotic findings in the carotid arteries and thoracic aorta in PAD patients justify these investments and improve patient care.

11.6.2 Thromboembolic Diseases

Arterial emboli originating from the heart (left atrial thrombi in atrial fibrillation, left ventricular thrombi, aor-

tic valve lesions) or the ascending aorta may affect the entire arterial system with the potential fatal consequences of stroke or limb ischemia. In these patients whole-body is the perfect procedure for further diagnostic workup. Rather than looking only at the vascular area that becomes symptomatic at first, whole-body MRA can display the embolic damage to the entire arterial system, discovering several other vascular regions that might become symptomatic in the future and can be treated in advance.

11.6.3 Screening for Atherosclerotic Disease

As the prevalence of atherosclerotic disease increases and thus has a higher socioeconomic impact, screening may appear reasonable, especially among patients at high risk such as smokers or diabetics. Although most atherosclerotic lesions are not completely reversible, lifestyle changes, reduction of risk factors, and pharmaceutical treatment can decelerate or even stop the progression of the disease.

Take home messages

- Up to now, invasiveness, radiation exposure, contrast dose limitations, and costs have been the most critical hurdles preventing an all-encompassing approach to arterial imaging.
- Whole-body MRA appears to be well-suited to visualize the systemic nature of atherosclerotic disease and allows the depiction of relevant concomitant disease affecting other arterial territories than the region that might become symptomatic first, without potentially harming the patient by applying ionizing radiation or high doses of iodinated CA.

- Non-invasiveness, three-dimensionality, extended coverage, and high contrast conspicuity are the characteristics of whole-body MRA.
- Intravascular contrast agents such as Vasovist® can further increase image quality and – by introducing new aspects to MR imaging techniques such as the differentiation of first pass and steady state vascular imaging – will most probably have a major impact on routine clinical imaging and image quality of whole-body MR angiography.

References

1. Adams MR, Celermajer DS (1999) Detection of presymptomatic atherosclerosis: a current perspective. Clin Sci (Lond) 97:615–624
2. Cahan MA, et al (1999) The prevalence of carotid artery stenosis in patients undergoing aortic reconstruction. Am J Surg 178:194–196
3. Diehm C, Kareem S, Lawall H (2004) Epidemiology of peripheral arterial disease. Vasa 33:183–189
4. Fowkes FG, et al (1991) Edinburgh Artery Study: prevalence of asymptomatic and symptomatic peripheral arterial disease in the general population. Int J Epidemiol 20:384–392
5. Goyen M, et al (2003) Detection of atherosclerosis: systemic imaging for systemic disease with whole-body three-dimensional MR angiography--initial experience. Radiology 227:277–282
6. Green D, Parker D (2003) CTA and MRA: visualization without catheterization. Semin Ultrasound CT MR 24:185–191
7. Leiner T, et al (2005) Peripheral arterial disease: comparison of color duplex US and contrast-enhanced MR angiography for diagnosis. Radiology 235:699–708
8. Prokop M (2000) Multislice CT angiography. Eur J Radiol 36:86–96
9. Steffens JC, et al (2003) Bolus-chasing contrast-enhanced 3D MRA of the lower extremity. Comparison with intraarterial DSA. Acta Radiol 44:185–192
10. Koelemay MJ, et al (1996) Diagnosis of arterial disease of the lower extremities with duplex ultrasonography. Br J Surg 83:404–409
11. Hirsch AT, et al (2006) ACC/AHA Guidelines for the Management of Patients with Peripheral Arterial Disease (lower extremity, renal, mesenteric, and abdominal aortic): a collaborative report from the American Associations for Vascular Surgery/Society for Vascular Surgery, Society for Cardiovascular Angiography and Interventions, Society for Vascular Medicine and Biology, Society of Interventional Radiology, and the ACC/AHA Task Force on Practice Guidelines (writing committee to develop guidelines for the management of patients with peripheral arterial disease) – summary of recommendations. J Vasc Interv Radiol 17:1383–1397; quiz 1398
12. Norgren L, et al (2007) Inter-society consensus for the management of peripheral arterial disease (TASC II). J Vasc Surg 45 [1 Suppl]:S5–S67
13. Gregor M, et al (2002) Peripheral run-off CE-MRA with a 1.0 molar gadolinium chelate (Gadovist) with intraarterial DSA comparison. Acad Radiol 9 [Suppl 2]:S398–400
14. Colquhoun I, et al (1992) The assessment of carotid and vertebral arteries: a comparison of CFM duplex ultrasound with intravenous digital subtraction angiography. Br J Radiol 65:1069–1074
15. Stanziale SF, et al (2005) Determining in-stent stenosis of carotid arteries by duplex ultrasound criteria. J Endovasc Ther 12:346–353
16. Rankin SC (1999) CT angiography. Eur Radiol 9: 297–310
17. Vasbinder GBC, De Haan MW, van Engelshoven JMA (2002) Accuracy of CTA and 3D contrast-enhanced MRA as compared to intra-arterial digital subtraction angiography for assessment of the number of renal arteries in 356 subjects. Radiology 225 (Proceedings): 400
18. Michaely HJ, et al (2007) Nephrogenic systemic fibrosis (NSF) – implications for radiology [in German]. Radiologe 47:785–793
19. Fenchel M, et al (2005) Whole-body MR angiography using a novel 32-receiving-channel MR system with surface coil technology: first clinical experience. J Magn Reson Imaging 21:596–603
20. Kramer H, et al (2005) Cardiovascular screening with parallel imaging techniques and a whole-body MR imager. Radiology 236:300–310
21. Goyen M, et al (2002) Whole-body three-dimensional MR angiography with a rolling table platform: initial clinical experience. Radiology 224:270–277
22. Shetty AN, et al (2002) Lower extremity MR angiography: universal retrofitting of high-field-strength systems with stepping kinematic imaging platforms initial experience. Radiology 222:284–291
23. Nael K, et al (2007) High-spatial-resolution whole-body MR angiography with high-acceleration parallel acquisition and 32-channel 3.0-T unit: initial experience. Radiology 242:865–872
24. Ruehm SG, et al (2000) Whole-body MRA on a rolling table platform (AngioSURF) [in German]. Rofo 172:670–674
25. Nael K, et al (2007) Multistation whole-body high-spatial-resolution MR angiography using a 32-channel MR system. AJR Am J Roentgenol 188:529–539
26. Vogt FM, et al (2004) Venous compression at high-spatial-resolution three-dimensional MR angiography of peripheral arteries. Radiology 233:913–920
27. Nikolaou K, et al (2006) High-spatial-resolution multistation MR angiography with parallel imaging and blood pool contrast agent: initial experience. Radiology 241:861–872
28. van Bemmel CM, et al (2003) Blood pool contrast-enhanced MRA: improved arterial visualization in the steady state. IEEE Trans Med Imaging 22:645–652
29. Klessen C, et al (2007) First pass whole-body magnetic resonance angiography (MRA) using the blood-pool contrast medium gadofosveset trisodium: comparison to gadopentetate dimeglumine. Invest Radiol 42:659–664
30. McGregor R, et al (2008) A multi-center, comparative, phase 3 study to determine the efficacy of gadofosveset-enhanced magnetic resonance angiography for evaluation of renal artery disease. Eur J Radiol 65(2):316-25. Epub 2007 May 17
31. Rapp JH, et al (2005) Aortoiliac occlusive disease in patients with known or suspected peripheral vascular disease: safety and efficacy of gadofosveset-enhanced MR angiography – multicenter comparative phase III study. Radiology 236:71–78

Endoleak Imaging

Sandra A.P. Cornelissen, Mathias Prokop, Hence J.M. Verhagen, and Lambertus W. Bartels

12.1 Introduction

Until 15 years ago, abdominal aortic aneurysm treatment involved major abdominal surgery in which a prosthetic graft was sewn into the aortic wall. As vascular surgeons were increasingly confronted with older patients with severe co-morbidity, attempts for less invasive aneurysm treatment were made. In 1991, Parodi et al. [1] were the first to report successful endovascular aortic aneurysm repair (EVAR) in human patients. Their technique involved cannulation of the common femoral artery and endovascular placement of a Dacron tubular graft with attached balloon expandable stents to anchor the graft to the aortic wall. Since then, this technique has become widely available and has emerged as a frequently used alternative for open aneurysm treatment. Today, many different types of endografts are available, and more varied and also more challenging anatomies can be treated endovascularly.

Due to the rapid development of endoprostheses, limited experience about long-term durability is available for most grafts. At present, life-long imaging follow-up is considered necessary in patients following EVAR. Imaging follow-up is needed to assess whether aneurysm size regresses, whether blood leaks out of the endograft into the aneurysm sac (endoleak), whether the endoprosthesis remains intact and at its original location, and whether the endoprosthesis remains patent.

Follow-up regimens differ worldwide but usually consist of a computed tomography angiography (CTA) examination shortly after the procedure, as well as repeated CTA examinations each year for the rest of the patient's life. Aneurysm size is an important parameter in this follow-up. In case of aneurysm growth, the danger of aneurysm rupture is still present, and repeat intervention is indicated. In case of aneurysm shrinkage, aneurysm treatment is considered successful.

12.2 Non-shrinking Aneurysms

Implantation of an endoprosthesis has the goal of excluding the aneurysm sac from the circulation. This will reduce pressure on the aneurysm wall and, through resorption of the ensuing thrombus, will lead to aneurysm shrinkage. In case of a non-shrinking or growing aneurysm, the etiology is not always clear, but endoleaks are the most frequent cause.

12.2.1 Endoleaks

Endoleaks are classified according to the source of leakage [2, 3]. Leakage via an attachment site is a type I endoleak and leads to markedly increased intra-aneurysmal pressure (high-pressure endoleak). Type II endoleaks originate from reversed flow in branch vessels, such as lumbar arteries or the inferior mesenteric artery, and lead to a pressure increase that depends on the amount of leakage. Type III endoleaks represent a defect in the graft material or a modular disconnection and usually cause a marked increase in intra-aneurysmal pressure. Type IV endoleak denotes leakage via porous graft fabric.

Accurate visualization and classification of endoleaks is needed to evaluate whether treatment of an endoleak is necessary. Especially high-pressure endoleaks, i.e., type I and III endoleaks which originate directly from the arterial circulation, seem to promote aneurysm growth and increase rupture risk. Type I or III endoleaks have been associated with a significantly greater risk of rupture than type II endoleaks [4]. This is why type I and III endoleaks are more aggressively treated than type II endoleaks. There is still controversy about whether treatment of type II endoleaks is needed. In general, type II endoleaks are treated in case of aneurysm growth, if possible by means of endovascular techniques.

12.2.2 The Endotension Problem

Endotension is a term used for increased pressure within the aneurysm sac that leads to aneurysm growth without evidence of endoleak (on CTA). Endotension has a prevalence of 1–3%. Because the aneurysm grows in patients with endotension, rupture risk is increased and treatment is indicated. However, because there is no visualized endoleak to direct treatment to, the main treatment option is currently conversion to surgery. For most patients, this is not an attractive alternative because of their cardiovascular co-morbidity.

The etiology of endotension is unknown. It could well be that the elevated intrasac pressure originates from an endoleak that was not diagnosed by CTA. This can be due to the slow flow rate of the endoleak or the intermittent leakage of an endoleak. Most likely, slow flow leaks are due to type II or type IV leakage. Type I or III leakage involves a direct communication with the arterial circulation and therefore has higher flow rates and should always be detectable by CTA.

Alternatively, the elevated intrasac pressure can originate from inside the aneurysm sac. Very little is known about the processes taking place inside the aneurysm sac following EVAR. Possibly, the intra-aneurysmal thrombus is not a static entity; rather, repeated liquefaction by fibrinolysis and clotting occurs. During fibrinolysis fluid accumulates inside the aneurysm sac, increasing the intrasac pressure. Other inflammatory reactions or graft infection can also cause fluid accumulation inside the aneurysm sac, resulting in intrasac pressure increase and aneurysm growth.

Nevertheless, a substantial number of endotension cases could represent missed endoleak. For further investigation, more sensitive techniques for visualizing endoleaks are needed, such as MRI. Here we postulate that the novel blood pool agent Vasovist® (Gadofosveset, Bayer Schering Pharma AG, Berlin, Germany) can play an important role in endoleak visualization because it has a high relaxivity and remains in the intravascular space for an extended period of time. This is interesting not only from a scientific point of view; accurate knowledge about endoleak in patients with endotension potentially provides more patient-specific – often endovascular – treatment alternatives to prevent future aneurysm growth. Adequate treatment of endotension potentially results in shrinkage of the aneurysm sac.

This chapter describes current strategies and questions in the follow-up after EVAR with special emphasis on the visualization of endoleak. Advantages and disadvantages of visualizing endoleaks with CT and magnetic resonance imaging (MRI) are described. Furthermore, the application of Vasovist®-enhanced MRI for endoleak visualization and MR protocols which can be used for endoleak imaging are described.

12.3 Challenges of Imaging Follow-up after EVAR

A substantial number of endotension cases and non-shrinking aneurysms probably represent endoleak not visualized by conventional imaging techniques. The challenge of radiologic follow-up after EVAR is to improve understanding of aneurysm sac behavior in such cases. As said before, lack of aneurysm shrinkage can be caused by slow flow endoleak or the intermittent leakage of an endoleak. If an endoleak has a slow flow rate, a longer time between injection and imaging is needed to allow for leakage of enhanced blood into the aneurysm sac (late-phase imaging). Increasing this delay gives rise to some problems. First of all, during late-phase imaging the images are not acquired during the first pass of a bolus of contrast material but at a later time, when contrast agent has mixed with the whole blood volume of a patient. Consequently, the contrast agent concentration in the blood volume is lower in late-phase imaging with respect to peak arterial-phase imaging, which results in lower intravascular enhancement. Additionally, almost all of the contrast agents used nowadays distribute to the extracellular space, which mean they leak into the interstitium during passage of tissue capillaries, which further decreases the intravascular contrast agent concentration.

12.3.1 CT and CTA

Pre-contrast combined with post-contrast CT imaging at different time points after injection of contrast fluid is currently the reference standard for endoleak detection.

The **pre-contrast CT** acquisition is used for differentiating calcium from endoleak [5]. For measurement of aneurysm diameter and for evaluating graft migration or kinking of the graft, the pre-contrast acquisition gives enough information.

Arterial-phase CTA is used for the detection of high-flow endoleaks and gives the best anatomic information regarding in-stent thrombus, patency of side branches, and dissections, which sometimes occur as a complication of EVAR. Iezzi et al. demonstrated that the combination of an initial pre-contrast and arterial acquisition 1 month after EVAR and only an arterial acquisition at subsequent follow-up moments is sufficient for endoleak detection [6]. In their opinion delayed-phase imaging to detect slow-flow endoleak is required only in case of an increase in aneurysm size.

Venous-phase (60 s after injection of contrast media) or delayed-phase CT (100 s after injection) acquisitions are used to visualize slow flow endoleaks [5]. Intravascular enhancement is far less compared with arterial CTA because the scan is acquired after the first pass of the injected bolus of contrast agent, so the contrast agent has been diluted in the whole intravascular blood volume and has leaked into the interstitium during its passage through capillaries. This is why the later this acquisition is acquired after contrast media injection, the lower the enhancement of the blood pool. Moreover, the amount of contrast medium needed for such an acquisition should be adjusted to patient weight (as approximation of the blood volume). Macari et al., however, argue that pre-contrast and venous acquisitions are sufficient for endoleak detection; arterial phase imaging is, in their point of view, not necessary for the routine detection of endoleaks [7].

The main problem with a delayed-phase scan is that it is always a compromise: the later the acquisition with regard to contrast media injection, the more contrast media is necessary or the lower the enhancement. If the blood is still sufficiently enhanced, the endoleak is better detected. If no endoleak is visualized on a late-phase acquisition, it is still not clear whether there is a true absence of endoleak. Delayed acquisitions are needed for the visualization of low-flow endoleaks. These acquisitions are less useful for imaging vascular anatomy. For diagnosing dissection or evaluating the patency of side branches arterial acquisitions are needed.

In summary, different protocols are used for endoleak detection. Obviously, in endoleak imaging with CT there is always a trade-off between the delay between injection and imaging and vascular enhancement. The delay between injection and imaging should be as long as possible to give contrast agent enough time to leak to achieve the accumulation of a detectable amount of contrast agent in the aneurysm sac. However, it should not be too long, because longer after injection the contrast agent already has disappeared from the blood, leaving only blood without contrast agent leaking into the aneurysm sac, which further deteriorates the visibility of the endoleak on CT images.

12.3.2 MR and MRA

Recent studies have shown that magnetic resonance imaging using Gd-DTPA is more sensitive for endoleak than CTA [8–11], so it is logical to use MRI to further investigate the role of endoleak in patients with endotension. Additionally, with dynamic MRA more endoleaks can be classified into one of the categories described before compared to CTA [12]. Improved endoleak classification primarily results from dynamic MRA acquisitions in which the same volume is scanned multiple times resulting in visualization of the contrast bolus flowing through the aortic trajectory in near real time. Lookstein et al. demonstrated that endoleak classification by dynamic MRA corresponded to the classification obtained by digital subtraction angiography [13]. Accurate endoleak classification is important for endoleak treatment. In case of a type II endoleak less aggressive treatment is indicated than for a type I or III endoleak.

Metal-related artifacts caused by the endoprosthesis can degrade the diagnostic value of MRI in patients after EVAR. Susceptibility artifacts, resulting from local field inhomogeneity caused by metal in the stent struts, give rise to geometrical distortions and local signal loss around the implant's metallic parts. The severity of these artifacts depends strongly on the susceptibility of materials used in the endograft. Endografts with stent struts of

MR compatible materials are MR-safe and result in diagnostic images in 1.5 T systems. In addition, MR imaging in the abdominal region is prone to artifacts. Care has to be taken to minimize ghosting artifacts originating from breathing. These artifacts can be prevented by placing a regional saturation slab ventrally on the subcutaneous fat of the abdomen.

Different scan types can be used for endoleak visualization. T1-weighted spin echo imaging and T1-weighted spoiled gradient echo (MR angiographic) protocols can be used. Spin echo imaging is preferred because the influence of the susceptibility artifacts caused by local field inhomogeneities of the stent struts is less compared to gradient echo imaging.

A typical imaging protocol for endoleak imaging [11, 12] with Gd-DTPA contains a:
1. Pre-contrast transverse T1-weighted spin echo acquisition
2. Coronal dynamic 3D contrast enhanced (CE)-MRA during injection of Gd-DTPA (Magnevist®, Bayer Schering Pharma AG, Berlin, Germany)
3. First pass Coronal 3D CE-MRA
4. Post-contrast transverse T1-weighted spin echo

Voxels inside the aneurysm sac, outside the lumen of the endograft with a high signal intensity on the post-contrast image and a low signal intensity on the pre-contrast image represent endoleak. The appearance of the aneurysm sac must be known before contrast administration. For this reason T1-weighted spin echo acquisitions are needed before and after contrast injection. In most patients the intra-aneurysmal thrombus appears dark before contrast injection on T1-weighted images, but in some cases the thrombus inside the aneurysm sac already has a high signal intensity before contrast injection. Presumably this is caused by the presence of methemoglobin in the aneurysm sac, which has a short T1, which should not be interpreted as endoleak. In ◗ Fig. 12.1 an example of an arterial CTA and delayed

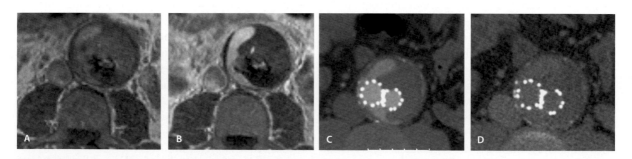

◗ **Fig. 12.1A–D. A** Pre-contrast and **B** post-contrast T1-weighted spin-echo images, **C** arterial CTA, and **D** delayed CT image of a patient with an endoleak. Hyperintense areas inside the aneurysm sac and outside the endograft on **B**, which are not this hyperintense on **A**, and hyperdense area on **C** represent endoleak

CT-image as well as the corresponding pre-contrast and post-contrast T1-weighted spin echo MR-images of a patient with endoleak are shown. The post-contrast MR-images were acquired approximately 3 min after injection of Gd-DTPA. The endoleak is hyperdense on CT-images with respect to the rest of the aneurysm sac. On the MR images a hyperintense area is present inside the endoleak on the post-contrast T1-weighted image which was less intense before contrast injection.

12.4 A new Approach to Endoleak Imaging: Vasovist®-enhanced MRA

12.4.1 General principle

Different classes of MR blood pool agents have been developed; coated iron particles and Gadolinium-based protein binding agents (of which Vasovist® is an example). Such agents remain in the intravascular space for a longer period compared to conventional contrast agents. Coated iron particles remain in the intravascular space because of their size and coating; Protein binding contrast agents remain intravascular by their reversible binding to human serum albumin [14]. In general, iron particles act as »negative« contrast agents, resulting in signal voids in the MR image caused by their local susceptibility effects which lead to dephasing of neighbouring spins. This phenomenon makes them mostly suitable for $T2^*$-weighted sequences [15]. However, when short echo times are used, iron particles can also be used as a positive contrast agent in T1-weighted protocols [16].

Vasovist® is a gadolinium-based protein binding contrast agent. For the visualization of endoleak, T1-weighted images before and after injection of Vasovist® can be used.

Vasovist® bound to albumin remains in the intravascular space for an extended period of time. Consequently, the delay between injection and imaging can be increased, allowing for the buildup of a higher concentration of contrast agent in slow-flow endoleaks. Intermittent endoleak also has a higher chance of being visualized in this way. The longer the delay between injection and imaging the higher the chance that during this time contrast agent leaks and accumulates in the aneurysm sac.

12.4.2 Examination Technique

Slight changes need to be made to the imaging protocol in order to adapt it to the use of Vasovist® instead of Gadolinium-DTPA. The first adaptation is the injection protocol. Because Vasovist® has a higher relaxivity than Gadolinium-DTPA, the injected dose is lower and it should be injected at a lower speed. The approved dose of Vasovist®, 0.12 ml/kg (0.03 mmol/kg) can be used and injected at 1 ml/s followed by a saline chaser of 30 ml with the same injection speed.

With this injection protocol the dynamic MRA protocol as used with gadolinium-DTPA can be used unchanged with Vasovist®. Subjectively, intravascular enhancement is higher with Vasovist® compared to gadolinium-DTPA. Dynamic acquisitions acquired during injection of Vasovist® typically show rapidly decreasing intravascular enhancement when the agent mixes with the whole blood volume (◘ Fig. 12.2).

After the dynamic series, late phase MRA images can be acquired. Because Vasovist® remains in the intravascular space for an extended period of time, MRA-images can be acquired much longer after injection than with Gd-DTPA. For acquiring late phase MRA acquisitions the flip angle of the steady state spoiled gradient echo imaging should be adjusted, e.g. lowered, to the expected T1 of blood. An example of two late phase MRA acquisitions acquired at 6 and 15 min after injection is shown in ◘ Fig. 12.3.

Additional postcontrast T1-weighted spin echo acquisitions can be added up to 1 hour after injection to fully utilize the longer intravascular residence time of Vasovist®. Examples of T1-weighted spin echo images acquired before and at different delays after administration of Vasovist® are shown in ◘ Figs. 12.4 and 12.5.

The T1 of blood is lowered during injection of Vasovist®. After injection, T1 rises again when the agent is diluted in the whole blood volume. The exact T1 of blood with contrast agent at different times after injection is not known. The development of blood T1 over time probably also depends on patient-related factors, like the concentration of albumin in the blood and renal function. Ideally the TR and the flip angle of MRA sequences should be adjusted to the T1 of blood expected at the specific post-injection delay. Longer after injection a longer T1 is expected and the TR should be increased and the flip angle should be adjusted to achieve maximal SNR. In the abdomen this is a problem because the scan should preferably fit in one breath hold.

12.4.3 Vasovist® for Detection of Slow-flow Endoleak

To investigate the possibility of visualizing slow flow endoleak, three patients were imaged with Vasovist® who did not have evidence of endoleak on CTA and delayed CT. All patients had been treated with the original Excluder endoprosthesis (W.L. Gore, Inc, Flagstaff, Arizona, USA).

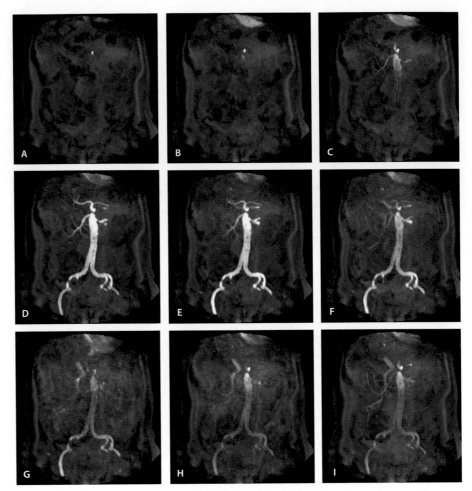

Fig. 12.2A–I. Maximum intensity projections of dynamic MRA acquisitions acquired (**A**) before and (**B to I**) following administration of Vasovist® 0.12 ml/kg at 1 ml/s

This endograft was changed in July 2004 by the manufacturer because it was associated with lower aneurysm shrinkage rates than other grafts. The cause was unclear but the manufacturer decided to incorporate an additional layer of ePTFE (expanded polytetrafluoroethylene) in the graft fabric because the low shrinkage rates were assumed to result from graft porosity. However, in human patients this had never been visualized.

Most probably, this graft porosity was not visualized using both CT or MR techniques due to the low flow rate, as explained above. In such cases it is useful to use Vasovist®. The scan protocol described above was used and late phase postcontrast T1-weighted spin echo acquisitions were added more than 30 min after injection. Using this protocol, endoleak was indeed visualized on the late phase images acquired more than 30 min after injection (◻ Fig. 12.6). The early postcontrast images acquired three min after injection did not show endoleak. On the late phase T1-w spin echo images, leakage of contrast agent into the aneurysm sac in the direct vicinity of a leg of the endoprosthesis was visualized. Because of this location,

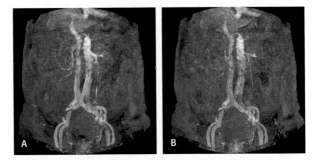

Fig. 12.3A,B. Maximum intensity projections of late-phase MRA acquisitions. Both acquisitions are steady state spoiled gradient echo acquisitions with a TR of 10 ms, TR of 2 ms and flip angle of 27 degrees. **A** was acquired 6 min and **B** 15 min following injection of Vasovist® in the standard dosage of 0.12 ml/kg at 1 ml/s

this leakage most probably arises from graft porosity. These images illustrate it is indeed possible to visualize slow-flow endoleaks by increasing the time window between injection and imaging when using the blood pool agent Gadofosveset [17].

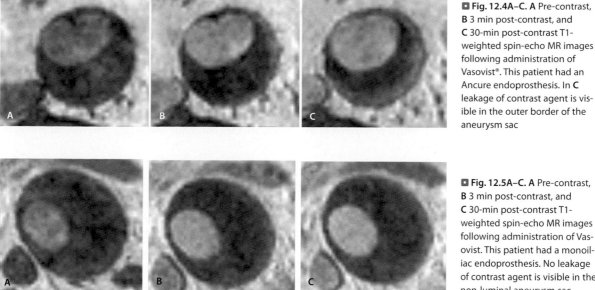

■ **Fig. 12.4A–C. A** Pre-contrast, **B** 3 min post-contrast, and **C** 30-min post-contrast T1-weighted spin-echo MR images following administration of Vasovist®. This patient had an Ancure endoprosthesis. In **C** leakage of contrast agent is visible in the outer border of the aneurysm sac

■ **Fig. 12.5A–C. A** Pre-contrast, **B** 3 min post-contrast, and **C** 30-min post-contrast T1-weighted spin-echo MR images following administration of Vasovist. This patient had a monoiliac endoprosthesis. No leakage of contrast agent is visible in the non-luminal aneurysm sac

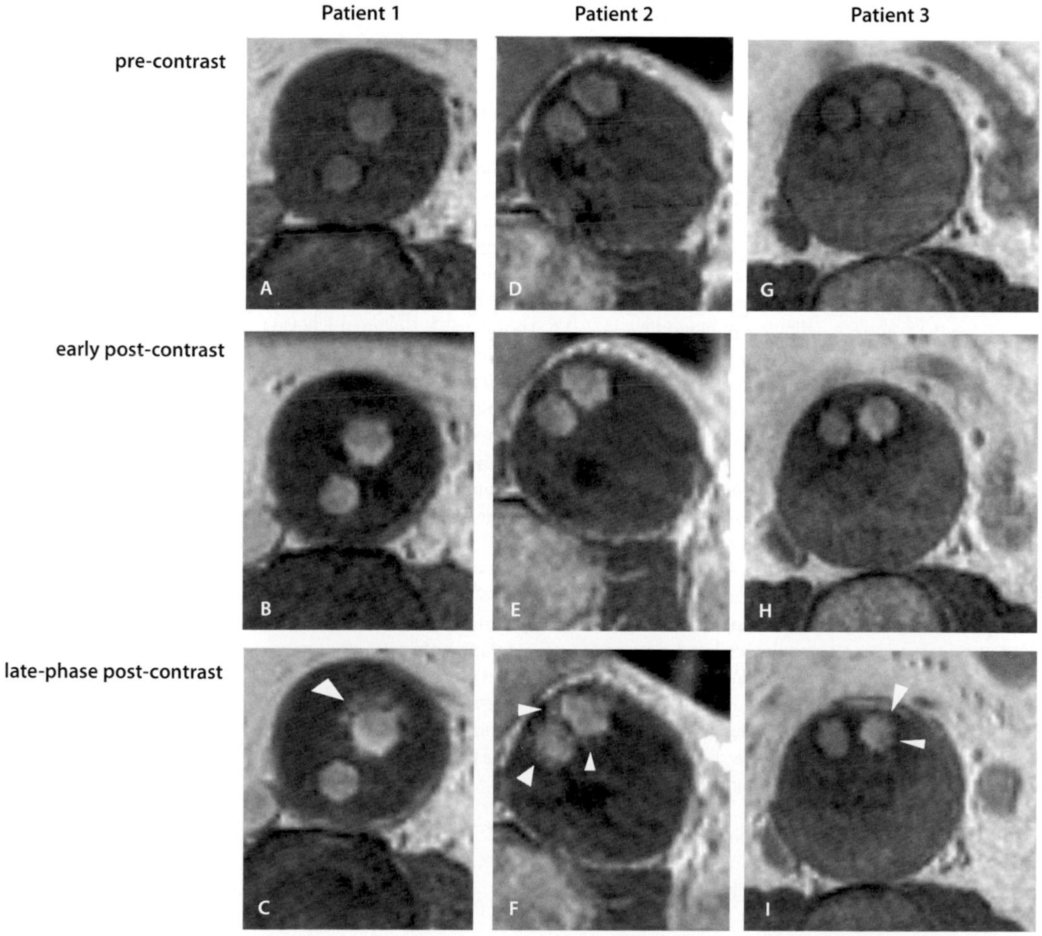

Patient 1   **Patient 2**   **Patient 3**

pre-contrast

early post-contrast

late-phase post-contrast

■ **Fig. 12.6A–I.** Transverse T1-weighted spin-echo MR images. **A,D,G** Pre-contrast, **B,E,H** early-phase post-contrast, **C,F,I** late-phase post-contrast T1-weighted images. Each column consists of images from the same patient and the same anatomical location. In the *bottom row*, endoleak (*arrowheads*) arising from graft porosity is visible. (Reused with permission from [17])

12.5   Summary

In the follow-up of EVAR, visualization of endoleak plays an important role, because endoleak hampers aneurysm shrinkage and promotes aneurysm growth, thus increasing rupture risk. It is currently not understood why not all aneurysms without evidence of endoleak on CTA shrink. Furthermore, some aneurysms grow without evidence of endoleak on CTA and delayed CT which is referred to as endotension. It could well be that in a substantial number of such cases endoleaks do play a role but are not visualized by the currently used imaging strategies due to the slow flow rate or intermittent nature of the endoleak. By using Vasovist® it is possible to increase the time window between contrast fluid injection and imaging to attain a higher accumulation of contrast agent in the endoleak. This improves visualization of slow flow endoleaks and increases the chance for visualizing intermittent endoleak.

> **Take home messages**
>
> - Patients who have undergone EVAR need life-long imaging to rule out endoleak and further growth of their aneurysm.
> - After EVAR, some aneurysms grow without evidence of endoleak on CTA and delayed CT. This is referred to as endotension.
> - With current CT and MRI imaging protocols endoleaks are not visualized in a substantial number of cases even when they are thought to be present.
> - Delayed-phase Vasovist®-enhanced MRI is a promising technique to detect suspected endoleak in cases where CT and convential MRI are negative.

References

1. Parodi JC, Palmaz JC, Barone HD (1991) Transfemoral intraluminal graft implantation for abdominal aortic aneurysms. Ann Vasc Surg 5:491–499

2. Veith FJ, Baum RA, Ohki T, Amor M, Adiseshiah M, Blankensteijn JD, et al (2002) Nature and significance of endoleaks and endotension: summary of opinions expressed at an international conference. J Vasc Surg 35:1029–1035

3. White GH, May J, Waugh RC, Chaufour X, Yu W (1998) Type III and type IV endoleak: toward a complete definition of blood flow in the sac after endoluminal AAA repair. J Endovasc Surg 5:305–309

4. van Marrewijk C, Buth J, Harris PL, Norgren L, Nevelsteen A, Wyatt MG (2002) Significance of endoleaks after endovascular repair of abdominal aortic aneurysms: The EUROSTAR experience. J Vasc Surg 35:461–473

5. Rozenblit AM, Patlas M, Rosenbaum AT, Okhi T, Veith FJ, Laks MP, et al (2003) Detection of endoleaks after endovascular repair of abdominal aortic aneurysm: value of unenhanced and delayed helical CT acquisitions. Radiology 227:426–433

6. Iezzi R, Cotroneo AR, Filippone A, Di Fabio F, Quinto F, Colosimo C, et al (2006) Multidetector CT in abdominal aortic aneurysm treated with endovascular repair: are unenhanced and delayed phase enhanced images effective for endoleak detection? Radiology 241:915–921

7. Macari M, Chandarana H, Schmidt B, Lee J, Lamparello P, Babb J (2006) Abdominal aortic aneurysm: can the arterial phase at CT evaluation after endovascular repair be eliminated to reduce radiation dose? Radiology 241:908–914

8. Cejna M, Loewe C, Schoder M, Dirisamer A, Hölzenbein T, Kretschmer G, et al (2002) MR angiography vs CT angiography in the follow-up of nitinol stent grafts in endoluminally treated aortic aneurysms. Eur Radiol 12:2443–2450

9. Haulon S, Lions C, McFadden EP, Koussa M, Gaxotte V, Halna P, et al (2001) Prospective evaluation of magnetic resonance imaging after endovascular treatment of infrarenal aortic aneurysms. Eur J Vasc Endovasc Surg 22:62–69

10. Pitton MB, Schweitzer H, Herber S, Schmiedt W, Neufang A, Kalden P, et al (2005) MRI versus helical CT for endoleak detection after endovascular aneurysm repair. AJR Am J Roentgenol 185:1275–1281

11. van der Laan MJ, Bartels LW, Viergever MA, Blankensteijn JD (2006) Computed tomography versus magnetic resonance imaging of endoleaks after EVAR. Eur J Vasc Endovasc Surg 32:361–365

12. van der Laan MJ, Bakker CJ, Blankensteijn JD, Bartels LW (2006) Dynamic CE-MRA for endoleak classification after endovascular aneurysm repair. Eur J Vasc Endovasc Surg 31:130–135

13. Lookstein RA, Goldman J, Pukin L, Marin ML (2004) Time-resolved magnetic resonance angiography as a noninvasive method to characterize endoleaks: initial results compared with conventional angiography. J Vasc Surg 39:27–33

14. Hartmann M, Wiethoff AJ, Hentrich HR, Rohrer M (2006) Initial imaging recommendations for Vasovist angiography. Eur Radiol 16 [Suppl 2]:B15–B23

15. Rohrer M, Bauer H, Mintorovitch J, Requardt M, Weinmann HJ (2005) Comparison of magnetic properties of MRI contrast media solutions at different magnetic field strengths. Invest Radiol 40:715–724

16. Ersoy H, Jacobs P, Kent CK, Prince MR (2004) Blood pool MR angiography of aortic stent-graft endoleak. AJR Am J Roentgenol 182:1181–1186

17. Cornelissen SA, Verhagen HJ, Prokop M, Moll FL, Bartels LW (2008) Visualizing type IV endoleak using magnetic resonance imaging with a blood pool contrast agent. J Vasc Surg 47:861–4

Gastrointestinal Bleeding

Joachim Lotz

Nuclear scans and angiography have their role in the detection of occult and obscure bleeding as a second-line modality. Usually this occurs in the setting of negative endoscopic evaluation of the colon and upper GI tract.

With massive bleeding angiography may be of advantage to rapidly diagnose and treat the origin of bleeding. This is true especially in altered anatomy due to extensive surgical procedures, where colonoscopy is difficult to perform. MSCT and MRI can be used for local and systemic staging and as a preparation for angiographic or surgical interventions [19].

13.5 Small Intestine

The diagnostic workup of bleeding originating from the small intestine is limited by the length and tortuosity of this part of the GI tract. Prior to the advent of capsule endoscopy, pathologies of the small intestine were the most challenging of all parts of the GI tract, usually requiring more than three different imaging modalities for sufficient diagnosis [1].

Conventional endoscopic equipment is limited to the exploration of the upper GI tract, including in some instances the duodenum up to the ligament of Treitz and up to the ileojejunal junction in a retrograde approach. Some technical variants of endoscopy have been introduced recently, the most promising being double-balloon endoscopy [20]. With this technique it is possible to evaluate the whole small intestine, usually in a combined antegrade (through the upper GI-tract) and retrograde (through the colon) approach. Even if performed by an experienced user, double-balloon endoscopy takes about 1.5–2 h to complete and requires patient immobilization and thorough patient preparation. Double-balloon endoscopes have an additional working channel for interventions. In a multimember approach, the diagnostic yield of double-balloon enteroscopy in LGIB was 52%. Examination-related morbidity tends to be around 1%. Failure to intubate the entire length of the small intestine occurs in about 31% of cases if a rectal approach is used [21].

Capsule endoscopy is a recent development that allows an endoluminal diagnosis of pathologies of the small intestine. Capsule endoscopy is an ambulatory procedure. Patients are asked to fast for 6 h prior to the examination. The capsule is swallowed by the patient and travels down the GI tract via natural peristalsis. During its passage through the GI tract a built-in camera takes a picture every 2 s for approximately 8 h (◘ Fig. 13.2). The images are transmitted wireless to a recorder attached to the patient's waist. Battery life usually suffices for the coverage of the small intestine. Most patients excrete the capsule naturally within 24–48 h. The sensitivity and specificity to

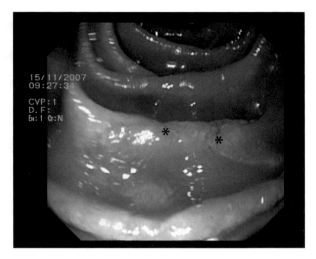

◘ **Fig. 13.2.** Image taken from a series of approximately 50 000 images acquired during a capsule endoscopy for obscure LGIB. Small mucosal changes are seen (*) that were judged responsible for bleeding. No further therapy was initiated

detect the sources of occult or obscure bleeding have been reported to be about 89% and 95%, respectively [22], with a diagnostic yield of 92% in another study [23]. There have been initial reports of 20% failure to reach the colon during reporting time [22]. Diagnostic accuracy is limited by food debris, fluid collections, and a limited field-of-view of 140° of the built-in optics. The most important complication of this technique is capsule entrapment in an unsuspected stenosis of the small bowl, in which case the capsule has to be retrieved by endoscopy or surgery. The incidence of this complication for the whole GI tract is about 0.75–5% [24]. If stenotic lesions are anticipated, a radiopaque dummy capsule can be used in advance that dissolves naturally within 2 days in the GI tract.

Capsule endoscopy is the primary diagnostic modality for obscure intestinal bleeding in the hemodynamically stable patient following initial upper and lower endoscopy. It is usually followed by an endoscopic examination if a target lesion has been identified and judged amendable to endoscopic therapy. Capsule endoscopy followed by double-balloon endoscopy seems to be the most promising diagnostic workup of obscure GI bleeding localized to the small intestine [25].

Scintigraphy was the mainstay of diagnosis for LGIB after negative upper and lower endoscopy until the introduction of capsule endoscopy. Active or intermittent active bleeding is necessary for the scan to yield diagnostic information. A blood sample is taken from the patient, the erythrocytes are labelled with 99m technetium, and 20 ml is reinjected into a peripheral vein. An abdominal 2D plane scan is done. Usually images are taken every 3 s for the first minute, every 5 min for the next 45 min, and then every 15–60 min depending on the clinical setting.

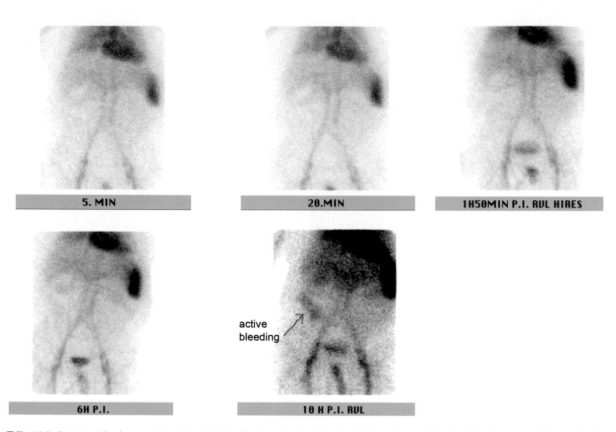

Fig. 13.3. Patient with obscure intermittent GI bleeding localized to the small intestine by upper and lower endoscopy. History of endoscopic cholecystectomy 2 weeks prior to the examination. 99m Tc Scintigraphy with labeled erythrocytes. Early scans are negative for bleeding. Eighteen hours following injection, an activity pooling is detectable in the upper right quadrant of the abdomen indicating active bleeding (*red arrow*). Patient was transferred to angiography for selective coil embolization

Table 13.2. Minimal bleeding rate detectable by different diagnostic modalities. No data are published for MRI, but it is estimated to be within the same range as CT with intravenous contrast. (rbc 99mTc: 99m Technetium-labeled erythrocytes)

Modality	Minimal bleeding rate
Angiography intra-arterial unselective	6 ml/min
Angiography i.a. selective	0.5 ml/min
Scintigraphy rbc 99m Tc	<0.1 ml/min
CT intra-arterial contrast	0.2 ml/min
CT intravenous contrast	6 ml/min
MRI	n/a

Activity accumulates in regions of intestinal bleeding, giving indirect clues about the site – but not the cause – of bleeding (**Fig. 13.3**). Additional tomographic scans (SPECT) can further improve the localization of a bleeding source. Scintigraphic scans are the most sensitive imaging technique for the detection of active bleeding (**Table 13.2**), with a diagnostic yield between 15% and 70% depending on the quantity and activity of bleeding [26]. The yield seems to be higher when an immediate pooling of activity is seen than when late pooling is present [27]. However, when definitive lesions are verified by other diagnostic modalities, the accuracy of a positive scan for lesion localization may be as low as 41% [28, 29]. Radionuclide scintigraphy still has its indication for obscure intermittent bleeding if endoscopy and other imaging modalities fail to localize a bleeding source.

Digital subtraction angiography (DSA) has frequently been used for obscure LGIB of the small intestine to detect and – if found – to embolize pathological vascular structures in the mesenteric territory. Angiography successfully detects pathologies with a rate of bleeding above 0.5 ml/min. Selective probing of the celiac trunk and the superior and inferior mesenteric artery is necessary. If the bleeding cannot be visualized, super-selective angiography of the different vascular territories must be done, focusing the efforts on the clinically most suspected areas. If the bleeding is not detectable on a super-selective angiogram, either the relevant vessel has not been catheterized or the rate of bleeding is too low to be detected. Sensitivity and specificity for super-selective angiography have been

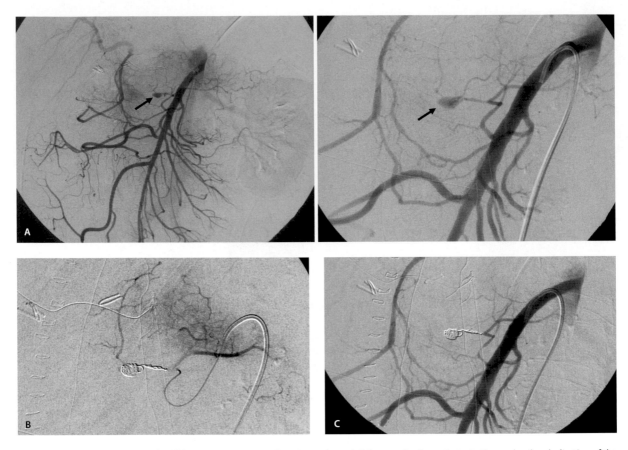

Fig. 13.4A–C. Digital angiography of the same patient as in Fig. 13.3. **A** Selective angiography of the superior mesenteric artery (SMA) depicts false aneurysm of a side branch of the middle colic artery (*arrow*). **B** Super-selective catheterization and coil embolization of the aneurysm. **C** Control series with the catheter placed in the SMA with successful embolization of the aneurysm

described as 89% and 100%, respectively, in the setting of occult bleeding [30]. Angiography remains important as a second-line modality when endoscopy, cross-sectional imaging modalities, and scintigraphy have failed to localize the site of bleeding. It is the next therapeutic modality for lesions identified but not amendable by endoscopy (Fig. 13.4). Variations such as arterial CT angiography have been used to improve sensitivity but have been replaced by and large by either capsule endoscopy or high-resolution MSCT or MRI.

Multiphase helical CT and MSCT have been described as useful in the detection of bleeding sources in the small intestine with or without the use of small bowel enteroclysis [31, 32]. The high resolution of up to isotropic 0.6 mm and speedy data acquisition qualify MSCT as the modality of choice, especially in the setting of massive active bleeding prior to angiographic or surgical interventions (Fig. 13.5). The minimal bleeding rate detectable by CT has been reported to be approximately 6 ml/min [33] though bleeding rates as low as 0.5 ml/min have been detected in animal models [34]. Various small studies, case reports, and reviews have described successful detection of various pathologies in GI bleeding [31, 32, 34, 35]. In 2003, Ernst et al. [36] published a series of 24 patients with acute bleeding. In this series triphasic helical CT was validated against colonoscopy, push enteroscopy, and surgery. CT accurately detected 15 (79%) of 19 bleeding sources. Filippone [35] recently published a review on a series of 32 patients with obscure GI bleeding using 4-slice MSCT and nasoduodenal tube enteroclysis in comparison to capsule endoscopy. The combination of capsule endoscopy and MSCT enteroclysis was able to detect a definitive cause of bleeding in 23 of the 32 patients, or an overall diagnostic yield of 72% as confirmed by surgery. In 16 of 23 patients, findings in both imaging modalities were consistent. In five of 23 patients capsule endoscopy depicted pathologies not seen on MSCT, whereas in two of 23 patients MSCT was able to detect neoplastic lesions not identified by capsule endoscopy. Pathologies not seen in the MSCT enteroclysis were mostly superficial mucosal lesions. This review is remarkable, as it gives MSCT a higher priority in the diagnostic pathway of overt obscure bleeding than capsule endoscopy in the evaluation of active obscure GI bleeding.

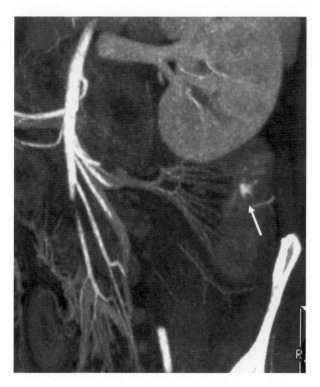

Fig. 13.5. MSCT of the abdomen in the evaluation of an intermittent obscure LGIB. Maximum intensity projection in coronal plane depicts active bleeding from angiodysplasia of the jejunum. Pathology was confirmed by endoscopy

Based on only a small number of cases, this review points to the potential of MSCT enteroclysis as an important first-line modality for the evaluation of obscure GI bleeding.

13.6   GI Bleeding and MRI

Magnetic resonance imaging (MRI) has not been a key modality in the diagnosis of GI bleeding irrespective of its source and location. There was a proof of concept for MRI in GI bleeding by Hilfiker in 1999 [37], and some case reports have been published on successful imaging of duodenal angiodysplasia [38] and varices in the ascending colon [39]. New techniques of 3D GRE imaging (VIBE, Thrive, LAVA) have been introduced since these reports that allow for reliable and high-resolution T1 imaging of the abdomen, usually within one breath hold. As has been shown in MSCT imaging, MRI enteroclysis is suited for the detection of intestinal tumors and inflammatory changes that might lead to GI bleeding, especially due to its lack of radiation and superior extramucosal contrast as compared with MSCT [40, 41].

Initial trials with high-resolution abdominal imaging using modified MRA sequences or inversion-recovery sequences similar to the 'late enhancement' sequences used for imaging of myocardial infarctions have been proposed for the detection of subtle vascular changes or subtle amounts of blood extravasation into the intestine. Though promising larger validation studies using these new imaging approaches with MRI have not yet been published, initial reports are promising.

As with MSCT, the diagnostic capabilities of MRI employing the latest imaging techniques have not yet been adequately evaluated for their role in the diagnostic workup of GI bleeding. Both modalities are underestimated in their diagnostic yield in this specific area and each institution will have to decide based on its local setting whether MRI or MSCT will be its primary cross-sectional modality for the diagnosis of GI bleeding.

13.7   Blood pool Contrast Agents

With the introduction of blood pool contrast agents, MRI has the potential to combine the solely morphological imaging of MSCT with the more functional imaging of scintigraphy. The high relaxivity of blood pool contrast agents such as Vasovist® (Gadofosveset, Bayer Schering Pharma AG, Berlin, Germany) is the basis for a high-resolution dynamic imaging that provides detailed morphological information about the vascular territory of the abdomen. Pathological vascular structures and active bleeding sites might be identified in these initial data sets, as has been shown with extracellular contrast agents [38]. The extended intravascular retention time unique to blood pool contrast agents can then be used to perform repeated scans over as long as 24 h. Similar to scintigraphy, these repeated scans help to detect extravascular contrast pooling as an indicator of extravasation of blood. This approach is most promising to localize the source of intermittent active bleeding to a specific part of the intestine. Repetitive scans might also provide evidence that an abnormal structure is the source of bleeding. This has been shown for intermittent bleeding from a gluteal aneurysm (Lotz, submitted).

The need for repetitive scans is a drawback to this approach, similar to scintigraphic scans. However, as the intestinal blood deposits are propelled by natural peristalsis, the exact timing of the scans is crucial to reliably define the source of bleeding. After initial dynamic images are acquired, we prefer to repeat coronal imaging every 60 min for 6 h and additional scans 12 h and 18–24 h after initial contrast administration (□ Table 13.3). Protocols and image characteristics are the same for 1.5- and 3-T systems once sequence parameters have been adapted to the longer T1 relaxation time in the 3-T environment. Artifacts from air within the intestine tend to be more relevant in a 3-T environment [42]. A bowel preparation

□ Table 13.3. Experimental protocol for diagnosis of intermittent obscure GI bleeding with MRI and Vasovist®. Whole abdomen is imaged with surface coils. Parallel imaging should be used if available to minimize acquisition times. Sequences are optimized for each system to be done in suspended respiration

Time	Sequences
12 h prior to scan	Small and large bowel preparation, same as for endoscopy: 4 l of fluid within 12 h Patients are to eat clear soup, no solid food for 12 h prior to and during the examination.

0	Butylscopolamin 20 mg*
	1. Transversal GRE T1
	2. Transversal GRE T1; fat suppression
	3. Transversal TSE T2; fat suppression
	4. Dynamic 3D GRE T1 coronal, fat suppression
	   a: w/o contrast
	   b: arterial phase
	   c: portalvenous phase (60 s p.i.)
	   d: venous phase (5 min p.i.)

20 min; 60 min; every 1 h for 6 h; Late scan after 12 h Late scan after 18–24 h	Butylscopolamin* 20 mg 1. Coronal 3D GRE T1; fat suppression 2. Transversal 3D GRE T1; fat suppression

p.i. post injection of contrast medium
*Butylscopolamin: be aware of possible contraindications and maximal dosage within 24 h

is crucial to avoid overlap with T1 hyperintense intestinal contents and to reduce the amount of air in the small intestine. We apply the same regimen for bowel preparation as is done for small-bowel endoscopy. Enteroclysis might be used in the initial scan, though its effect will not last for the duration of the whole exam of 12 h and more. During the time of examination patients should avoid solid food as well as any food or liquid that might interfere with the T1 hyperintense signal of Vasovist®. Intravenous butylscopolamin is mandatory to reduce artifacts from bowel movement and to achieve higher image quality. Patients are imaged in a supine position, although prone positioning might improve image quality if patients are able to cooperate. Extravasation of blood is seen as a hyperintense signal within the intestine not seen in the initial scans (□ Fig. 13.6).

There are no valid data on the sensitivity and specificity of this MRI approach to detect and localize GI bleeding, and no reliable information is available about the minimal bleeding rate detectable with this technique. These data will have to be derived from forthcoming studies.

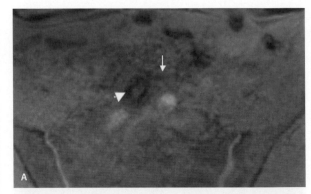

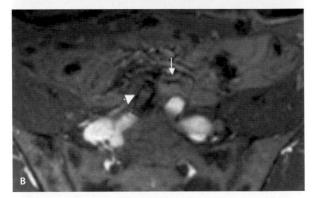

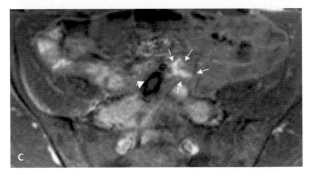

□ Fig. 13.6A–C. MRI done in a patient with obscure massive intermittent LGIB caused by an aortoileal fistula. Contrast extravasation to an ileal loop is seen 6 h after initial application of 10 ml Vasovist® (*arrows*). Origin of bleeding was defined to be at the upper end of a stent placed at the aortic bifurcation into the right common iliac artery (*arrowhead*)

13.8   Summary

The diagnostic approach to GI bleeding depends on its suspected location and the intensity of bleeding. The ability to combine primary diagnosis with the option of local treatment has made endoscopic techniques the first-line diagnostic tool in the workup of GI bleeding. These include classic push endoscopy as well as double-balloon endoscopy and colonoscopy. Capsule endoscopy has emerged as a valuable modality for obscure bleeding from the small intestine.

Cross-sectional imaging modalities are an important second option, if endoscopic techniques alone are not diagnostic or an extraintestinal pathology is suspected to be the primary cause of bleeding. Scintigraphy is well-established for intermittent obscure bleeding, although additional cross-sectional imaging usually is employed to better characterize the causative lesion found on the radionuclide scans. Angiography nowadays is usually performed with the aim of treatment. Diagnostic angiography is the last resort if all other imaging modalities cannot identify the underlying pathology in serious GI bleeding. Intraoperative endoscopy has the highest diagnostic yield of all modalities but is restricted to patients with serious blood loss from obscure bleeding sites.

In abdominal imaging, MRI has been inferior to MSCT in terms of speed of data acquisition and spatial resolution. MSCT is the modality of choice for the diagnostic evaluation of massive acute bleeding within the small intestine in unstable patients. Recent 3D GRE sequences optimized for abdominal imaging have made MRI an alternative to MSCT in case of stable intermittent bleeding not amendable by endoscopy. The combination of MRI with blood pool contrast agents promises to broaden the indications for MRI in GI bleeding. Though it still has to be proven in adequate studies, MRI in combination with Vasovist® has the potential to combine the high-resolution morphological imaging of traditional MRI with the functional information usually derived from scintigraphy about the origin and activity of bleeding.

Take home messages

- Endoscopic techniques including capsule endoscopy are the primary imaging tools for GI bleeding.
- Cross-sectional imaging modalities are second-line options if endoscopy is inconclusive.
- Up to now MRI has not been the preferred imaging modality for the diagnostic workup of GI bleeding.
- MRI with blood pool contrast agents promises to close the gap between morphological imaging

and functional information usually derived from scintigraphy.
- The main benefit of MRI in GI bleeding, therefore, might be in the workup of intermittent obscure bleeding.
- Further studies are needed to provide evidence of efficiency and reliability of MRI in the diagnosis of GI bleeding.

References

1. Prakash C, Zuckerman GR (2003) Acute small bowel bleeding: a distinct entity with significantly different economic implications compared with GI bleeding from other locations. Gastrointest Endosc 58:330–335
2. Rubin TA, Murdoch M, Nelson DB (2003) Acute GI bleeding in the setting of supratherapeutic international normalized ratio in patients taking warfarin: endoscopic diagnosis, clinical management, and outcomes. Gastrointest Endosc 58:369–373
3. Peura DA, Lanza FL, Gostout CJ, Foutch PG (1997) The American College of Gastroenterology Bleeding Registry: preliminary findings. Am J Gastroenterol 92:924–928
4. Velayos FS, Williamson A, Sousa KH, et al (2004) Early predictors of severe lower gastrointestinal bleeding and adverse outcomes: a prospective study. Clin Gastroenterol Hepatol 2:485–490
5. van Leerdam ME, Vreeburg EM, Rauws EA, et al (2003) Acute upper GI bleeding: did anything change? Time trend analysis of incidence and outcome of acute upper GI bleeding between 1993/1994 and 2000. Am J Gastroenterol 98:1494–1499
6. Vreeburg EM, Snel P, de Bruijne JW, Bartelsman JF, Rauws EA, Tytgat GN (1997) Acute upper gastrointestinal bleeding in the Amsterdam area: incidence, diagnosis, and clinical outcome. Am J Gastroenterol 92:236–243
7. Longstreth GF (1995) Epidemiology of hospitalization for acute upper gastrointestinal hemorrhage: a population-based study. Am J Gastroenterol 90:206–210
8. Longstreth GF (1997) Epidemiology and outcome of patients hospitalized with acute lower gastrointestinal hemorrhage: a population-based study. Am J Gastroenterol 92:419–424
9. Boonpongmanee S, Fleischer DE, Pezzullo JC, et al (2004) The frequency of peptic ulcer as a cause of upper-GI bleeding is exaggerated. Gastrointest Endosc 59:788–794
10. Strate L (2005) Lower GI bleeding: epidemiology and diagnosis. Gastroenterol Clin North Am 34:643–664
11. Segal WN, Cello JP (1997) Hemorrhage in the upper gastrointestinal tract in the older patient. Am J Gastroenterol 92:42–46
12. Palmer K (2004) Management of haematemesis and melaena. Postgrad Med J 80:399–404
13. Landi B, Tkoub M, Gaudric M, et al (1998) Diagnostic yield of push-type enteroscopy in relation to indication. Gut 42:421–425
14. Lewis BS (1999) The history of enteroscopy. Gastrointest Endosc Clin N Am 9:1–11
15. Jensen DM, Kovacs TO, Jutabha R, et al (2002) Randomized trial of medical or endoscopic therapy to prevent recurrent ulcer hemorrhage in patients with adherent clots. Gastroenterology 123:407–413
16. Laine L, Peterson WL (1994) Bleeding peptic ulcer. N Engl J Med 331:717–727
17. Zuckerman GR, Prakash C (1998) Acute lower intestinal bleeding. I: Clinical presentation and diagnosis. Gastrointest Endosc 48:606–617
18. Schuetz A, Jauch KW (2001) Lower gastrointestinal bleeding: therapeutic strategies, surgical techniques and results. Langenbecks Arch Surg 386:17–25

19. Lee EW, Laberge JM (2004) Differential diagnosis of gastrointestinal bleeding. Tech Vasc Intervent Radiol 7:112–122

20. Yamamoto H, Sugano K (2003) A new method of enteroscopy – the double-balloon method. Can J Gastroenterol 17:273–274

21. Mehdizadeh S, Ross A, Gerson L, et al (2006) What is the learning curve associated with double-balloon enteroscopy? Technical details and early experience in 6 U.S. tertiary care centers. Gastrointest Endosc 64:740–750

22. Pennazio M, Santucci R, Rondonotti E, et al (2004) Outcome of patients with obscure gastrointestinal bleeding after capsule endoscopy: report of 100 consecutive cases. Gastroenterology 126:643–653

23. Apostolopoulos P, Liatsos C, Gralnek IM, et al (2007) Evaluation of capsule endoscopy in active, mild-to-moderate, overt, obscure GI bleeding. Gastrointest Endosc 66:1174–1181

24. Pennazio M (2004) Small-bowel endoscopy. Endoscopy 36:32–41

25. Rondonotti E, Villa F, Mulder CJ, Jacobs MA, de Franchis R (2007) Small bowel capsule endoscopy in 2007: indications, risks and limitations. World J Gastroenterol 13:6140–6149

26. Howarth DM, Tang K, Lees W (2002) The clinical utility of nuclear medicine imaging for the detection of occult gastrointestinal haemorrhage. Nucl Med Commun 23:591–594

27. Ng DA, Opelka FG, Beck DE, et al (1997) Predictive value of technetium Tc 99m-labeled red blood cell scintigraphy for positive angiogram in massive lower gastrointestinal hemorrhage. Dis Colon Rectum 40:471–477

28. Hunter JM, Pezim ME (1990) Limited value of technetium 99m-labeled red cell scintigraphy in localization of lower gastrointestinal bleeding. Am J Surg 159:504–506

29. Chamberlain SA, Soybel DI (2000) Occult and obscure sources of gastrointestinal bleeding. Curr Probl Surg 37:861–916

30. Vernava AM, 3rd, Moore BA, Longo WE, Johnson FE (1997) Lower gastrointestinal bleeding. Dis Colon Rectum 40:846–858

31. Jain TP, Gulati MS, Makharia GK, Bandhu S, Garg PK (2007) CT enteroclysis in the diagnosis of obscure gastrointestinal bleeding: initial results. Clin Radiol 62:660–667

32. Paulsen SR, Huprich JE, Hara AK (2007) CT enterography: noninvasive evaluation of Crohn's disease and obscure gastrointestinal bleed. Radiol Clin North Am 45:303–315

33. Ettorre GC, Francioso G, Garribba AP, Fracella MR, Greco A, Farchi G (1997) Helical CT angiography in gastrointestinal bleeding of obscure origin. AJR Am J Roentgenol 168:727–731

34. Kuhle WG, Sheiman RG (2003) Detection of active colonic hemorrhage with use of helical CT: findings in a swine model. Radiology 228:743–752

35. Filippone A, Cianci R, Milano A, Valeriano S, Di Mizio V, Storto ML (2007) Obscure gastrointestinal bleeding and small bowel pathology: comparison between wireless capsule endoscopy and multidetector-row CT enteroclysis. Abdom Imaging

36. Ernst O, Bulois P, Saint-Drenant S, Leroy C, Paris JC, Sergent G (2003) Helical CT in acute lower gastrointestinal bleeding. Eur Radiol 13:114–117

37. Hilfiker PR, Weishaupt D, Kacl GM, et al (1999) Comparison of three dimensional magnetic resonance imaging in conjunction with a blood pool contrast agent and nuclear scintigraphy for the detection of experimentally induced gastrointestinal bleeding. Gut 45:581–587

38. Erden A, Bozkaya H, Turkmen Soygur I, Bektas M, Erden I (2004) Duodenal angiodysplasia: MR angiographic evaluation. Abdom Imaging 29:12–14

39. Chevallier P, Motamedi JP, Demuth N, Caroli-Bosc FX, Oddo F, Padovani B (2000) Ascending colonic variceal bleeding: utility of phase-contrast MR portography in diagnosis and follow-up after treatment with TIPS and variceal embolization. Eur Radiol 10:1280–1283

40. Fidler J (2007) MR imaging of the small bowel. Radiol Clin North Am 45:317–331

41. Ryan ER, Heaslip IS (2008) Magnetic resonance enteroclysis compared with conventional enteroclysis and computed tomography enteroclysis: a critically appraised topic. Abdom Imaging 33:34–37

42. Barth MM, Smith MP, Pedrosa I, Lenkinski RE, Rofsky NM (2007) Body MR imaging at 3.0 T: understanding the opportunities and challenges. Radiographics 27:1445–1462; discussion 1462–1444

43. Esrailian E, Gralnek IM (2005) Nonvariceal upper gastrointestinal bleeding: epidemiology and diagnosis. Gastroenterol Clin North Am 34:589–605

44. Schmulewitz N, Fisher DA, Rockey DC (2003) Early colonoscopy for acute lower GI bleeding predicts shorter hospital stay: a retrospective study of experience in a single center. Gastrointest Endosc 58:841–846

45. Strate LL, Syngal S (2003) Timing of colonoscopy: impact on length of hospital stay in patients with acute lower intestinal bleeding. Am J Gastroenterol 98:317–322

46. Ohyama T, Sakurai Y, Ito M, Daito K, Sezai S, Sato Y (2000) Analysis of urgent colonoscopy for lower gastrointestinal tract bleeding. Digestion 61:189–192

47. Mujica VR, Barkin JS (1996) Occult gastrointestinal bleeding. General overview and approach. Gastrointest Endosc Clin North Am 6:833–845

Part IV New Horizons in Vascular Diagnostics

Vasovist® for Imaging Ischemic and Congenital Heart Disease

Sebastian Kelle, Gerald Greil, Reza Razavi, and Eike Nagel

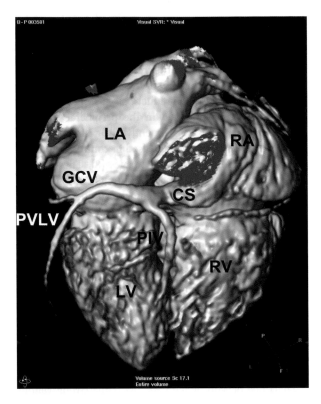

Fig. 14.3. Vasovist® enhanced 3D reconstruction of the heart. *LA* left atrium; *RA* right atrium; *LV* left ventricle; *RV* right ventricle. The presence of the following veins at the crux cordis is demonstrated: *CS* coronary sinus; *PIV* posterior interventricular vein; *GCV* = great cardiac vein; *PVLV* = posterior vein of the left ventricle. (Courtesy of Dr. Amedeo Chiribiri)

tients it can be difficult to access the cardiac veins with the guidewire. In these cases it helps to have detailed information on the venous anatomy including side branches available.

In a first study we demonstrated the capability of CMR to depict the complex anatomy of the venous system of the heart in vivo through the combined use of 3D whole-heart imaging and the injection of blood pool contrast agents (16 volunteers and seven patients (Gadofosveset and Gadomer-17) [21]. We used the whole-heart approach to cover a three-dimensional volume. This imaging technique was described formerly for the visualization of the whole coronary artery tree [22]. The strong venous enhancement with BPCA allowed us to visualize the coronary veins from 2–10 min up to 2 h post injection (Fig. 14.3).

Thus, CMR may be proposed as the method of choice for the evaluation of patients who are candidates for cardiac resynchronization therapy and LV lead positioning, not only as a method to identify scar tissue, as proposed by van de Veire [23], but as a method capable of simultaneously evaluating the presence of scar, the LV function and viability in combination with identifying a suitable

cardiac vein for LV lead placement, thus helping to optimize the implantation strategy [21].

14.4 Detection of Myocardial Perfusion Defects with Vasovist®

The wash-in kinetics and the local T1/T2 shortening in the myocardial tissue depend on the concentration of the contrast agent, the flow rate, diffusion of the contrast agent into the interstitial tissue, relative tissue volume fractions, contrast bolus duration, and recirculation effects [24]. For perfusion imaging, intravascular contrast agents differ from conventional agents in several ways. (a) The quantification of blood volume may be possible from T1 values. (b) Due to the small distribution volume (only 5–10% of the myocardial volume consists of blood) [25] intravascular contrast agents result in a lower contrast effect, which may reduce their efficacy for perfusion imaging. (c) The higher relaxivity of intravascular versus extracellular contrast agents may compensate for the smaller distribution volume [26]. (d) In addition, there is a potential for full quantification with minimal reliance on complex models, since the diffusion component of the contrast agent is smaller than that of conventional agents. However, since a small fraction of Vasovist® still diffuses into the interstitium, quantification will be more complex than with truly intravascular macromolecules such as gadomer-17 or gadomelitol.

Several animal studies have shown that the detection of perfusion defects during vasodilatation is feasible with intravascular contrast agents [3, 27–29]. The first study to detect myocardial perfusion defects with Vasovist® first pass stress-induced (dipyridamol) perfusion was compared with SPECT in an animal model of coronary artery stenosis. The authors reported a prolonged hypointense signal and lower peak signal intensity in ischemic myocardium during stress. An MRI defect, classified as 75% reduction in peak myocardial signal intensity in the affected territory, was detected in 92.3% of the animals. In the presence of mild coronary stenosis, there was uniform enhancement with MRI and tracer uptake by SPECT. The concordance of MRI and SPECT for detecting perfusion defects was 85%. In addition, three animals with myocardial infarction (i.e., triphenyltetrazolium chloride [TTC] non-staining regions by postmortem analysis) had hypoenhancing lesions on MR images. Only two of these three animals with myocardial infarction also had perfusion defects in SPECT images [30].

In a different study by Jerosch-Herold et al. in pigs, Vasovist® was used to determine the relation between the rate of myocardial signal enhancement during the first pass (upslope) and myocardial blood flow (MBF) and to derive and validate a corrected perfusion reserve (PR)

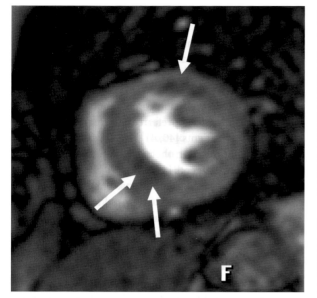

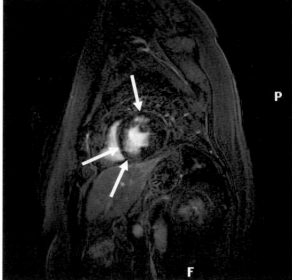

Fig. 14.4. Perfusion MRI using MS-325: equatorial short-axis view. There are clear perfusion defects in the anterior and septal segment (*arrows*)

Fig. 14.5. Short-axis view post injection of MS-325 in a dosage of 0.05 mmol/kg body weight in a patient with chronic myocardial infarction demonstrated delayed enhancement in the anterior and septal segment (*arrows*)

index from the upslope parameter. This was done with an intravascular BPCA, because the characteristic time for the vascular transit cannot be determined as easily for an extracellular tracer as for an intravascular tracer [31].

First applications of Vasovist® in patients with chronic myocardial infarctions have shown promising results for first pass perfusion imaging. The capability to detect chronic myocardial infarction with a combination of dynamic perfusion at rest and delayed enhancement was demonstrated (**Fig. 14.4**). In a direct comparison, a larger number of infarcted segments showed perfusion defects with Vasovist® than with the extracellular contrast agent [32].

14.5 Late Gadolinium Enhancement

There are only few reports about delayed enhancement with BPCA. In an animal study in pigs using a combined protocol for myocardial perfusion and viability with P792 (Vistarem®, Guerbet Group, Paris, France) in comparison to an extracellular contrast agent in a non-reperfused infarction model, Peukert and co-workers reported that the BPCA allowed evaluation of myocardial viability [33]. From a pig study, Saeed et al. reported a similar visualization of acute myocardial infarction with both intravascular and extracellular contrast. However, chronic infarctions enhanced only with the extracellular but not the intravascular agents [34]. In coronary occlusion and coro-

nary stenosis, intravascular MR contrast agents provide longer delineation of the area at risk than extracellular agents [35]. In small-animal models, intravascular agents were shown to be more suitable than extracellular agents for the prolonged delineation of no-reflow zones and for defining small (few pixels) microvascular obstruction areas. Thus, BPCAs may be useful for delineating microembolization in human beings. Furthermore, these agents have been used to demonstrate the progressive growth in the size of the no-reflow zone in mild, moderate, and severe myocardial injury [36] and the effect of the duration of reperfusion on the size of the no-reflow zone (up to 24 h following reperfusion) [37].

In an animal study with pigs it was demonstrated that Vasovist® provided a robust visualization of acute myocardial infarction over a time-period of at least 2 h without the need to change the inversion recovery time [38]. Our group showed that Vasovist® allows for a detection of chronic myocardial infarction in patients (**Fig. 14.5**). However, in a direct comparison to extracellular contrast agent, the transmurality of the scar and the number of scarred left ventricular segments were smaller with Vasovist® [32]. This is most likely due to a slower diffusion of the contrast agent because of its albumin binding. However, the unbound fraction should behave similar to conventional contrast agents. Potentially, one could wait much longer (on the order of hours) to allow sufficient time for the contrast agent to diffuse. However, no data on this question are currently available.

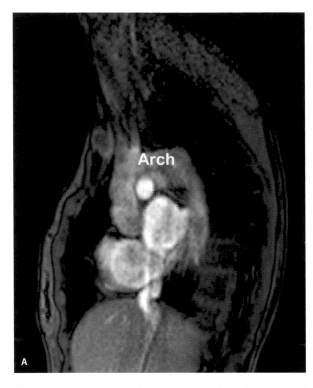

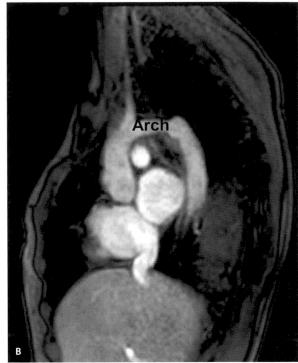

□ **Fig. 14.8A,B.** The magnitude images of in-plane phase-encoded images of the previously shown 22-year-old patient following i.v. administration of Magnevist® (**A**) and Vasovist® (**B**). Signal and contrast are more homogeneous after administration of Vasovist® compared with Magnevist®. *Arch* narrowed aortic arch after repair of coarctation of the aorta

First promising clinical applications in these patients have been performed [60, 61]. Even though through-plane phase-contrast imaging does not seem to benefit from contrast agents, our preliminary experience shows increased in-plane signal in phase-contrast imaging (□ Fig. 14.8).

In summary, Vasovist® would allow a standardized and comprehensive imaging protocol in patients with acquired and congenital heart disease. After a single injection of Vasovist® a first pass high temporal resolution sequence would allow assessment of different enhancement kinetics of the arterial and venous vascular systems. An SSFP (1.5-T) or gradient echo (3-T) sequence with an inversion recovery prepulse and navigator gating for prospective slice correction to compensate for respiratory motion, in combination with ECG triggering, would then be added. This would provide high spatial resolution images with high SNR and CNR values of intra- and extracardiac vascular structures. Qualitative and quantitative functional information of the ventricles will be obtained using 3D time-resolved high-resolution imaging of the heart and vessels. Multidimensional phase-contrast imaging will provide important qualitative and quantitative flow information of the heart and vessels.

14.7   Conclusion

Vasovist® provides advantages in enhanced depiction of blood vessels as well as intracardiac structures, due to greater relaxivity and shortening of the intravascular T_1 than extracellular contrast agents. It offers the possibility to minimize background signal, as the T_1 changes remain confined mainly to the intraluminal spaces. Vasovist® seems to be effective in dynamic and steady state MR angiography. Further future applications may be established with contrast-enhanced angiography in the 3-T environment using gradient echo sequences. Also in reduced data acquisition methods the increased intraluminal contrast can be used for shortening of acquisition time for quantitative evaluation of cardiac volumes and function. Its usefulness for assessing myocardial perfusion, microvascular permeability, and viability has been shown in preliminary small studies and animal experiments. However, its true value remains to be assessed. Vasovist® may further allow the design of highly standardized and reproducible MRI examination protocols in patients with acquired and congenital heart disease. This is of particular importance, as these patients require regular follow-up examinations throughout their life.

14

Take home messages

- Vasovist® allows enhanced depiction of blood vessels and intracardiac structures due to greater relaxivity and shortening of the intravascular T1 than extracellular contrast agents. It offers the possibility to minimize background signal, as the T1 changes remain confined mainly to the intraluminal spaces.
- Vasovist® seems to be effective in dynamic and steady state MR angiography at 1.5 T. Further future applications may be established with contrast-enhanced angiography in the 3-T environment using gradient echo sequences.
- The increased intraluminal contrast can be used for reduced data acquisition methods to shorten acquisition times at 1.5 T and 3 T.

- Its usefulness for assessing myocardial perfusion, microvascular permeability, and viability has been shown in preliminary small studies and animal experiments. Larger clinical trials are needed for further evaluation.
- The previously shown advantages of Vasovist® allow the design of highly standardized and reproducible MRI examination protocols in patients with acquired and congenital heart disease. This is of particular importance, as these patients require regular follow-up examinations throughout their life.

References

1. Pennell DJ, et al (2004) Clinical indications for cardiovascular magnetic resonance (CMR): Consensus Panel report. Eur Heart J 25:1940–1965
2. Hendel RC, et al (2006) ACCF/ACR/SCCT/SCMR/ASNC/NASCI/SCAI/SIR 2006 appropriateness criteria for cardiac computed tomography and cardiac magnetic resonance imaging: a report of the American College of Cardiology Foundation Quality Strategic Directions Committee Appropriateness Criteria Working Group, American College of Radiology, Society of Cardiovascular Computed Tomography, Society for Cardiovascular Magnetic Resonance, American Society of Nuclear Cardiology, North American Society for Cardiac Imaging, Society for Cardiovascular Angiography and Interventions, and Society of Interventional Radiology. J Am Coll Cardiol 48:1475–1497
3. Kroft LJ, de Roos A (1999) Blood pool contrast agents for cardiovascular MR imaging. J Magn Reson Imaging 10:395–403
4. Herborn CU, et al (2003) Coronary arteries: contrast-enhanced MR imaging with SH L 643A – experience in 12 volunteers. Radiology 229:217–223
5. Herborn CU, et al (2004) 2MR coronary angiography with SH L 643 A: initial experience in patients with coronary artery disease. Radiology 33:567–573
6. Paetsch I, et al (2004) Improved three-dimensional free-breathing coronary magnetic resonance angiography using gadocoletic acid (B-22956) for intravascular contrast enhancement. J Magn Reson Imaging 20:288–293
7. Paetsch I, et al (2006) Detection of coronary stenoses with contrast enhanced, three-dimensional free breathing coronary MR angiography using the gadolinium-based intravascular contrast agent gadocoletic acid (B-22956). J Cardiovasc Magn Reson 8:509–516
8. Klein C, et al (2003) Improvement of image quality of non-invasive coronary artery imaging with magnetic resonance by the use of the intravascular contrast agent Clariscan (NC100150 injection) in patients with coronary artery disease. J Magn Reson Imaging 17:656–662
9. Kelle S, et al (2007) Whole-heart coronary magnetic resonance angiography with MS-325 (gadofosveset). Med Sci Monit 13:CR469–474
10. Parmelee DJ, et al (1997) Preclinical evaluation of the pharmacokinetics, biodistribution, and elimination of MS-325, a blood pool agent for magnetic resonance imaging. Invest Radiol 32:741–747
11. Lauffer RB, et al (1998) MS-325: albumin-targeted contrast agent for MR angiography. Radiology 207:529–538
12. Bluemke DA, et al (2001) Carotid MR angiography: phase II study of safety and efficacy for MS-325. Radiology 219:114–122
13. Grist TM, et al (1998) Steady state and dynamic MR angiography with MS-325: initial experience in humans. Radiology 207:539–544
14. Mohs AM, Lu ZR (2007) Gadolinium (III)-based blood-pool contrast agents for magnetic resonance imaging: status and clinical potential. Expert Opin Drug Deliv 4:149–164
15. Jahnke C, et al (2004) Coronary MR angiography with steady state free precession: individually adapted breath-hold technique versus free-breathing technique. Radiology 232:669–676
16. Stuber M, et al (1999) Contrast agent-enhanced, free-breathing, three-dimensional coronary magnetic resonance angiography. J Magn Reson Imaging 10:790–799
17. Nassenstein K, et al (2006) MR coronary angiography with MS-325, a blood pool contrast agent: comparison of an inversion recovery steady state free precession with an inversion recovery fast low angle shot sequence in volunteers [in German]. Rofo 178:508–514
18. Nassenstein K, et al (2007) Magnetic resonance coronary angiography with MS-325: in-vivo T1-measurements to improve image quality of navigator and breath-hold techniques. Eur Radiol (Epub ahead of print)
19. Abraham WT, Hayes DL (2003) Cardiac resynchronization therapy for heart failure. Circulation 108:2596–2603
20. Puglisi A, et al (2004) Limited thoracotomy as a second choice alternative to transvenous implant for cardiac resynchronisation therapy delivery. Eur Heart J 25:1063–1069
21. Chiribiri A, et al (2008) Visualization of the cardiac venous system using cardiac magnetic resonance. Am J Cardiol 101:407–412
22. Jahnke C, et al (2005) Rapid and complete coronary arterial tree visualization with magnetic resonance imaging: feasibility and diagnostic performance. Eur Heart J 26:2313–2319
23. Van de Veire NR, et al (2006) Non-invasive visualization of the cardiac venous system in coronary artery disease patients using 64-slice computed tomography. J Am Coll Cardiol 48:1832–1838

15.1   Introduction

Vasovist® (Gadofosveset, Bayer Schering Pharma AG, Berlin, Germany) represents a third generation of contrast agents. It is the first approved MR contrast medium with a pronounced and reversible protein binding, resulting in a long blood half-life. The agent is categorized as an intravascular or blood pool agent and was developed for MR angiographic applications, allowing imaging in a submillimeter resolution range in the equilibrium phase.

There are a growing number of reports about the role of Vasovist® in MR angiography [1–4]. Although several potential alternative applications were investigated, the extravascular behavior of the agent and its potential for imaging tissue pathologies have not yet been systematically explored and reported.

In this chapter we will present the first clinical experience with the extravascular contrast behavior of Vasovist® in patients with brain tumors. All cases presented were seen within exploratory examinations on an off-label basis with written informed consent of the patients.

In order to explain the potential of Vasovist® as an extravasal contrast agent, the specific pharmacodynamics and kinetics of the agent have to be evaluated. Quite different from conventional extracellular MRI-CM, the pharmacokinetics of Vasovist® need to be understood. As described in detail in ► Chap. 1, its pharmacokinetics are characterized not only by a single, dominating elimination half-life time $t_{1/2}$, but rather by an initial (»distribution phase«) half-life time $t_{1/2\alpha}$, followed by a later (»disposition phase«) half-life time $t_{1/2\beta}$. The resulting bi-exponential pharmacokinetics can be easily rationalized by a relatively high local concentration immediately post i.v. injection (first pass), during which the fraction of protein-bound CM molecules increases, depending on the relative local concentrations of human serum albumin and Vasovist® molecules, respectively. During this initial phase, the larger fraction of unbound molecules leads both to a more pronounced extravasation rate and to a more pronounced glomerular filtration rate, compared with the following equilibrium state. Hence, an averaged initial $t_{1/2\alpha}$ is obtained in the order of 0.5 h, not significantly exceeding the $t_{1/2}$ of conventional extracellular MRI-CM [5].

However, after a few circulation cycles of the contrast medium, the contrast agent molecules remaining in the vascular system can be regarded as homogeneously distributed in the entire blood volume and are found in a rather stable equilibrium state, characterized by approximately 85–90% of the molecules in the protein-bound state. Consequently, both rates of extravasation and renal elimination are substantially reduced, but the remaining 10–15% of unbound molecules are still able to extravasate. But even if the agent is bound to serum albumin it might be speculated that the complex is able to extravasate into pathologic tissue if the gap between the vessel wall cells is large enough.

On the second effect, binding affinity to albumin in the extravascular space leads to a significant extension of T1 and T2 relaxivities and hence to changes in MR contrasting. The T1 relaxivity, a measure of the paramagnetic property, is about five times higher (at 1.5 T) compared with the unbound state and with conventional, Gd-chelate-containing contrast agents with a direct effect on the contrast properties. This effect is even higher at lower field strength [6]. This causes a rise in enhancement with a direct influence particularly on the vascular signal in MRA but also on the contrast behavior in tissue.

With respect to the brain the situation is even easier. Because of the presence of the blood-brain barrier (BBB), represented mainly by endothelial tight junctions, all currently available MR contrast media do not leak into the brain tissue. The BBB blocks all molecules except those that cross cell membranes by means of lipid solubility (such as oxygen, carbon dioxide, ethanol, and steroid hormones) and those that are allowed in by specific transport systems (such as sugars and some amino acids). Substances with a molecular weight higher than 180 Daltons (Da), which include all available imaging contrast media, generally cannot cross the BBB [7, 8]. Therefore, the degree of enhancement in CNS neoplasm depends on several factors, including the leakage of the BBB, the intravascular CM concentration and its magnetic properties, the vascularity of the lesion, the blood flow in the vessels supplying the tumor, and the degree of edema, as well as on technical and contrast media-specific parameters, mainly the relaxivity [8, 9].

In intra-axial primary tumors, mainly gliomas, the BBB can be compromised by neovascularization and direct tumor-related damage. Since non-neoplastic astrocytes are required to induce BBB features of cerebral endothelial cells, it is conceivable that malignant astrocytes have lost this ability due to dedifferentiate. Alternatively, glioma cells might actively degrade previously intact BBB tight junctions [10, 11]. In secondary tumors, mainly metastases and extra-axial tumors, the lesion vessels are different from normal cerebral vasculature and have no, or a strongly disturbed, BBB [12, 13].

In both primary and secondary neoplasms, a high albumin concentration has been described in the interstitial space of the pathologic tissue [14, 15]. This theoretically enables the extravasated Vasovist® molecules to bind to albumin in the interstitial space, which substantially increases the relaxivity and consequently the enhancement characteristics of the agent.

In an early rat glioma model, Adzamali et al. [16] first described the use of two different intravascular contrast agents for imaging brain neoplasms. Although the bind-

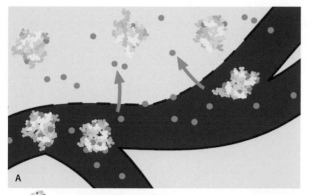

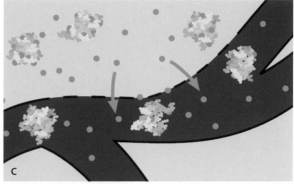

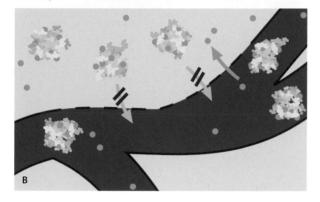

Albumin loaded with Gadofosveset

■ **Fig. 15.1A–C.** Mechanism of parenchymal contrast enhancement with Vasovist®. Early after injection (**A**) the molecules are only partially bound to albumin (approximately 50–75%), which allows for an extravasation of the unbound molecules (*green dots*) into the interstitial space. The bound molecules are not able to pass the disrupted blood brain barrier. In the second parenchymal phase (**B**) the Vasovist® molecules bind to albumin present in high concentration in tumors, which keeps them from redistributing into the intravascular space. Since there is a stable equilibrium between bound (85%) and unbound (15%) molecules, there is a trapping of contrast medium in the interstitial space, causing an increase of enhancement over time. After approximately 12 h the gradient changes toward the redistribution from the interstitium into the vascular compartment (**C**); however, the contrast enhancement can last for more than 24 h

ing capabilities of Vasovist® are different in mice, the authors found a two- to threefold stronger enhancement based on the applied contrast dose. They explained the greater effectiveness of the albumin-bound agents by an increased systemic persistence. While the standard agents used peaked within the first 5 min after administration, the intravascular agents showed a slower kinetics, requiring about 30 min to reach a maximum which then lasted for about 3 h. Despite the species dependence of the biophysical properties of Vasovist®, which indicates strongly reduced protein-binding capabilities in rodents compared with human beings [17], these findings in animal models already suggest a very interesting and promising pharmacokinetic mode of action, which cannot be obtained with conventional extracellular MRI-CM and may have a significant additional diagnostic potential in cerebral tumor perfusion MRI using protein-binding blood pool agents such as Vasovist® [18]: The hypothesis includes a »trapping effect« of contrast agent molecules after their passage of the diseased BBB in the unbound state, followed by protein-binding in the tumor compartment leading to both strongly reduced back-flow rates and increased relaxivity (■ Fig. 15.1). This mechanism is suggested to be responsible for the contrast enhancement as observed in our initial patient studies, which are described in the following examples.

15.2 First Experience with Vasovist® in Human Brain Tumor Imaging

To assess the early post-contrast imaging capabilities of Vasovist®, ten consecutive patients with different types of intracerebral tumors were examined in a pilot study using the standard dose of 0.03 mmol/kg body weight.

All MR examinations were performed on standard clinical 1.5-T systems (Magnetom Avanto® and Magnetom Symphony®, Siemens, Erlangen, Germany) using a circular polarized head coil or an eight-channel head coil. Eight patients were referred for follow-up MRI after radiotherapy, two patients in the pretherapeutic workup. For all patients, data from previous MR examinations with a standard extracellular contrast agent (1.5 years to 2 weeks prior to the Vasovist® examination) were available and served as a reference.

The imaging protocol included a T1-SE, T2-FSE and FLAIR prior contrast and contrast-enhanced T1-SE in axial and coronal orientation. In patients with skull-base tumors, an additional fat-suppression T1-SE was performed. The time between contrast medium administration and imaging was about the same for all patients at 3 min after application.

Compared with the standard agents, the intensity of the enhancement was rated equal for Vasovist® despite

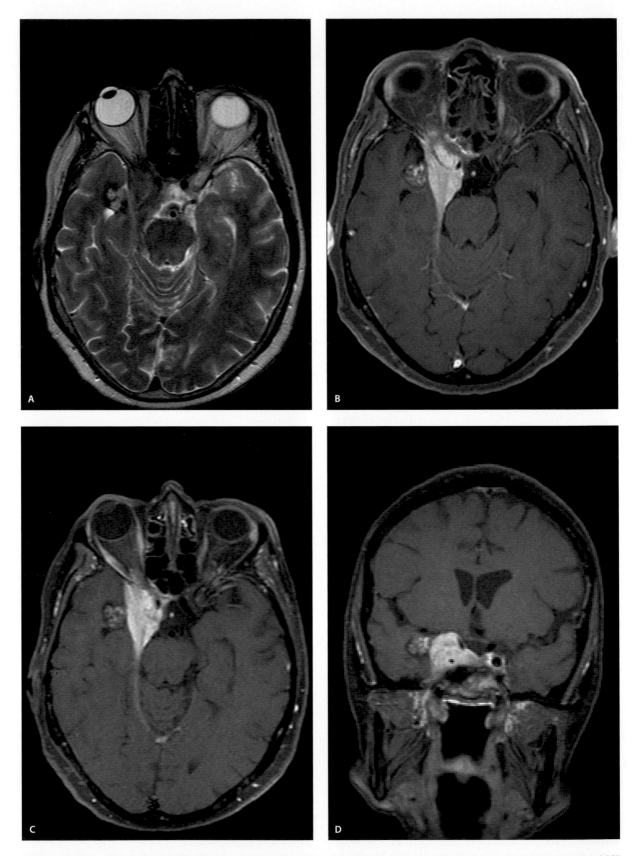

■ Fig. 15.2A–D. Vasovist®-enhanced MRI study in a 55-year-old patient with meningioma. Intraindividual comparision with a conventional ECF agent-enhanced study the substantially lower gadolinium concentration, which is less than 1/6 of the gadolinium dosage for standard extracellular agents used with 0.1 mmol/kg body wt dosage. The significantly higher relaxivity seems to compensate for the lower concentration. In the following we present two examples of early post-contrast imaging with Vasovist®.

In the first case, a 55-year-old female patient with histologically confirmed meningioma of the left skull base was examined in an intraindividual comparative manner using a standard ECF agent for the first scan and for the second Vasovist®. The tumor, presenting the typical MR imaging characteristics of a meningioma, was initially diagnosed in 2000 and treated with stereotactic conformal radiotherapy. The patient presented for a routine yearly follow-up without clinical symptoms. The initial examination showed an unchanged meningioma at the right medial middle cerebral fossa (■ Fig. 15.2A,B) presenting a typical homogeneous enhancement with dural tail using a standard contrast medium (■ Fig. 15.2C). In the examination with Vasovist® (■ Fig. 15.2D) the tumor is displayed in the same extension as in the previous examinination, with visually identical tumor contrast. The dural tail and the infiltration of the cavernous sinus are clearly visible.

Meningiomas as primary extra-axial tumors present tumor vessels without a BBB, allowing the unbound and part of the bound fraction of Vasovist® to extravasate into the extracellular space, which causes an enhancement comparable to that of standard MR contrast media 5 min after contrast medium administration.

The second example is of an intra-axial brain tumor: a 67-year-old patient with malignant glioma and clinical symptoms of seizures and minor neurologic deficits. The examination was performed with a standard dose of Vasovist® for diagnostic work and biopsy planning. Unenhanced T1 (■ Fig. 15.3A) and FLAIR imaging (■ Fig. 15.3B) presents a large mass lesion in the right temporal lobe with strong enhancement (■ Fig. 15.3C,D). The enhancement pattern and intensity was rated equal to a previous exam only 1 week previously. Vasovist® was in this case able to achieve a strong tumor enhancement with clear delineation of the enhancing tumor parts, which allows for biopsy and treatment planning both for neurosurgery and for radiotherapy. Note the increasing enhancement from the axial scans to the coronal scans acquired 3 min later.

Anaplastic and malignant gliomas typically present with a disrupture of the integrity of the BBB, which causes an early enhancement as observed after Vasovist® injection. The reason for the strong enhancement with the blood pool agent might be twofold in this case: first, the extravasation of the unbound fraction and the significantly higher relaxivity; second the extravastion of bound molecules via the severely disrupted BBB.

Depiction and better quantification of the BBB disruption is essential for the grading of such lesions. This further enables treatment decision and improved biopsy planning in these heterogeneous lesions. Since the enhancing tumor parts are the target of neurosurgical resection, the information about the extension of a BBB disruption substantially influences the neuronavigation-assisted resection.

Because of the very promising experience and based on the previous work in animals, a second study was started to assess the time dependence of the enhancement properties of Vasovist®. In a small series of only five patients, the participants were asked to return for follow-up examinations at 5, 12, and 24 h after a single injection (0.03 mmol/kg body weight) of Vasovist®. The studies were performed with a 1.0 T MR system using a standard circular head coil. In only one patient was a comparative study with standard extracellular agents obtained. Following Vasovist® injection the enhancement gradually increased over the first 12 h (■ Fig. 15.4) and lasted more than 24 h. Follow-up studies on a larger series of patients will systematically assess the potential of this new agent and the exact time course of enhancement.

In the following we present two cases which show the potential of Vasovist® in late-enhanced imaging.

A 62-year-old patient suffering from renal cell carcinoma with a fast progressive left-sided hemiparesis and epileptic seizures was referred for contrast enhanced MRI to rule out cerebral metastasis. We found multiple intracerebral lesions of different sizes and with blurred borders. The greatest metastasis left frontal was manifold lobulated (■ Fig. 15.4A).

Following intravenous administration of Vasovist® in a typical dosage there was a clear signal increase in T1-weighted images related to the BBB leakage. Even small lesions, e.g., a few millimeter-sized lesions left frontobasal, showed a comparable contrast uptake pattern (■ Fig. 15.4B). Even 8 h after a single dosage (0.03 mmol/kg body wt) of Vasovist® there was a persistent signal increase within the lesions (■ Fig. 15.4C,D). After 24 h this signal increase was diminishing but remained evident (■ Fig. 15.4E,F).

In the second case, a 65-year-old patient suffered from a recurrent glioblastoma with solid and cystic compartments. The clinical course was slowly progressive after surgery. The initial images after intravenous administration of Vasovist® demonstrated a left temporal mass lesion with BBB leakage resulting in a strongly enhancing cystic tumor appearance (■ Fig. 15.5A,B). Early imaging, acquired immediately after injection of the contrast medium, revealed a multilocular tumor with a second, more solid and nodular emerging signal increase in projection of the dorsal corpus callosum. Further images were acquired after 5 min (■ Fig. 15.5C,D). Besides the lesion in

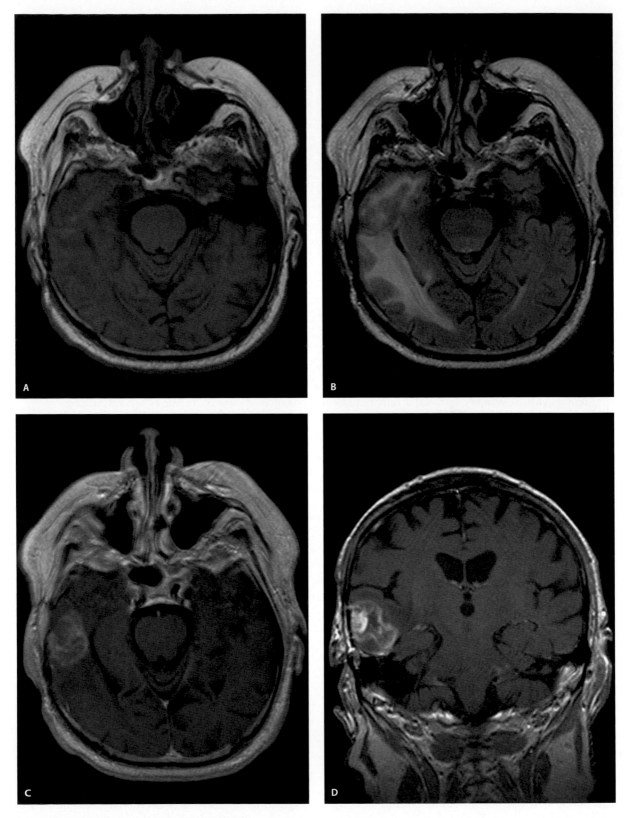

Fig. 15.3A–D. Vasovist®-enhanced MRI study in a 67-year-old patient with glioblastoma

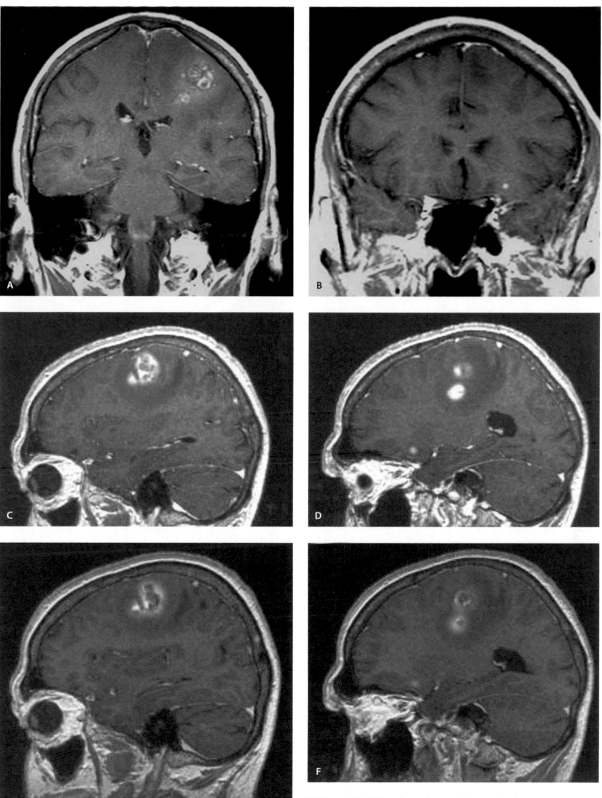

Fig. 15.4A–F. Time dependence of Vasovist® enhancement in a patient with cerebral metastases of renal cell carcinoma

16.1   Introduction

Nodal tumor spread in cancer patients is associated with a poor prognosis [1–3]. Multimodality treatment in cancer – combining surgery with pre- and/or postoperative systemic +/- radiation therapy – aims at eradicating microscopic tumor deposits in the surgical bed and locoregional nodes, as well as at sterilizing occult metastases in distant organs and distant lymph nodes. The effectiveness of multimodality treatment for the high-risk groups has been shown in multiple cancer treatment trials [4]. Combined preoperative modality treatment, however, carries a considerable perioperative morbidity and mortality [5–7] and it is questioned whether, with multimodality treatment of all cancer patients, the overall increased morbidity will outweigh the clinical effectiveness. The Dutch TME trial has shown in rectal cancer surgery that when rectal tumor nodes were involved, the local recurrence rate at 5 years was significantly lower for patients who received standard preoperative radiation therapy compared with patients who underwent immediate surgery. However, this was at the expense of radiotherapy toxicity and a significant increase in perioperative morbidity in terms of perineal wound leakage [8]. Furthermore, long-term complications such as bowel dysfunction were also described [9]. The trial also proved that subgroups of patients with early-stage rectal tumors without nodal involvement (stage I), did not significantly benefit from radiotherapy in addition to surgery, because these patients were already at low risk for local failure. If it were possible to select these patients from the higher risk patients with bulky tumors and nodal involvement, then a more individually based stratification of a multimodality treatment regime could be introduced, restricting the more aggressive combined preoperative treatment for the »ugly« cases and omitting preoperative irradiation in the »good« early tumors. Likewise, in patients with a head and neck squamous cell carcinoma (HNSCC), the choice of workup and management depends on the extent of lymph node metastases from the primary tumor to the different levels in the neck, as the presence of lymph node metastases (N+ neck) here is also an important prognostic factor.

As with rectal cancer, it is of clinical relevance for head and neck cancer whether any imaging tool can reliably confirm the findings of a neck without lymph node metastases at clinical examination (the clinically palpable N0 neck). Weiss et al. performed a sensitivity analysis to determine the optimal threshold for treatment of the neck. Patients with a primary HNSCC with a clinically N0 neck should be observed by a wait-and-see policy if the probability of occult cervical lymph node metastasis is less than 20%. The calculated risk is based mainly on the histopathological features, location, and extent of the primary tumor as assessed by clinical and imaging findings. If the probability exceeds 20%, the neck should be treated. Treatment consists either of a single modality of therapy, such as a neck dissection or radiation therapy, or a combination of both in which the decision will be driven by the treatment of the primary tumor [10]. Predictive models based on the histological and clinical behavior patterns of the tumor to assess which of the patients are at low and which are at high risk for local treatment failure as with HNSCC, are presently being used mainly because imaging tools to reliably identify pN0 patients are lacking. A substantial number of patients with HNSCC and an N0 neck as predicted by the presently available imaging methods are known to be understaged, because metastases in small cervical nodes remain beyond the detection levels of presently available imaging tools. As with rectal cancer patients, in HNSCC patients the development of accurate imaging methods to reliably distinguish between the N0 and N+ necks could help clinicians to more confidently and accurately stratify their patients into a tailored individually based treatment.

So far, no imaging tool has been reliable for detecting nodal metastases. A recent meta-analysis of all endoluminal ultrasonography (EUS), computed tomography (CT), and magnetic resonance imaging (MRI) studies on nodal detection in rectal cancer patients has confirmed that identifying nodal disease using the presently available noninvasive imaging techniques is not accurate enough for clinical decision-making [11]. Distinction between malignant and benign nodes with noninvasive imaging tools has been done only using morphological criteria such as size for CT and in addition to size, border contour, and heterogeneity for EUS and MRI, consequently leaving small malignant nodes undetected. For example, in rectal cancer treatment using the 9-mm cut-off to differentiate benign from malignant nodes would lead to a considerable understaging of patients with nodal involvement because more than half of the malignant rectal cancer nodes are between 2 and 5 mm [12].

According to the literature for head and neck cancers, MRI is infrequently used for the assessment of lymph node metastases, despite its superior contrast resolution, and this again concerns the detection of metastases in very small lymph nodes [13]. The criterion used at present of an at least 10-mm cut-off short axial diameter for malignant nodes will result in misclassification of malignant nodes as normal.

Consequently, if imaging is to develop into a more powerful predictor for confident stratification of the higher-risk cancer patients to a more aggressive treatment and the lower-risk cancer patients to surgery only or even a wait-and-see policy, further research needs to be done to investigate advanced imaging techniques to improve nodal staging. In this pursuit radiologists are aided by new developments in lymph-node-specific contrast agents. MR blood pool contrast agents, such as ultrasmall super paramagnetic iron oxide (USPIO), have shown better sensitivities and specificities for the detection of malignant nodes in various studies (concerning lymphoma, colon, rectum, lung, breast, head and neck, prostate, uterus, endometrial, ovarian, testicles, kidney, bladder, cervical, and vulval cancer). Another blood pool MR contrast agent approved for MR angiography is now on the market which is also promising for visualization of lymph nodes: Vasovist® (Gadofosveset, Bayer Schering Pharma AG, Berlin, Germany) [14].

This chapter describes the present status of modern imaging techniques for identifying nodal disease in high-risk patients, focusing on colorectal and head and neck cancer, and the promising new techniques and novel contrast agents that may help radiologists to improve the selection of oncology patients with lymph node metastases using non-invasive procedures.

16.2 Lymph Node Anatomy and Physiology

Knowledge of the anatomy and physiology of the lymphatic system and lymph nodes is important in order to have a basic understanding of lymph node imaging. Lymph nodes are small, bean-shaped structures that are usually less than 2.5 cm in length. Lymph nodes are distributed largely in the drainage areas of body sites most exposed to the external environment like limbs, gastrointestinal tract, lungs, and the pharyngeal axis. The lymphatic system is an essential first line of defense against pathogens.

The normal lymph node is separated into compartments called lymph nodules and surrounded by a connective-tissue capsule (◻ Fig. 16.1). In these lymph nodules, dense masses of macrophages and lymphocytes are situated and separated by spaces called lymph sinuses. Through these lymph sinuses the lymph fluid passes, on its way from the numerous afferent lymphatic vessels towards an efferent lymphatic vessel. The efferent vessel leaves the node at a concave area called the hilum. The lymph fluid consists of chyle, proteins, fat and white blood cells, primarily lymphocytes. The lymph fluid flow to lymph nodes is anatomically defined by the lymphatic vessels and the lymph node pattern. Metastasis can follow this structured lymph flow to spread to the next lymph node. Cabanas et al. demonstrated the existence of a specific lymph node center, the so-called sentinel lymph node (SLN), which was the primary site of metastases in penile cancer [15]. When biopsy of the SLN is negative for metastatic disease, the other lymph nodes downstream are likely to also be benign. Thus, a specific node can be the doorway for cancer to spread to other regional nodes. It is possible for a metastasis in a sentinel node to grow and block the lymphatic flow, thus redirecting lymph and tumor cells to other, possibly not ordinarily sequential nodes. This hypothesis of a sentinel node has been firmly established in such malignancies as breast cancer, penile cancer, and melanoma, but not in several other malignancies such as thyroid, head and neck, gastric, colorectal, cervical, and endometrial cancers.

16.3 EUS and Ultrasound for Lymph Node Staging

During the past decades radiologists have gained a great deal of experience in lymph node imaging by means of EUS and/or ultrasound [16, 17]. Several morphological

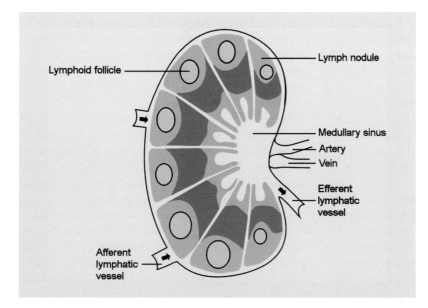

◻ **Fig. 16.1.** The anatomy of a normal lymph node

characteristics are assessed to distinguish malignant from benign lymph nodes. Characteristics suggesting tumoral lymph node involvement are: enlargement, round shape, irregular border, loss of the central hilum, and hypoechogeneity [18].

However, none of these morphological characteristics is accurate enough to identify a malignant node and therefore (E)US alone, without fine-needle aspiration cytology (FNAC), cannot be relied on for clinical decision-making in the staging of either head and neck cancer or gastrointestinal tract cancer such as of the esophagus and rectum. In rectal cancer EUS was slightly, although not significantly, better than CT or MRI in a large meta-analysis evaluating the diagnostic performance for nodal staging. However, large variations can be found in the accuracy of EUS for nodal detection (62–85%), illustrating its operator dependency [19–22]. Controversial reports on the performance of EUS-FNAC exist. Harewood et al. found no benefit from EUS-FNAC staging as compared with EUS staging alone [17], while Shami et al. showed significant improvement for EUS-FNAC compared with EUS alone, with a sensitivity of 93% [23].

Regarding lymph node staging in head and neck cancer, with the introduction of ultrasound-guided fine-needle aspiration cytology (USg-FNAC), sensitivity and specificity ranging from 63–97% and 69–100%, respectively have been obtained [24–26]. The associated diagnostic odds ratio (DOR) for US alone was 40 whereas the DOR for USg-FNAC was significantly higher, up to 260, which means an enormous improvement in the performance of preoperative cervical lymph node staging [13]. A drawback of ultrasound in general is that the performance depends on the experience of the sonographer, and in rectal cancer multicenter trials, EUS staging accuracy has been shown to drop by 30% when non-expert centers are doing the examination [27]. The operator dependency has also been shown to impact cervical nodal US staging [28]. A further drawback of USg-FNAC in head and neck cancer staging is the poor accessibility of cervical nodes deeply located in anatomical regions such as the retropharynx, and for the evaluation of these nodes other cross-sectional imaging such as CT or MRI is recommended nowadays. Therefore, the recommendations in the guidelines for diagnostic workup of head and neck cancer is to stage primarily with planar imaging techniques such as CT and limit US staging of head and neck cancer patients to experienced centers only.

The drawbacks regarding operator dependency of the Usg-FNAC performance, combined with generally restricted availability, its inability to accurately access some anatomical cervical regions at risk, and its inherently invasive nature makes USg-FNAC a staging tool that is unlikely to gain general acceptance in head and neck cancer diagnostic workup. Likewise, in rectal cancer EUS-FNAC

has been introduced but not widely adopted. First, beside the fact that the technique is highly operator dependent and invasive, it is limited in that many nodes outside the reach of the endosonography probe remain undetected. Second, if nodes adjacent to the tumor are suspected based on their EUS appearance, cytological aspiration of these nodes, which can be done only by direct penetration of the needle through the tumoral wall, contaminates the needle with tumor cells, leading to false-positive results [31]. Finally, there is the high probability of sampling errors, especially when small nodes of less than 5 mm have to be aspirated. In rectal cancer these nodes have a 20–50% chance of harboring tumor cells.

New ultrasound techniques such as Doppler-ultrasound combined with micro-bubble contrast agents or 3D EUS are being studied with promising results, although reports are limited mostly to experience at single centers, and the real question is whether advanced noninvasive EUS techniques in rectal cancer will gain widespread acceptance if they turn out to be operator dependent in future multicenter studies [32–34].

16.3.1 Computed Tomography

Computed tomography has long been adopted as a tool for identifying malignant retroperitoneal lymph nodes in several cancers. On CT imaging, mesorectal nodes measuring >5 mm can be identified as oval structures of soft tissue density within the fatty mesorectum [35]. Conventional single and 4- to 16-slice CT machines demonstrated accuracies varying between 22% and 77% for nodal staging in rectal cancer [22, 36–38]. In contrast to EUS, CT has a much larger field of view and is less reader/operator dependent. However, due to its low contrast resolution, conventional computed tomography techniques have relied primarily on size criteria. Size on its own is insufficient for a reliable distinction between malignant and benign lymph nodes, and the high frequency of malignant nodes between 2 and 5 mm in rectal cancer patients would only further limit CT in its ability to identify rectal nodal disease.

For the same reason, prediction of cervical lymph node metastases in head and neck cancer by means of conventional single and 4- to 16-slice CT techniques remains low in specificity. The main criterion for the assessment of cervical lymph node involvement using CT (and MRI) is the short axial diameter, and several studies have been undertaken to determine the optimal cut-off size of the short axial diameter for discrimination between metastatic and non-metastatic lymph nodes. In general, 10 mm is a commonly used cut-off size but a range varying from 9 to 15 mm has been described [39, 40]. Other criteria, such as the presence of necrosis or extranodal tumor spread, are used but less valuable [26, 41]. Necrosis is seen mainly in lymph nodes exceeding 10 mm, and those lymph nodes will already be classified as malignant in the first instance based on their large size. In the neck, with its densely packed structures of vessels and muscles, it is very difficult to achieve an acceptable soft tissue contrast resolution with conventional CT techniques, and it remains to be seen whether 64-slice CT with improved contrast and spatial resolution will lead to better results in this regard.

Advances in MDCT techniques with 64-slice CT being introduced in patient clinics could theoretically mean an upgrading of CT for nodal disease detection, but so far no studies exist on 64-slice CT for evaluating rectal cancer nodes except for one, which indeed showed an improvement with an 85% accuracy [42].

16.3.2 FDG-PET

^{18}Fluorodeoxyglucose (FDG) positron emission tomography (PET) has proven to be of additional value in the search for distant metastases in a wide variety of tumor types. Cancer cells have an increased glycolytic rate compared with normal cells, which ^{18}FDG-PET is able to detect. Although FDG-PET has proven its value for the detection of distant extrahepatic disease in rectal cancer patients, the results were unsatisfactory for locoregional staging of the primary rectal tumor. An important limitation of the currently available human PET scanners is their low spatial resolution and consequent inaccuracy for the detection of low-bulk tumor, requiring at least 1 cm^3 tumor volume before it can be depicted by PET. Furthermore, the uptake of ^{18}FDG within the primary tumor and urinary bladder obscures the visualization of approximate mesorectal nodes in rectal cancer, because of the scatter artifacts. This may explain why in primary rectal cancer staging with FDG-PET more than half of the malignant nodes go undetected, resulting in an unacceptably low sensitivity of 21–29% [43, 44].

For patients presenting with a head and neck tumor, it is of utmost importance to accurately predict lymph node metastases in the lower cervical levels (level IV and VI), because lymph node involvement at these levels implies a significantly higher prevalence of distant metastases, mainly to the lungs. In these patients a chest CT has so far been recommended in the workup as a first-line staging tool [29].

A recent study of patients presenting with cervical lymph node metastases, in which FDG-PET was employed to search for the unknown primary tumor and distant metastases, showed it to be superior to conventional CT staging, and FDG-PET is now recommended for this group of patients [30, 46].

However, only few reports are available on the use of FDG-PET for locoregional staging in primary head and neck cancer. The low spatial resolution of presently available PET machines may be the reason why interpretation of PET images in the complex anatomy of the head and neck remains very difficult for staging of both the clinically N+ neck as well as the N0 neck [40]. Despite these shortcomings, Myers et al. reported a trend in increased accuracy for FDG-PET compared with CT for the detection of cervical metastases in the N0 neck in HNSCC (PPV 100%, NPV 88%, accuracy 92% for PET versus PPV 80%, NPV 75% and accuracy 76% for CT) [45]. This study was performed in only a very small series of 14 patients with HNSCC in the oral cavity, oropharynx, and hypopharynx. Therefore, further and larger studies are needed to validate these results, also for other tumor sites in the head and neck.

The introduction of hybrid techniques for whole-body staging such as PET-CT, combining anatomical and functional information, might lead to better results than with PET or CT only as a single staging tool, but to date no substantial evidence exists to support this assertion [47]. In fact, to date a single study of 53 rectal cancer patients has been reported, showing a disappointing accuracy of 72% for nodal staging using PET-CT [48].

16.4   Magnetic Resonance Imaging

In general, conventional MR techniques with 0.5- to 1.5-Tesla systems are not accurate for the detection of nodal metastases in cancer patients, despite the superior contrast resolution of MR imaging as compared with all other existing conventional imaging techniques. Two meta-analyses in the literature report a similar ROC curve for the detection of nodal metastases with conventional MRI, both showing insufficient performance for clinical decision-making [11, 22, 49–55]. Most of these studies used size criteria to distinguish malignant from benign nodes. Only studies that investigated new criteria in addition to size, such as a border contour and signal homogeneity, demonstrated higher sensitivities and specificities for the prediction of lymph node involvement in patients with rectal cancer, yet only large metastases, over 5 mm in size, could be accurately evaluated with regard to border and MR signal intensity [54, 55] (◘ Fig. 16.2). The introduction of higher field MR systems into clinical practice could improve the disappointing performance of conventional MRI. So far, two studies on rectal cancer staging with 3-Tesla MRI have reported promising accuracies of 91–95% for predicting nodal metastases in rectal cancer [56, 57], but larger studies are necessary before the role of high-field MR machines for staging rectal cancer can be established.

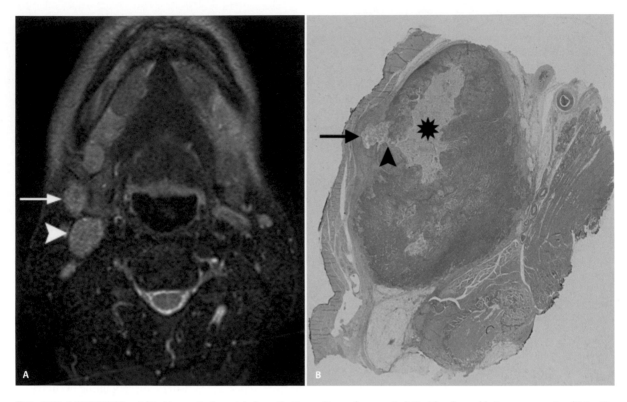

◻ Fig. 16.2. A SPIR TSE T2-weighted image in the axial plane. On the right side of the neck in level II an enlarged lymph node (*arrowhead*) with a short axial diameter of 12 mm would be classified as malignant based on the size criterion; however, cytology revealed no metastasis. Another, smaller lymph node (*arrow*) with a short axial diameter of only 8 mm shows an indistinct border and heterogeneous signal intensity. Cytology confirmed the diagnosis of a metastasis. **B** At histological examination (H&E) of this latter lymph node, the region of heterogeneous signal intensity corresponds to a metastasis (*asterisk*) with extranodal spread (*arrow*). Note disruption of the lymph node capsule (*arrowhead*)

In the staging of head and neck cancer MRI remains of limited use for malignant lymph node detection, as shown in a recent meta-analysis in which MRI was the least-performing noninvasive diagnostic modality [13]. This is probably primarily due to the use of the short axis diameter as a criterion whether a lymph node is benign or malignant. In addition to the size, other morphological aspects, such as necrosis or enhancement pattern, are used as criteria in daily practice, but the diagnostic performances still have to be established in future studies.

16.5   Lymph-node-specific MR Contrast Agents

During the past decade, new MR contrast agents such as ultrasmall super paramagnetic iron oxide (USPIO), Gadofluorine M, and Vasovist® have been developed and have proven in preclinical as well as clinical studies to be promising for oncology patients [14, 58, 59]. Of these, USPIO is at present the agent that has shown the largest evidence of being effective in the nodal staging of cancer patients.

16.5.1   Ultrasmall Superparamagnetic Iron Oxide

USPIO is a contrast agent that undergoes phagocytosis by the reticuloendothelial system in the liver but also by macrophages located in benign lymph nodes. Uptake of USPIO within the node results in a decrease of signal intensity on T2*-weighted images due to increased susceptibility artifacts. This means that benign regions in a node appear hypointense on T2*-weighted images (◻ Fig. 16.3). In malignant nodes macrophages are displaced by tumor deposits. In these regions no uptake of USPIO will occur (◻ Fig. 16.4) and they will be depicted as regions within the node with high signal intensity (white regions). Weissleder et al. were the first to distinguish malignant from benign nodes in an animal model using USPIO [59]; they were followed by Anzai et al., who demonstrated in a study with healthy volunteers that the uptake of USPIO reached its peak after 24 h [60]. Harisinghani et al. published the results of a study in 80 patients with prostate cancer and showed that USPIO MRI distinguished malignant from benign nodes with 100% sensitivity and 95.7% specificity [61]. A recent meta-analysis of 19 USPIO MR studies showed that USPIO MRI has a sensitivity and specificity of

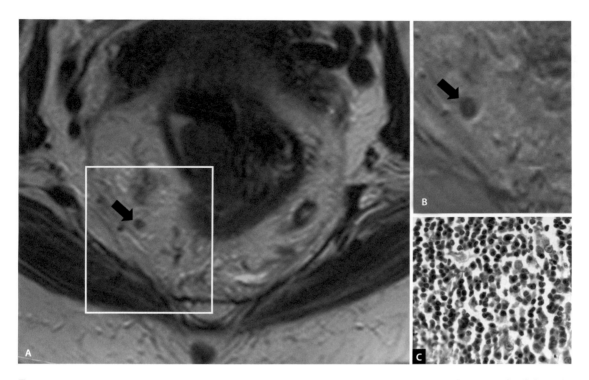

☐ **Fig. 16.3A–C. A** T2-weighted TSE image in the axial plane of the pelvis of a rectal cancer patient. On the conventional T2-weighted image it is difficult to predict whether this 5-mm lymph node (*arrow*) is malignant or benign. (**B**) On the corresponding USPIO-enhanced T2*-weighted image the same node in more detail showed general low signal intensity, indicating a normal USPIO uptake pattern within the node. (**C**) At histological examination (H&E) this node showed a normal nodal architecture and no metastasis

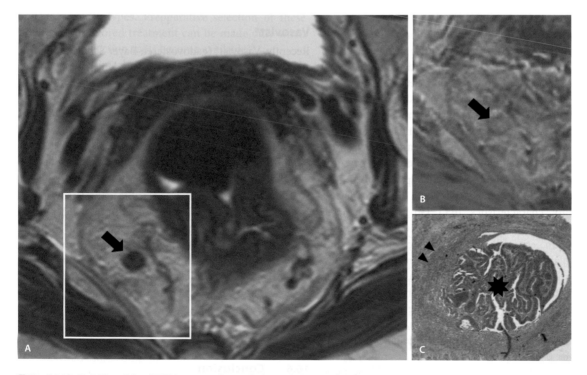

☐ **Fig. 16.4A–C. A** T2-weighted TSE image in the axial plane of the pelvis of a rectal cancer patient with a 7-mm mesorectal lymph node (*arrow*). **B** On the corresponding USPIO-enhanced T2*-weighted image the same lymph node (*arrow*) showed central high signal intensity, indicating no USPIO uptake. At the border of the lymph node there is still uptake of USPIO. **C** This correlated at histological examination (H&E) with the centrally located tumor deposit (*asterix*) and the remaining surrounding normal lymphoid tissue (*arrowheads*)

References

1. Herrera L, Brown MT (1994) Prognostic profile in rectal cancer. Dis Colon Rectum 37 [Suppl 2]:S1–5
2. Jakobsen J, Hansen O, Jorgensen KE, Bastholt L (1998) Lymph node metastases from laryngeal and pharyngeal carcinomas – calculation of burden of metastasis and its impact on prognosis. Acta Oncol 37:489–493
3. Ono I, Ebihara S, Saito H, Yoshizumi T (1985) Correlation between prognosis and degree of lymph node involvement in carcinoma of the head and neck. Auris Nasus Larynx 12 [Suppl 2]:S85–89
4. Sauer R (2002) Adjuvant and neoadjuvant radiotherapy and concurrent radiochemotherapy for rectal cancer. Pathol Oncol Res 8:7–17
5. Valentini V, Coco C, Cellini N, Picciocchi A, Fares MC, Rosetto ME, Mantini G, Morganti AG, Barbaro B, Cogliandolo S, et al (2001) Ten years of preoperative chemoradiation for extraperitoneal T3 rectal cancer: acute toxicity, tumor response, and sphincter preservation in three consecutive studies. Int J Radiat Oncol Biol Phys 51:371–383
6. Taylor JM, Mendenhall WM, Lavey RS (1991) Time-dose factors in positive neck nodes treated with irradiation only. Radiother Oncol 22:167–173
7. Newman JP, Terris DJ, Pinto HA, Fee WE, Jr., Goode RL, Goffinet DR (1997) Surgical morbidity of neck dissection after chemoradiotherapy in advanced head and neck cancer. Ann Otol Rhinol Laryngol 106:117–122
8. Marijnen CA, Kapiteijn E, van de Velde CJ, Martijn H, Steup WH, Wiggers T, Kranenbarg EK, Leer JW (2002) Acute side effects and complications after short-term preoperative radiotherapy combined with total mesorectal excision in primary rectal cancer: report of a multicenter randomized trial. J Clin Oncol 20:817–825
9. Peeters KC, van de Velde CJ, Leer JW, Martijn H, Junggeburt JM, Kranenbarg EK, Steup WH, Wiggers T, Rutten HJ, Marijnen CA (2005) Late side effects of short-course preoperative radiotherapy combined with total mesorectal excision for rectal cancer: increased bowel dysfunction in irradiated patients – a Dutch colorectal cancer group study. J Clin Oncol 23:6199–6206
10. Weiss MH, Harrison LB, Isaacs RS (1994) Use of decision analysis in planning a management strategy for the stage N0 neck. Arch Otolaryngol Head Neck Surg 120:699–702
11. Lahaye MJ, Engelen SM, Nelemans PJ, Beets GL, van de Velde CJ, van Engelshoven JM, Beets-Tan RG (2005) Imaging for predicting the risk factors--the circumferential resection margin and nodal disease--of local recurrence in rectal cancer: a meta-analysis. Semin Ultrasound CT MR 26:259–268
12. Monig SP, Baldus SE, Zirbes TK, Schroder W, Lindemann DG, Dienes HP, Holscher AH (1999) Lymph node size and metastatic infiltration in colon cancer. Ann Surg Oncol 6:579–581
13. de Bondt RB, Nelemans PJ, Hofman PA, Casselman JW, Kremer B, van Engelshoven JM, Beets-Tan RG (2007) Detection of lymph node metastases in head and neck cancer: a meta-analysis comparing US, USgFNAC, CT and MR imaging. Eur J Radiol 64(2):266–72
14. Herborn CU, Lauenstein TC, Vogt FM, Lauffer RB, Debatin JF, Ruehm SG (2002) Interstitial MR lymphography with MS-325: characterization of normal and tumor-invaded lymph nodes in a rabbit model. AJR Am J Roentgenol 179:1567–1572
15. Cabanas RM (1977) An approach for the treatment of penile carcinoma. Cancer 39:456–466
16. Vassallo P, Wernecke K, Roos N, Peters PE (1992) Differentiation of benign from malignant superficial lymphadenopathy: the role of high-resolution US. Radiology 183:215–220
17. Harewood GC, Wiersema MJ, Nelson H, Maccarty RL, Olson JE, Clain JE, Ahlquist DA, Jondal ML (2002) A prospective, blinded assessment of the impact of preoperative staging on the management of rectal cancer. Gastroenterology 123:24–32
18. Tregnaghi A, De Candia A, Calderone M, Cellini L, Rossi CR, Talenti E, Blandamura S, Borsato S, Muzzio PC, Rubaltelli L (1997) Ultrasonographic evaluation of superficial lymph node metastasis in melanoma. Eur J Radiol 24:216–221
19. Rifkin MD, Ehrlich SM, Marks G (1989) Staging of rectal carcinoma: prospective comparison of endorectal US and CT. Radiology 170(2):319-322
20. Herzog U, von Flue M, Tondelli P, Schuppisser JP (1993) How accurate is endorectal ultrasound in the preoperative staging of rectal cancer? Dis Colon Rectum 36:127–134
21. Akasu T, Sugihara K, Moriya Y, Fujita S (1997) Limitations and pitfalls of transrectal ultrasonography for staging of rectal cancer. Dis Colon Rectum 40 [Suppl 10]:S10–15
22. Kwok H, Bissett IP, Hill GL (2000) Preoperative staging of rectal cancer. Int J Colorectal Dis 15:9–20
23. Shami VM, Parmar KS, Waxman I (2004) Clinical impact of endoscopic ultrasound and endoscopic ultrasound-guided fine-needle aspiration in the management of rectal carcinoma. Dis Colon Rectum 47:59–65
24. Knappe M, Louw M, Gregor RT (2000) Ultrasonography-guided fine-needle aspiration for the assessment of cervical metastasis. Arch Otolaryngol Head Neck Surg 126:1091–1096
25. Takes RP, Righi P, Meeuwis CA, Manni JJ, Knegt P, Marres HA, Spoelstra HA, de Boer MF, van der Mey AG, Bruaset I, et al (1998) The value of ultrasound with ultrasound-guided fine-needle aspiration biopsy compared to computed tomography in the detection of regional metastases in the clinically negative neck. Int J Radiat Oncol Biol Phys 40:1027–1032
26. van den Brekel MW, Castelijns JA, Stel HV, Golding RP, Meyer CJ, Snow GB (1993) Modern imaging techniques and ultrasound-guided aspiration cytology for the assessment of neck node metastases: a prospective comparative study. Eur Arch Otorhinolaryngol 250:11–17
27. Marusch F, Koch A, Schmidt U, Zippel R, Kuhn R, Wolff S, Pross M, Wierth A, Gastinger I, Lippert H (2002) Routine use of transrectal ultrasound in rectal carcinoma: results of a prospective multicenter study. Endoscopy 34:385–390
28. Zenk J, Bozzato A, Hornung J, Gottwald F, Rabe C, Gill S, Iro H (2007) Neck lymph nodes: prediction by computer-assisted contrast medium analysis? Ultrasound Med Biol 33:246–253
29. Plaat RE, de Bree R, Kuik DJ, van den Brekel MW, van Hattum AH, Snow GB, Leemans CR (2005) Prognostic importance of paratracheal lymph node metastases. Laryngoscope 115:894–898
30. Regelink G, Brouwer J, de Bree R, Pruim J, van der Laan BF, Vaalburg W, Hoekstra OS, Comans EF, Vissink A, Leemans CR, et al (2002) Detection of unknown primary tumours and distant metastases in patients with cervical metastases: value of FDG-PET versus conventional modalities. Eur J Nucl Med Mol Imaging 29:1024–1030
31. Bhutani MS (2007) Recent developments in the role of endoscopic ultrasonography in diseases of the colon and rectum. Curr Opin Gastroenterol 23:67–73
32. Kim JC, Kim HC, Yu CS, Han KR, Kim JR, Lee KH, Jang SJ, Lee SS, Ha HK (2006) Efficacy of 3-dimensional endorectal ultrasonography compared with conventional ultrasonography and computed tomography in preoperative rectal cancer staging. Am J Surg 192:89–97
33. Hunerbein M, Schlag PM (1997) Three-dimensional endosonography for staging of rectal cancer. Ann Surg 225:432–438
34. Hünerbein, Pegios W, Rau, Vogl, Felix, Schlag P (2000) Prospective comparison of endorectal ultrasound, three-dimensional endorectal ultrasound, and endorectal MRI in the preoperative evaluation of rectal tumors. Preliminary results. Surg Endosc 14:

35. Kim NK, Kim MJ, Yun SH, Sohn SK, Min JS (1999) Comparative study of transrectal ultrasonography, pelvic computerized tomography, and magnetic resonance imaging in preoperative staging of rectal cancer. Dis Colon Rectum 42:770–775

36. Netri G, Coco C, Valentini V, Fioravanti PM, Aronne O, Cellini N, Puglionisi A (1985) Clinical staging of rectal cancer. Results of a prospective continuing study. Ital J Surg Sci 15:169–174

37. Zheng G, Johnson RJ, Eddleston B, James RD, Schofield PF (1984) Computed tomographic scanning in rectal carcinoma. J R Soc Med 77:915–920

38. Balthazar EJ, Megibow AJ, Hulnick D, Naidich DP (1988) Carcinoma of the colon: detection and preoperative staging by CT. AJR Am J Roentgenol 150:301–306

39. Curtin HD, Ishwaran H, Mancuso AA, Dalley RW, Caudry DJ, McNeil BJ (1998) Comparison of CT and MR imaging in staging of neck metastases. Radiology 207:123–130

40. McGuirt WF, Williams DW 3rd, Keyes JW jr., Greven KM, Watson NE jr., Geisinger KR, Cappellari JO (1995) A comparative diagnostic study of head and neck nodal metastases using positron emission tomography. Laryngoscope 105:373–375

41. Steinkamp HJ, Zwicker C, Langer M, Mathe M, Ehritt C, Neumann K, Felix R (1992) Reactive enlargement of cervical lymph nodes and cervical lymph node metastases: sonography (M/Q quotient) and computed tomography [in German]. Aktuelle Radiol 2:188–195

42. Sinha R, Verma R, Rajesh A, Richards CJ (2006) Diagnostic value of multidetector row CT in rectal cancer staging: comparison of multiplanar and axial images with histopathology. Clin Radiol 61:924–931

43. Abdel-Nabi H, Doerr RJ, Lamonica DM, Cronin VR, Galantowicz PJ, Carbone GM, Spaulding MB (1998) Staging of primary colorectal carcinomas with fluorine-18 fluorodeoxyglucose whole-body PET: correlation with histopathologic and CT findings. Radiology 206:755–760

44. Llamas-Elvira JM, Rodriguez-Fernandez A, Gutierrez-Sainz J, Gomez-Rio M, Bellon-Guardia M, Ramos-Font C, Rebollo-Aguirre AC, Cabello-Garcia D, Ferron-Orihuela A (2007) Fluorine-18 fluorodeoxyglucose PET in the preoperative staging of colorectal cancer. Eur J Nucl Med Mol Imaging 34:859–867

45. Myers LL, Wax MK, Nabi H, Simpson GT, Lamonica D (1998) Positron emission tomography in the evaluation of the N0 neck. Laryngoscope 108:232–236

46. Bohuslavizki KH, Klutmann S, Sonnemann U, Thoms J, Kroger S, Werner JA, Mester J, Clausen M (1999) F-18 FDG PET for detection of occult primary tumor in patients with lymphatic metastases of the neck region [in German]. Laryngorhinootologie 78:445–449

47. Schwartz DL, Ford E, Rajendran J, Yueh B, Coltrera MD, Virgin J, Anzai Y, Haynor D, Lewellyn B, Mattes D, et al (2005) FDG-PET/CT imaging for preradiotherapy staging of head-and-neck squamous cell carcinoma. Int J Radiat Oncol Biol Phys 61:129–136

48. Tateishi U, Maeda T, Morimoto T, Miyake M, Arai Y, Kim EE (2007) Non-enhanced CT versus contrast-enhanced CT in integrated PET/CT studies for nodal staging of rectal cancer. Eur J Nucl Med Mol Imaging 34:1627–1634

49. Will O, Purkayastha S, Chan C, Athanasiou T, Darzi AW, Gedroyc W, Tekkis PP (2006) Diagnostic precision of nanoparticle-enhanced MRI for lymph-node metastases: a meta-analysis. Lancet Oncol 7:52–60

50. Thaler W, Watzka S, Martin F, La Guardia G, Psenner K, Bonatti G, Fichtel G, Egarter-Vigl E, Marzoli GP (1994) Preoperative staging of rectal cancer by endoluminal ultrasound vs. magnetic resonance imaging. Preliminary results of a prospective, comparative study. Dis Colon Rectum 37:1189–1193

51. McNicholas MM, Joyce WP, Dolan J, Gibney RG, MacErlaine DP, Hyland J (1994) Magnetic resonance imaging of rectal carcinoma: a prospective study. Br J Surg 81:911–914

52. Hodgman CG, MacCarty RL, Wolff BG, May GR, Berquist TH, Sheedy PF 2nd, Beart RW jr., Spencer RJ (1986) Preoperative staging of rectal carcinoma by computed tomography and 0.15T magnetic resonance imaging. Preliminary report. Dis Colon Rectum 29:446–450

53. Schnall M, Furth E, Rosato E, Kressel H (1994) Rectal tumor stage: correlation of endorectal MR imaging and pathologic findings. Radiology 190:709–714

54. Kim JH, Beets GL, Kim MJ, Kessels AG, Beets-Tan RG (2004) High-resolution MR imaging for nodal staging in rectal cancer: are there any criteria in addition to the size? Eur J Radiol 52:78–83

55. Brown G, Richards CJ, Bourne MW, Newcombe RG, Radcliffe AG, Dallimore NS, Williams GT (2003) Morphologic predictors of lymph node status in rectal cancer with use of high-spatial-resolution MR imaging with histopathologic comparison. Radiology 227):371–377

56. Winter L, Bruhn H, Langrehr J, Neuhaus P, Felix R, Hanninen LE (2007) Magnetic resonance imaging in suspected rectal cancer: determining tumor localization, stage, and sphincter-saving resectability at 3-Tesla-sustained high resolution. Acta Radiol 48:379–387

57. Kim CK, Kim SH, Chun HK, Lee WY, Yun SH, Song SY, Choi D, Lim HK, Kim MJ, Lee J, et al (2006) Preoperative staging of rectal cancer: accuracy of 3-Tesla magnetic resonance imaging. Eur Radiol 16:972–980

58. Misselwitz B, Platzek J, Weinmann HJ (2004) Early MR lymphography with gadofluorine M in rabbits. Radiology 231:682–688

59. Weissleder R, Elizondo G, Wittenberg J, Lee AS, Josephson L, Brady TJ (1990) Ultrasmall superparamagnetic iron oxide: an intravenous contrast agent for assessing lymph nodes with MR imaging. Radiology 175:494–498

60. Anzai Y, McLachlan S, Morris M, Saxton R, Lufkin RB (1994) Dextran-coated superparamagnetic iron oxide, an MR contrast agent for assessing lymph nodes in the head and neck. AJNR Am J Neuroradiol 15:87–94

61. Harisinghani MG, Barentsz J, Hahn PF, Deserno WM, Tabatabaei S, van de Kaa CH, de la Rosette J, Weissleder R (2003) Noninvasive detection of clinically occult lymph-node metastases in prostate cancer. N Engl J Med 348:2491–2499

62. Koh D-M, Brown G, Temple L, Raja A, Toomey P, Bett N, Norman AR, Husband JE (2004) Rectal cancer: mesorectal lymph nodes at MR imaging with USPIO versus histopathologic findings – initial observations. Radiology 231:91–99

63. Kvistad KA, Rydland J, Smethurst HB, Lundgren S, Fjosne HE, Haraldseth O (2000) Axillary lymph node metastases in breast cancer: preoperative detection with dynamic contrast-enhanced MRI. Eur Radiol 10:1464–1471

64. Fischbein NJ, Noworolski SM, Henry RG, Kaplan MJ, Dillon WP, Nelson SJ (2003) Assessment of metastatic cervical adenopathy using dynamic contrast-enhanced MR imaging. AJNR Am J Neuroradiol 24:301–311

65. de Lussanet QG, Backes WH, Griffioen AW, Padhani AR, Baeten CI, van Baardwijk A, Lambin P, Beets GL, van Engelshoven JM, Beets-Tan RG (2005) Dynamic contrast-enhanced magnetic resonance imaging of radiation therapy-induced microcirculation changes in rectal cancer. Int J Radiat Oncol Biol Phys 63:1309–1315

66. Liney GP, Gibbs P, Hayes C, Leach MO, Turnbull LW (1999) Dynamic contrast-enhanced MRI in the differentiation of breast tumors: user-defined versus semi-automated region-of-interest analysis. J Magn Reson Imaging 10:945–949

67. Choi SH, Han MH, Moon WK, Son KR, Won JK, Kim JH, Kwon BJ, Na DG, Weinmann HJ, Chang KH (2006) Cervical lymph node metastases: MR imaging of gadofluorine M and monocrystalline iron oxide nanoparticle-47 in a rabbit model of head and neck cancer. Radiology 241:753–762

Vasovist® for Breast Cancer Recognition

Joan C. Vilanova and Klaus Wasser

17.1   Introduction

Radiological imaging of the breast using mammography and ultrasound has well-defined roles which are currently central to the diagnosis, assessment of treatment response, and follow-up of breast cancer. During the past decade interest in breast imaging by MR has grown and it is meanwhile the most import imaging technique in support of mammography and ultrasound. Dynamic contrast-enhanced MRI (DCE-MRI) is the technique generally used for breast imaging, and the diagnosis is based primarily on the quantitative or semiquantitative evaluation of signal-intensity curves. DCE-MRI has proved to be a suitable tool for breast imaging in patients with metastatic disease of unknown primary cancer [1]. Furthermore it is used to distinguish scar tissue from local tumor recurrence after breast-conserving therapy [2] and to follow up primary chemotherapy of breast cancer [3]. Several studies have shown that DCE-MRI is a powerful screening tool in women with an increased risk of breast cancer [4]. Therefore, the American Cancer Society recently recommended the annual application of DCE-MRI for women at high risk [5]. All these developments indicate that breast MRI will play an ever-increasing role in the future and that a large amount of innovative work has to be focused on this technique. However, it is generally known that DCE-MRI has a limited specificity for the characterization of breast lesions, although specificity has been somewhat increased within the past few years due to optimized morphological imaging.

17.2   Vasovist® for Breast MRI

One approach to improving the validity of breast MRI might be found in the use of recently accepted blood pool contrast agents. Vasovist® (Gadofosveset, Bayer Schering Pharma AG, Berlin, Germany), originally known as MS 325, is a small gadolinium chelate (957 Da), which binds reversibly to circulating albumin, forming a macromolecular complex [6]. The percentage of binding varies with species and is approximately 85% in human beings. Despite the presence of small unbound molecules diffusing into the interstitial space, Vasovist® produces a strong vascular enhancement and has proved to be excellent in MR angiography studies [7]. So far, studies on Vasovist® for imaging and characterization of tumors have been rare. Turetschek et al. [8] investigated Vasovist® in experimental breast tumors. No significant correlations were found between MRI-estimated characteristics and pathological tumor grade or microvascular count, a marker of angiogenesis; the lack of correlation was attributed in part to the inability to resolve the kinetics of the small-unbound Vasovist® and the larger protein-bound

complex. As the agent is about 85% bound and 15% free, the models describing signal change on dynamic MRI and its relationship with microvascular parameters such as capillary permeability would need to be more complex than those currently used. Perhaps also the semiquantitative findings of signal-intensity curves require a new interpretation. What can we really expect, therefore, from Vasovist® for breast MRI? Given the inadequate data currently available, we can only speculate. One advantage might be found in the strong vascular enhancement and a detailed vascular mapping after administration of Vasovist®. Using current extracellular small molecular gadolinium chelates, Sardanelli et al. [9] were the first to evaluate vascular maps of the breast by maximum intensity projections and they introduced a semiquantitative vascularity score. They found that one-sided increased vascularity is an MRI finding frequently associated with ipsilateral invasive breast cancer. Schmitz et al. [10] demonstrated that the diagnostic accuracy of contrast-enhanced 3.0-T breast MRI increased significantly when the vascularity score was added to the standard morphological and kinetic data analysis. As shown at ◘ Fig. 17.1, the vascular mapping can be further improved by the administration of Vasovist®. Furthermore, it might be of interest to determine whether changes in vascular mapping are an indicator of response during neoadjuvant chemotherapy. However, one should consider that the vascular mapping does not directly correspond with the microvascular level of breast tumors.

17.3   Additional Benefits

Another benefit of Vasovist® may be found in an improved morphological imaging of breast lesions. Using standard protocols, depiction of morphological details of a lesion is best during the early post-contrast phase, before the wash-out in cancers occurs. Due to the kinetic features of Vasovist®, a measurement with high spatial resolution would be possible in a strongly enhanced phase of steady state (◘ Fig. 17.2). In the meantime, however, a high spatial resolution can be attained by current DCE-MRI protocols, e.g., an in-plane resolution of 0.8 x 0.6 mm was described by Kuhl et al. [11]. There would be a questionable benefit of a further improvement in morphological imaging.

The measurement during the steady state after administration of Vasovist® could provide another important benefit. Based on our previous experience, contrast enhancement of diffuse mastopathic breast parenchyma is less pronounced in the steady state, when vascularized lesions still show a stronger enhancement (◘ Fig. 17.3). Using current protocols, the enhancement of mastopathic tissue is still a limiting factor in breast MRI [12].

As mentioned above, one might expect that we need a new understanding of the dynamic contrast enhance-

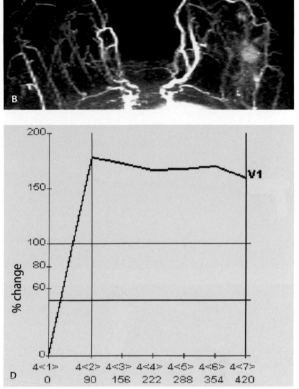

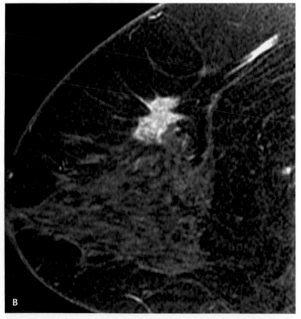

□ Fig. 17.1A–D. Standard dynamic protocol following administration of Gadopentetate dimeglumine (A, C) and Vasovist® (B, D) in the same patient with invasive ductal carcinoma (MIP). The examination by the standard protocol (A, C) shows a slight depiction of vessels and a type III kinetic curve after ROI analysis of the tumor. The examination by Vasovist® (B) depicts a more detailed vascular map and the similar type III kinetic curve after ROI analysis of the tumor (D)

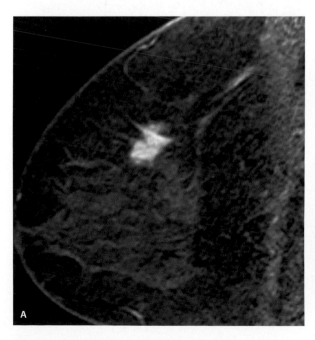

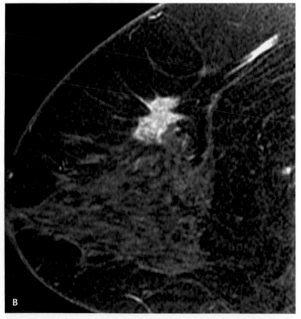

□ Fig. 17.2A,B. Early (A) and delayed post-contrast phase (B) following administration of Vasovist®. The delineation of morphological details of the tumor is somewhat improved in the delayed post-contrast phase of steady state due to a higher spatial resolution (0.5 x 0.5 mm in-plane resolution)

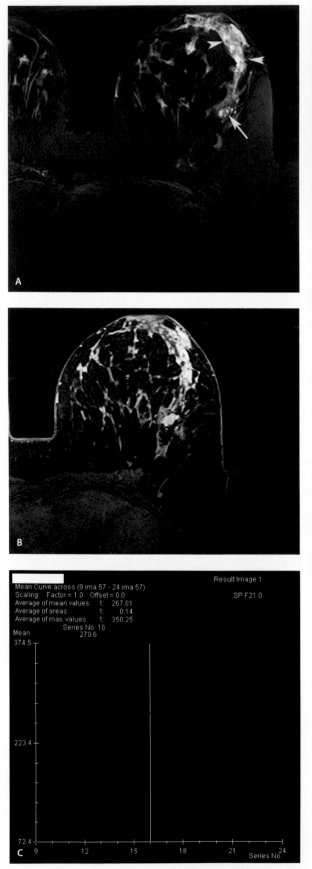

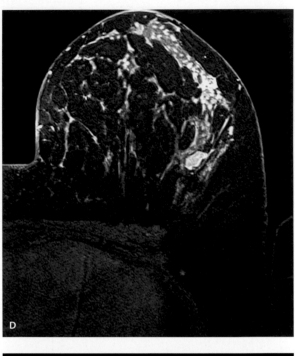

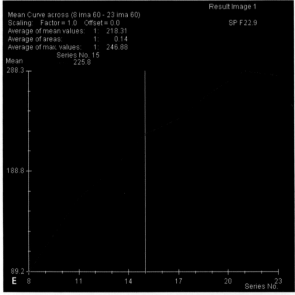

Fig. 17.3A–E. Breast MRI of a 42-year-old woman. The STIR sequence (**A**) shows a histologically confirmed fibroadenoma (*long arrow*) and mastopathic breast parenchyma (*arrowheads*). Following administration of Gd-DOTA the fibroadenoma is well-defined in the delayed post-contrast phase (**B**) (T1wfl3D with 0.6-mm isotropic imaging), and a type I kinetic curve is generated by dynamic evaluation (**C**). Following administration of Vasovist® the fibroadenoma is sharply defined in the delayed post-contrast phase (**D**), (T1wfl3D with 0.5-mm isotropic imaging) and dynamic evaluation shows the same type I kinetic curve (**E**). Note the less-enhanced mastopathic breast parenchyma using Vasovist® (**D**) compared with Gd-DOTA (**B**)

17

ment of breast lesions because of the complex distribution kinetics of Vasovist®. So far, however, our personal investigations show no substantial differences between signal-intensity curves based on Vasovist® or current small molecular gadolinium chelates (■ Figs. 17.1 and 17.3).

17.4 Conclusion

Given the inadequate data currently available, one should consider the pros and cons of Vasovist® for breast MRI with great care. Previous experience shows that there are at least no substantial disadvantages of Vasovist® compared with current small molecular gadolinium chelates. Hypothetically, improved vascular mapping and morphological imaging, as well as a decreased enhancement of mastopathic breast parenchyma, could improve the validity of breast MRI. However, all these hypotheses have to be confirmed by fundamental studies in the future.

Take home messages

- Vasovist® improves the vascular map for breast MRI
- Vasovist® might be beneficial for breast morphological evaluation
- Further investigation is needed to validate the use of Vasovist® for breast MR

References

1. Schorn C, Fischer U, Luftner-Nagel S, Westerhof JP, Grabbe E (1999) MRI of the breast in patients with metastatic disease of unknown primary. Eur Radiol 9:470–473
2. Gilles R, Guinebretière JM, Shapeero LG, Lesnik A, Contesso G, Sarrazin D, Masselot J, Vanel D (1993) Assessment of breast cancer recurrence with contrast-enhanced subtraction MR imaging: preliminary results in 26 patients. Radiology 188: 473–478
3. Wasser K, Klein SK, Fink C, Junkermann H, Sinn HP, Zuna I, Knopp MV, Delorme S (2003) Evaluation of neoadjuvant chemotherapeutic response of breast cancer using dynamic MRI with high temporal resolution. Eur Radiol 13:80–87
4. Kriege M, Brekelmans CT, Boetes C, Besnard PE, Zonderland HM, Obdeijn IM, Manoliu RA, Kok T, Peterse H, Tilanus-Linthorst MM, Muller SH, Meijer S, Oosterwijk JC, Beex LV, Tollenaar RA, de Koning HJ, Rutgers EJ, Klijn JG; Magnetic Resonance Imaging Screening Study Group (2004) Efficacy of MRI and mammography for breast-cancer screening in women with a familial or genetic predisposition. N Engl J Med 351:427–437
5. Saslow D, Boetes C, Burke W, Harms S, Leach MO, Lehman CD, Morris E, Pisano E, Schnall M, Sener S, Smith RA, Warner E, Yaffe M, Andrews KS, Russell CA; American Cancer Society Breast Cancer Advisory Group (2007) American Cancer Society guidelines for breast screening with MRI as an adjunct to mammography. CA Cancer J Clin 57:75–89
6. Kroft LJ, de Roos A (1999) Blood pool contrast agents for cardiovascular MR imaging. J Magn Reson Imaging 10: 395–403
7. Bluemke DA, Stillman AE, Bis KG, Grist TM, Baum RA, D'Agostino R, Malden ES, Pierro JA, Yucel EK (2001) Carotid MR angiography: phase II study of safety and efficacy for MS-325. Radiology 219:114–122
8. Turetschek K, Floyd E, Helbich T, Roberts TP, Shames DM, Wendland MF, Carter WO, Brasch RC (2002) MRI assessment of microvascular characteristics in experimental breast tumors using a new blood pool contrast agent (MS-325) with correlations to histopathology. J Magn Reson Imaging 14:237–242
9. Sardanelli F, Iozzelli A, Fausto A, Carriero A, Kirchin MA (2005) Gadobenate dimeglumine-enhanced MR imaging breast vascular maps: association between invasive cancer and ipsilateral increased vascularity. Radiology 235:791-7
10. Schmitz AC, Peters NH, Veldhuis WB, Fernandez Gallardo AM, van Diest PJ, Stapper G, van Hillegersberg R, Mali WP, van den Bosch MA (2008) Contrast-enhanced 3.0-T breast MRI for characterization of breast lesions: increased specificity by using vascular maps. Eur Radiol 18:355–64
11. Kuhl CK, Schild HH, Morakkabati N (2005) Dynamic bilateral contrast-enhanced MR imaging of the breast: trade-off between spatial and temporal resolution. Radiology 236: 789–800
12. Kuhl CK, Seibert C, Sommer T, Kreft B, Gieseke J, Schild HH (1995) Focal and diffuse lesions in dynamic MR-mammography of healthy probands. Rofo 163:219–224

Vasovist® for Multiple Sclerosis Recognition

Michael Forsting

18.1 Introduction

Multiple sclerosis is the most common immune-mediated inflammatory demyelinating disease of the CNS. The exact etiology of MS is still unknown. All we do know is that it is a chronic inflammatory disease, perhaps based on genetic factors, environmental factors, and cellular pathogen factors. In familial studies it was shown that family members of MS patients do have a markedly increased risk: in twins the risk is 250-fold, in siblings 30-fold and in half-brothers and -sisters tenfold. So the lifetime risk of a twin of an MS patient is 20–40%, the risk of a sibling is 3–5%, and that of a half-brother and -sister approximately 1%.

The incidence of MS per 100 000 inhabitants is in Germany around 3. This results in around 1500 new MS patients per year in Germany. However, since average life expectancy is not dramatically shortened, the prevalence of MS is high, i.e., about 130 patients per 100 000 inhabitants. There are approximately 2.5 million MS patients worldwide. It is not known why women are much more at risk for MS than men; the ratio ranges from 1.5:1 up to 3:1. Additionally, it is not clear why MS is more frequently found in Scandinavia and less frequent around the equator and in Japan.

Pathologically, MS is defined as an inflammatory demyelinating disease, characterized by perivenous inflammation and disseminated primary demyelinating plaques with reactive gliosis. Within the brain this is typically the white matter, specifically around the ventricles. Other areas with a high incidence are the optic tract, the cerebellar peduncles, and cerebellar white matter. The spinal cord is often not extensively involved; the majority of plaques are located within the cervical spine.

18.2 Diagnostic Criteria

Decades ago, the diagnosis of MS was based mainly on clinical findings. Today, the diagnostic decision is based additionally on so-called paraclinical results. Besides clinical signs and symptoms, the McDonald criteria [5] take into account the results of MRI, neurophysiological examination (evoked potentials), and the presence of oligoclonal bands in the cerebrospinal fluid (CSF).

Table 18.1. Diagnostic criteria according to McDonald et al. [5]

Subgroup	Diagnosis
Multiple sclerosis	At least two clinical attacks and two or more objective lesions. Clinically proven dissemination in time and space.
	At least two clinical attacks and only one objective lesion. Clinically proven dissemination in time. Dissemination in space demonstrated by MRI (»positive MRI«*, or positive CSF** and two more MRI lesions consistent with MS). No other, better explanations for clinical features.
	Only one clinical attack and two or more objective lesions. Clinically proven dissemination in space. Dissemination in time demonstrated by MRI*** or further clinical attack. No other, better explanations for clinical features.
	No attack (progression from onset) and one objective lesion. Primary progressive MS. Dissemination in time demonstrated by MRI or continued progression for 1 year and dissemination in space demonstrated by MRI or MRI and VEP and positive CSF² (criteria according to McDonald et al. [2] and Thomson et al. [4]).
Possible MS	At least two clinical attacks and only one objective lesion. Additional investigations not sufficient for the diagnosis of MS, criteria not completely met.
	Only one clinical attack and two or more objective lesions. Additional investigations not sufficient for the diagnosis of MS, criteria not completely met.
	Only one clinical attack and one objective lesion. Additional investigations not sufficient for the diagnosis of MS, criteria not completely met.
	No attack (progression from onset) and one objective lesion. Additional investigations not sufficient for the diagnosis of MS, criteria not completely met.

*As recommended by McDonald et al. [5] and given in detail in the text
**Oligoclonal bands or raised immunoglobulin G index
***A Gd-enhancing lesion demonstrated in a scan done at least 3 months following onset of clinical attack at a site different from attack or in absence of Gd-enhancing lesions at a 3-month scan, follow-up scan after an additional 3 months showing Gd-lesion or new T2 lesion (2).
MRI magnetic resonance imaging; *MS* multiple sclerosis; *CSF* cerebrospinal fluid

18.3   Radiological Examinations

MRI is the method of choice to support the clinical diagnosis of MS. Typically, MS plaques are located within the periventricular region, the corpus callosum, the centrum semiovale, and – although less frequently – in deep structures of the white matter and the basal ganglia. MS plaques are mostly ovoid, and many lesions are arranged in a rectangular manner around the corpus callosum (◘ Fig. 18.1A–C). Plaques are hyperintense on PD and T2-weighted images and hypointense on T1-weighted images. Rarely, MS plaques can be slightly hyperintense on T1-weighted images. Patients with confirmed MS do have typical white matter lesions in more than 90% of the cases. On the other hand, CNS lesions in other diseases such as ischemia, systemic lupus erythematosus, Behçet's disease, vasculitis, and sarcoidosis can exactly mimic MS (◘ Fig. 18.2A,B). This is specifically true for ischemic lesions, e.g. small-vessel disease, and led to the conclusion that MS criteria are less reliable for patients older than 50 years. MRI is more predictive for the prognosis regarding the development of clinically proven MS than any other examination such as CT, CSF, or evoked potentials. Patients progressing to clinically proven MS do have a higher lesion load on the first MRI compared with patients who do not develop MS. In addition, an increased lesion load correlates with a shorter time to the development of clinical MS.

On the other hand, the number of cranial MS plaques does not necessarily correlate with the degree of the clinical handicap. Patients with a low number of MS lesions can be severely handicapped, and vice versa.

For a diagnosis of MS, three of the four McDonald criteria have to be met:

1. One gadolinium-enhancing-lesion or nine T2-hyperintense lesions if there is no gadolinium-enhancing lesion
2. At least one infratentorial lesion
3. At least one cortical lesion and/or
4. At least three periventricular lesions

In general, one spinal lesion replaces one cerebral lesion. These criteria reflect the spatial dissemination of MRI findings. The dissemination in time is defined by McDonald as follows: if the first MR is performed within 3 months after the onset of clinical symptoms, dissemination in time can be shown via a second MR 3 months or more after the clinical incident, if there is a new gadolinium-enhancing lesion. If there is no new gadolinium-enhancing lesion in this second MR, the diagnosis can be confirmed with another MR after 3 additional months showing a new T2-lesion or a gadolinium-enhancing lesion.

A specific clinical finding is the so-called clinically isolated syndrome (CIS). Approximately 90% of all patients with MS did initially have a CIS with an acute onset. The most frequent clinical manifestations of CIS are neuritis of the optic nerve and brainstem or spinal cord symptoms. In 50–70% of these patients cranial MR reveals disseminated lesions with a typical MS appearance. The presence of such lesions increases the probability for definite MS dramatically.

18.4   Classical Findings in MRI

For the diagnostic workup of MS MRI plays an important, if not the most important role. With characteristic

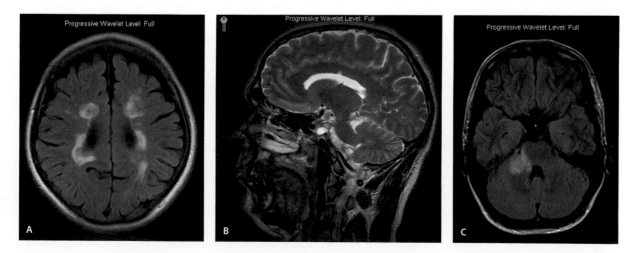

◘ **Fig. 18.1A–C. A** Typical white matter lesions in FLAIR-MR. **B** Sagittal T2-weighted image with typical MS plaques within the corpus callosum. **C** FLAIR-MRI with a typical MS plaque within the cerebellar peduncle

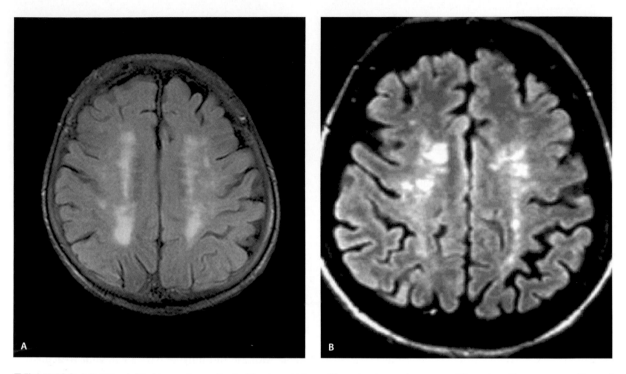

◻ Fig. 18.2A,B. A FLAIR-weighted image in a patient with a long history of hypertension and a severe white-matter disease on a small-vessel basis. **B** FLAIR-weighted image with multiple hyperintense lesions in the subcortical area of both hemispheres due to vasculitis

MR findings at the time of the first clinical symptoms, the probability of developing manifest MS during the next 10 years is greater than 80%. If the MR is normal, the probability is only around 10%. However, MR imaging alone is not specific enough to allow a diagnosis of MS. This can be done only together with clinical symptoms and/or other findings. An illustration will show how »dangerous« it can be if one relies just on MR: In 2005 Carmosino figured out that of 300 patients who where referred to a hospital with a diagnosis of MS only 1% really had MS according to the McDonald criteria. Among those patients for whom the diagnosis of MS was based only on MR the diagnosis was correct in just 11%. Turing this around, if the diagnosis of MS is based only on MR findings you can be wrong in up to 90% of cases.

18.5   Recommendations with Regard to MR Technique

To reveal supratentorial plaques, fluid attentuated inversion recovery (FLAIR) sequences are optimal. However, smaller demyelinating plaques can be missed infratentorially. The reasons are the well-known artifacts of FLAIR at this level. The best way to also visualize subclinical plaques is a combination of dual echo with proton-density and T2-weighted images and FLAIR images. All images should be acquired in at least two planes, the sagittal plane being recommended as most important in daily practice. The sagittal view should be planned such that not only the brain, but also the upper cervical spine is visible. In 98% of patients with MS periventricular plaques will be found, mainly around the posterior part of the ventricles and at the level of the sella media. In over 90% of patients the corpus callosum is affected, best seen on sagittal images; these are the so-called Dawson fingers. Typically, MS plaques are found along the venules, explaining relatively well why plaques are found periventricularly. Infratentorially, brainstem plaques and plaques within the cerebellar peduncles are typical. In chronic MS patients plaques present very frequently on T1 images as so-called black holes. In addition, many patients suffer from very severe brain atrophy.

Generally, for a patient with established MS, I recommend the following imaging protocol: cranial MRIs should contain at least a double-echo sequence (proton and T2-weighted images) and contrast-enhanced T1-weighted images. It's important to use standardized and not frequently changing protocols and to try to position the patient more or less identically during all follow-up examinations. Post-contrast images should be obtained at least 5–7 min following injection of the contrast-agent.

18.6   Role of Contrast Agents

Acute MS lesions exhibit an increased permeability of the blood-brain barrier. MS contrast-enhanced MR increases the sensitivity for new lesions compared with T2-weighted images alone, specifically for small subcortical lesions. However, one can find a 5- to 10-fold frequency of blood-brain-barrier disruption compared with clinical deterioration, indicating substantial subclinical inflammatory activity. In about 70% of the enhancing lesions the contrast-enhancement pattern is nodular, in around 20% it is ring-like (◘ Fig. 18.3A–C). This different behavior of the contrast agent is not completely explained. The nodular pattern reflects, however, more an acute plaque. Really new MS plaques obviously enhance for 4–6 weeks, and fewer than 10% of the lesions reveal contrast enhancement for more than 6 months. It is important to realize that corticosteroids repair the blood-brain barrier within 2 days following intravenous administration and the disrupted blood-brain barrier is no longer seen. Overall, the disruption of the blood-brain barrier as an MRI parameter of activity is limited, however, because there can be inflammatory plaques without disruption of the blood-brain barrier and then the contrast-enhanced MRI will not show any enhancement. Despite this limitation, the detection of acute contrast-enhancing plaques side by side with obviously non-enhancing plaques is a very important diagnostic criterion for the dissemination in time of the plaques. Spinal plaques also enhance in the acute phase.

On a second view, the role of contrast agents is much more complex than initially thought. The number of MS plaques in which a disruption of the blood-brain barrier can be found is dependent mainly on the examination technique. With conventional extracellular contrast media the doubling of the contrast-agent dose leads almost always to a doubling of the so-called active, meaning contrast-enhancing, plaques. Tripling the extracellular contrast-agent dose leads to a fourfold increase in the number of contrast-enhancing plaques. Additionally, the number of enhancing plaques is dependent on the scanner field strength, the spatial resolution of the sequence, the relaxivity of the contrast agent, and the delay between contrast injection time and starting of the scans. Increasing the delay leads to an increased number of detectable enhancing plaques.

At present, the role of intravascular contrast agents such as Vasovist® (Gadofosveset, Bayer Schering Pharma AG, Berlin, Germany) is not clear. Nevertheless, there are case reports that demonstrate signal-increased enhancing lesions up to 8 h following a single-dose administration of Vasovist®. However, delayed imaging techniques obviously reveal that Vasovist® penetrates into the plaques and can thus show at least the blood-brain-barrier disruption as extracellular agents can.

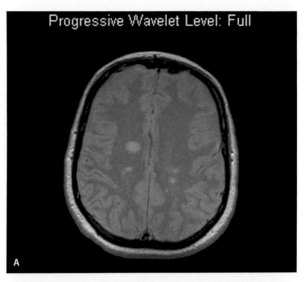

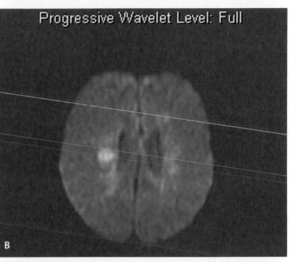

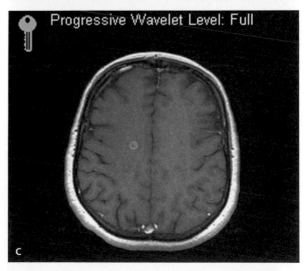

◘ **Fig. 18.3A–C.** **A** PD-weighted MR with typical MS-lesions. **B** The DWI reveals one of the plaques as an acute plaque within restricted diffusion. **C** T1-weighted contrast-enhanced image matches exactly with the DWI. The lesion with a restricted diffusion enhances the contrast agent

18.7   Variants of MS

Concentric sclerosis of Baló is a very rare demyelinating disease that in general is a variant of MS. The clinical course is monophasic and very rapidly progressing: In most patients the disease progresses within weeks or months. MR reveals concentric rings on T2- and T1-weighted images.

Another monophasic disease is the so-called Marburg disease, which is MS with a very rapid clinical progression. In general, it has an aggressive clinical course with very large demyelinating plaques in both hemispheres. Owing to their size, the plaques are commonly misinterpreted as brain tumors, and in these patients brain biopsies are usually performed. However, there is an agreement within the literature today that brain biopsy is not necessary when the patient's history, the CSF findings and serial MRIs are suspicious for MS. After administration of cortical steroids a dramatic reduction in the size of the plaques is always visible on MR.

In 1994, Devic for the first time described a 45-year-old woman with bilateral optic neuritis and myelitis transversa. This disease was later called neuromyelitis optica or Devic syndrome. The typical finding for the Devic syndrome is the bilateral involvement of the optic nerve and plaques within the spinal cord, mostly the cervical spine. Typical white-matter lesions in Devic syndrome will almost never be found, however.

ADEM is an acute disseminating encephalomyelitis. It is rare and occurs mostly in children and young adults. An infectious disease, usually measles, typically precedes the acute phase. Sometimes vaccination has been performed 1 or 2 weeks earlier. Clinically, there is a typical acute onset of multifocal neurological deficits.

18.8   Differential Diagnosis

The most common differential diagnosis includes mainly »small-vessel disease« in elderly patients and variants thereof (◘ Fig. 18.2A). Specifically in those patients with a »borderline age«, between 45 and 55, it can sometimes be difficult to differentiate MS plaques from the ischemic lesions of small-vessel disease. One hint can be to look at the cervical spine. In many patients with multiple sclerosis MS plaques can be seen within the cervical spine. On the other hand, spinal ischemic lesions are very rare in patients with a typical small-vessel disease. Additionally, it can help to perform T2*-gradient echo images, which will reveal hemorrhagic lesions in around 30% of patients with small-vessel disease and almost never in patients with MS (◘ Fig. 18.4A,B). If the lesion shows contrast-enhancement, the highest probability then is MS again.

Another similar disease is called CADASIL (cerebral autosomal dominant arteriopathy with subcortical inf-

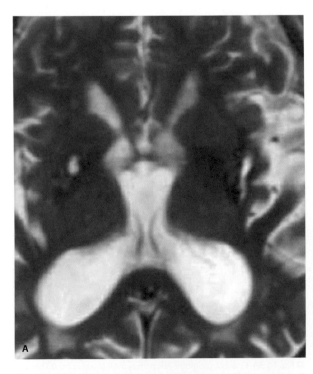

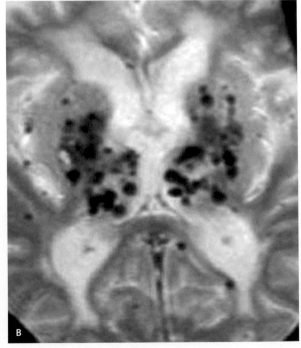

◘ Fig. 18.4A,B. MRI in a patient with a long history of hypertension. A Lacunar lesions on a T2-weighted image. B T2* reveals multiple hemorrhagic lesions. The T2-sequence should be obtained in all patients with the suspicion of small vessel disease. MS patients never have these hemorrhagic plaques

arcts and leukoencephalopathy), first described in 1991. This disease has an autosomal dominant inheritance pattern with the genetic problem on chromosome 19. Clinically, middle-aged patients without vascular risk factors present with repetitive ischemic symptoms and subcortical infarcts. Over the years, most of these patients develop vascular dementia. Very often they also develop depression. In CADASIL patients there is never a lesion in the optic nerve or the spinal cord, not clinically and not radiologically. From an imaging point of view, the extension of the white-matter lesion into the temporal lobe and particularly the temporal pole is very specific. As always, vasculitis behaves like a chameleon and can mimic MS perfectly, both clinically and on MRI. On MR multifocal infarcts in different vascular territories can be seen. However, in these patients vasculitis does cause cortical lesions as well. Sometimes in lupus patients the differentiation between MS plaques and the typical lupus lesions can be very difficult.

18.9   Conclusion

In summary, MR is the most important diagnostic tool for the diagnostic workup of multiple sclerosis. However, MR should never be the only diagnostic tool; a careful clinical examination is as least as important as the radiological imaging. Contrast enhancement is important to visualize the activity of plaques. Therapeutic strategies today depend on these MR-findings. Another important message of this chapter should be that not all white spots on T2-weighted images are MR plaques. Following the McDonald criteria will clearly reduce the number of false-positive MS reports.

Take home messages

- There are MR criteria that allow to establish the diagnosis of MS with a high sensitivity and specificity
- There are typical MR findings in patients with MS
- Contrast enhancement of plaques indicates active plaques
- There are certain variants of MS

References

1. Carmosino MJ, et al (2005) Initial evaluations for multiple sclerosis in a university multiple sclerosis center: outcomes and role of magnetic resonance imaging in referral. Arch Neurol 62:585–590
2. Diener HC, Hacke W, Forsting M (2005) Schlaganfall. Thieme, Stuttgart
3. Kesselring J (2005) Multiple Sklerose, 4th edn. W. Kohlhammer, Stuttgart
4. McDonald WI (2003) Multiple sclerosis. 2. Blue Books of Practical Neurology. Butterworth-Heinemann, Elsevier Science
5. McDonald WI, et al (2001) Recommended diagnostic criteria for multiple sclerosis: guidelines from the International Panel on the diagnosis of multiple sclerosis. Ann Neurol 50:121–127
6. Olek MJ (2005) Multiple sclerosis. Etiology, diagnosis, and new treatment strategies. Humana Press, Totowa, NJ
7. Osborn AG (2004) Diagnostic neuroradiology. Mosby, St. Louis

Interventional MR Imaging

Michael Bock and Frank Wacker

nodes. Several of these limitations might be overcome with recently developed T1-shortening agents including polymeric gadolinium compounds and liposomal encapsulated gadubutrol [14, 15]. At this time, however, their use remains confined to the pre-clinical stage.

20.8 Indirect Interstitial MR Lymphography

The interstitial injection of gadolinium chelates results in nodal enhancement in both animals and human beings. For animal studies, Vasovist®-enhanced interstitial MR lymphography is feasible and permits differentiation of normal from metastatic lymph nodes [16]. Based on its affinity to albumin, the interstitially administered small dose of Vasovist® is rapidly taken up into the lymphatic system. Marked T1 shortening associated with the agent allows for the display of the lymphatic system encompassing both lymph vessels and nodes from the feet to the chest in animals. Since enhancement is limited to normal lymphatic tissues, the technique permits differentiation of normal and tumor-infiltrated lymph nodes. Further investigation will be required to optimize the administered dose and determine the efficacy of Vasovist® for interstitial MR lymphography in human beings.

Compared with an intravenous approach, interstitial MR lymphography permits a more select and more comprehensive display of the lymphatic system. Thus, a small dose of 0.03 mmol/kg of Vasovist® (0.5 ml), injected subcutaneously into the dorsal foot pads of the rabbits, has been shown to be sufficient for striking contrast enhancement of the draining lymphatic vasculature and successive lymph node groups. Maximum intensity projections (MIP) provided a comprehensive display of the entire lymph system encompassing nodal structures as well as afferent and efferent lymphatic vessels of the hind legs and the abdomen (◘ Fig. 20.2). The applied dosage rendered homogeneous enhancement of normal nodes. Although the signal is uniform in the early phase, nodal uptake of Vasovist® is likely to vary between paracortical and medullary regions. Tagged probes may elucidate such distribution patterns in further studies.

The feasibility of interstitial MR lymphography has been successfully shown with commercially available extracellular paramagnetic agents also in human beings [2]. Without the protein-binding affinity inherent to Vasovist, the interstitially administered extracellular contrast agent was taken up in large part in by the capillary system, reducing the ability to delineate the lymphatic system. The presented data point to a far better contrast agent for interstitial MR lymphography: Vasovist®. The agent has successfully passed clinical evaluations as an intravenously administered blood pool contrast agent [17–19]. The same albumin-binding affinity which assures the agent's prolonged presence in the vascular system is responsible for its suitability as an agent for interstitial MR lymphography.

The interstitial application of Vasovist® appears safe. Regarding the inertness of the agent, murine experiments have shown extravasated Vasovist® not to be associated with inflammatory reactions within the subcutaneous tissues [20, 21]. Furthermore, the applied volume is very low. Extrapolated to human standard weights, the volume of Vasovist® for interstitial MR lymphography would range

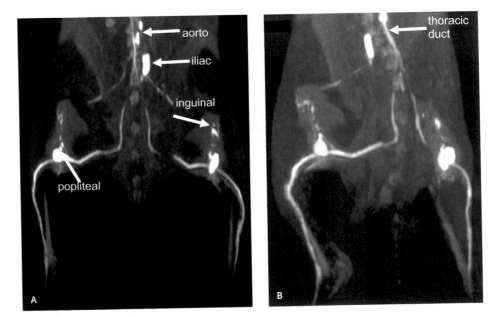

◘ **Fig. 20.2A,B. A** Maximum intensity projection (MIP) of a rabbit without any implanted tumor 15 min after subcutaneous injection of Vasovist® into dorsal foot pads of both hind legs. Popliteal, inguinal, iliac, and para-aortic lymph nodes can be delineated. **B** Oblique view on 3D dataset facilitates delineation of the thoracic duct

between 5 and 10 ml. The determined increase of signal-to-noise on T1-weighted images suggests a considerable potential for a dose reduction. Even these volumes should be well-tolerated, however. For display of the uptake of Vasovist® within the lymphatic system the volumetric interpolated breath-hold examination (VIBE) [22] was valuable for the structural display of lymph nodes with regard to considerable fat suppression and sensitivity for T1-shortening compounds. Following the interstitial administration of Vasovist®, this permitted accurate delineation of the lymphatic anatomy and especially of lymph nodes. The inherent three-dimensionality aided in the morphological analysis of individual nodes.

Following the subcutaneous administration of Vasovist® the lymphatic vasculature, together with popliteal and inguinal lymph nodes, markedly enhanced within 15 min (◻ Fig. 20.3). The aortoiliac lymph nodes and inferior parts of the thoracic duct were best visualized 30 min after injection of the compound. Washout of Vasovist® occurred quickly and was comparable in time to that observed with Gadoterate meglumine [3], gadofluorine,

and gadofluoramide [14] with signal intensities reaching almost baseline values within 2 h after the injection.

The exact means of Vasovist® uptake into the lymphatic system have not been determined. The process is likely to be driven by a combination of osmosis and pressure [23]. Lack of enhancement of lymphoid tissue within a node following the subcutaneous injection of Vasovist® is likely to correspond to the presence of tumor infiltration, as displayed by the histological examination of the lymph node specimen. At the same time, the enhancement of normal lymph nodes remains remarkably homogeneous. With this technique, metastases as small as 3 mm can be detected by the absence of contrast enhancement within the node (◻ Fig. 20.4).

Clearly, more studies of the lympholytic properties of Vasovist® are warranted. At this time, the potential of Vasovist®-enhanced MR lymphography lies within the interstitial administration of the agent and the consequent enhancement of normal lymph nodes. The technique promises not merely to display the entire lymphatic system, but also to permit the differentiation

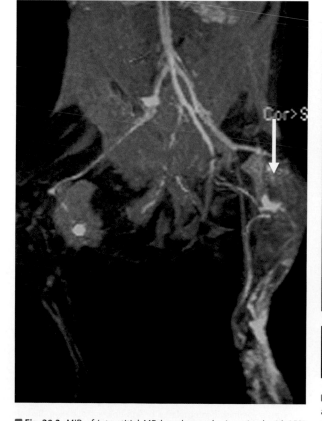

◻ **Fig. 20.3.** MIP of interstitial MR lymphography in animal with VX2 tumor in left hind leg. The invasion of tumor cells to the popliteal lymph node can be assessed by signal void of tumor-invaded lymph node (*arrow*). Popliteal lymph node on right side appears round and with homogeneous enhancement

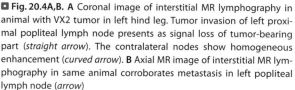

◻ **Fig. 20.4A,B. A** Coronal image of interstitial MR lymphography in animal with VX2 tumor in left hind leg. Tumor invasion of left proximal popliteal lymph node presents as signal loss of tumor-bearing part (*straight arrow*). The contralateral nodes show homogeneous enhancement (*curved arrow*). **B** Axial MR image of interstitial MR lymphography in same animal corroborates metastasis in left popliteal lymph node (*arrow*)

between normal and tumor-infiltrated lymph nodes. This potential might gain more clinical impact with further improvements of high-resolution MR imaging techniques, especially on MR machines operating at higher field strength.

In comparison to the potential of other paramagnetic or superparamagentic contrast agents, the use of Vasovist® for MR lymphographic purposes might be advantageous with regard to the albumin binding within the lymph and the consequentially increased relaxivity of the agent. This allows for smaller doses of the agent, which is highly desirable especially for interstitial administration.

20.9   Conclusion

Recent advances in the fields of contrast agents and MRI have clearly shown that lymphatic imaging no longer relies exclusively on conventional lymphography. Lymph nodes can be easily analyzed with indirect MR lymphography following the interstitial injection of gadolinium chelates, such as Vasovist®. The respective role of this technique remains to be determined in human beings; however, the potential impact of nodal imaging with Vasovist® could set a new standard in diagnostic staging for malignant tumors with lymphatic spread.

> **Take home messages**
>
> ▬ Reflecting the results from preclinical studies, Vasovist® might be used for MR lymphography as the agent is drained by the lymphatic system after interstitial administration.
> ▬ Vasovist® accumulates in normal lymph node tissue while necrotic tumor components remain spared out by the contrast material
> ▬ Rapid spoiled gradient echo sequences as used for MR angiography permit the display of lymphatic vessels and lymph nodes following the interstitial injection of Vasovist®

References

1. Moghimi SM, Bonnemain B (1999) Subcutaneous and intravenous delivery of diagnostic agents to the lymphatic system: applications in lymphoscintigraphy and indirect lymphography. Adv Drug Deliv Rev 37:295–312
2. Ruehm SG, Schroeder T, Debatin JF (2001) Interstitial MR lymphography with gadoterate meglumine: initial experience in humans. Radiology 220:816–821
3. Ruehm SG, Corot C, Debatin JF (2001) Interstitial MR lymphography with a conventional extracellular gadolinium-based agent: assessment in rabbits. Radiology 218:664–669
4. Moskovic E, Fernando I, Blake P, Parsons C (1991) Lymphography – current role in oncology. Br J Radiol 64:422–427
5. Cserni G (1999) Metastases in axillary sentinel lymph nodes in breast cancer as detected by intensive histopathological work up. J Clin Pathol 52:922–924
6. Dowlatshahi K, Fan M, Snider HC, Habib FA (1997) Lymph node micrometastases from breast carcinoma: reviewing the dilemma. Cancer 80:1188–1197
7. Rety F, Clement O, Siauve N, et al (2000) MR lymphography using iron oxide nanoparticles in rats: pharmacokinetics in the lymphatic system after intravenous injection. J Magn Reson Imaging 12:734–739
8. Mumtaz H, Hall-Craggs MA, Davidson T, et al (1997) Staging of symptomatic primary breast cancer with MR imaging. AJR Am J Roentgenol 169:417–424
9. Luciani A, Dao TH, Lapeyre M, et al (2004) Simultaneous bilateral breast and high-resolution axillary MRI of patients with breast cancer: preliminary results. AJR Am J Roentgenol 182:1059–1067
10. Weissleder R, Elizondo G, Wittenberg J, Lee AS, Josephson L, Brady TJ (1990) Ultrasmall superparamagnetic iron oxide: an intravenous contrast agent for assessing lymph nodes with MR imaging. Radiology 175:494–498
11. Bellin MF, Roy C, Kinkel K, et al (1998) Lymph node metastases: safety and effectiveness of MR imaging with ultrasmall superparamagnetic iron oxide particles--initial clinical experience. Radiology 207:799–808
12. Taupitz M, Wagner S, Hamm B, Dienemann D, Lawaczeck R, Wolf KJ (1993) MR lymphography using iron oxide particles. Detection of lymph node metastases in the VX2 rabbit tumor model. Acta Radiol 34:10–15
13. Weissleder R, Stark DD, Engelstad BL, et al (1989) Superparamagnetic iron oxide: pharmacokinetics and toxicity. AJR Am J Roentgenol 152:167–173
14. Misselwitz B, Platzek J, Raduchel B, Oellinger JJ, Weinmann HJ (1999) Gadofluorine 8: initial experience with a new contrast medium for interstitial MR lymphography. Magma 8:190–195
15. Staatz G, Nolte-Ernsting CC, Adam GB, et al (2001) Interstitial T1-weighted MR lymphography: lipophilic perfluorinated gadolinium chelates in pigs. Radiology 220:129–134
16. Herborn CU, Lauenstein TC, Vogt FM, Lauffer RB, Debatin JF, Ruehm SG (2002) Interstitial MR lymphography with MS-325: characterization of normal and tumor-invaded lymph nodes in a rabbit model. AJR Am J Roentgenol 179:1567–1572
17. Goyen M, Edelman M, Perreault P, et al (2005) MR angiography of aortoiliac occlusive disease: a phase III study of the safety and effectiveness of the blood-pool contrast agent MS-325. Radiology 236:825–833
18. Goyen M, Shamsi K, Schoenberg SO (2006) Vasovist-enhanced MR angiography. Eur Radiol 16 [Suppl 2]:B9–14
19. Goyen M, Grand DJ (2006) Gadofosveset: viewpoints. Drugs 66:858–859
20. Parmelee DJ, Walovitch RC, Ouellet HS, Lauffer RB (1997) Preclinical evaluation of the pharmacokinetics, biodistribution, and elimination of MS-325, a blood pool agent for magnetic resonance imaging. Invest Radiol 32:741–747
21. Straub V, Donahue KM, Allamand V, Davisson RL, Kim YR, Campbell KP (2000) Contrast agent-enhanced magnetic resonance imaging of skeletal muscle damage in animal models of muscular dystrophy. Magn Reson Med 44:655–659
22. Rofsky NM, Lee VS, Laub G, et al (1999) Abdominal MR imaging with a volumetric interpolated breath-hold examination. Radiology 212:876–884
23. Ikomi F, Hanna GK, Schmid-Schonbein GW (1995) Mechanism of colloidal particle uptake into the lymphatic system: basic study with percutaneous lymphography. Radiology 196:107–113

Part V   Image Processing

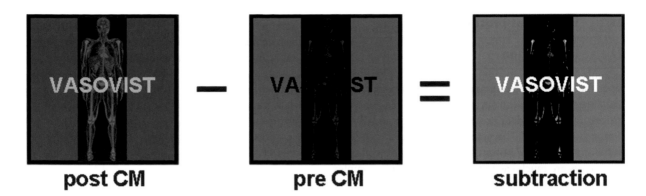

Fig. 21.3. Principle of subtraction: post-contrast minus pre-contrast

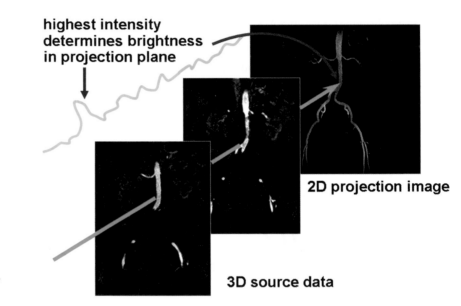

Fig. 21.4. The maximum intensity projection (MIP) principle

21.2.3 MIP and Thin MIP

The MIP [2, 3] is the most important tool used for post-processing MR angiograms. An MIP image delivers an impression similar to a conventional X-ray angiogram. The MIP data can be presented in positive contrast (bright lumen, dark background) or inverted (dark lumen, bright background).

The MIP technique extracts the vessels by casting parallel rays through the 3D dataset along the required viewing direction on a 2D projection plane. Each ray collects the intensities of the voxels along its path into a curve (histogram-like), and the highest intensity found is assigned to the corresponding pixel on the projection plane (□ Fig. 21.4). The result is an image with suppressed background signal.

Arbitrary projections of the 3D volume can be generated by rotating the ray direction. The radial projections are typically generated along the main axes (right–left, anterior–posterior, inferior–superior) in the prescribed number and orientation. For example, to project aneurysms without superposition, free adjustment of the projection direction is required. Superficial superpositions can also be eliminated by manually reducing the volume to be projected with cuboid or elliptical boundaries. This method also allows projections for each side separately (right and left carotid artery, lower extremities). The option of freely cutting out interfering structures lying within the volume (full bladder) represents other means of improving the quality of MR angiograms. Regional editing by combining both of these techniques produces MIP images almost free of artifacts (□ Fig. 21.5).

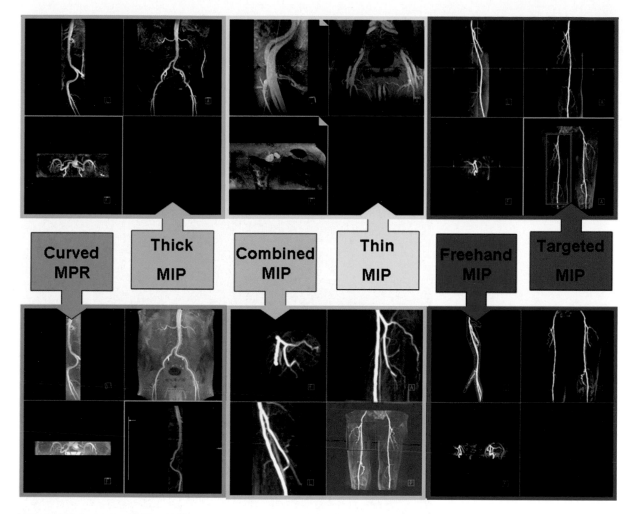

☐ Fig. 21.5. Refinements of MIP and MPR

21.2.4 MPR and Thick MPR

Starting with a certain viewing direction towards the basic dataset, which is ideally isotropic, the multiplanar reconstruction (MPR) generates parallel, radial or, as far as the section thickness and section gap are concerned, extended series, as well as parallel curved stacks of slices. The main view is in the three main orientations with the best possible resolution in each case (☐ Fig. 21.6). The orthogonal reconstructions can also be produced with thicker slices with variable overlap (thick MPR) to reduce the amount of data and to improve visualization. Curved parallel cuts in a thick MPR view can project tortuous vessel courses into one plane for easier inspection (☐ Fig. 21.5, lower left, and ☐ Fig. 21.7). Careful drawing of the cutline is essential to avoid misinterpretation.

21.2.5 SSD, VRT, Thin VRT, and 4D Viewing

The 3D imaging techniques surface-shaded display (SSD) or surface rendering (SR) are based on the extraction of gray levels lying between two predefined threshold values (☐ Fig. 21.8). SSD images are three-dimensional reconstructions of surface structures. The threshold values are less selective for MR series than for CT data, which causes residual tissue superposition.

The VRT (☐ Fig. 21.9) supplements SSD with a more precise depiction and separation of different tissue types and intensity regions. The impression made by the image becomes more three-dimentional by assigning color, opacity, and transparency for the respective intensity groups. These parameter settings can also be approximated for MR series in the form of an image gallery,

21

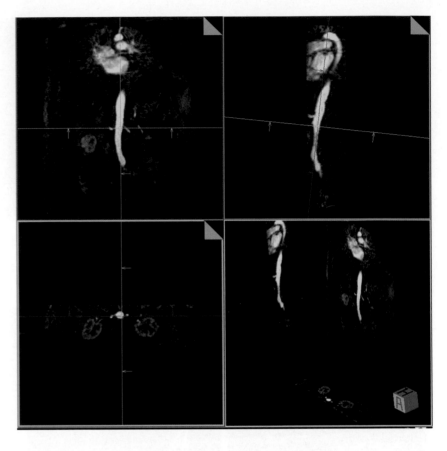

□ Fig. 21.6. Multiplanar reconstructions (MPR) of the three main planes

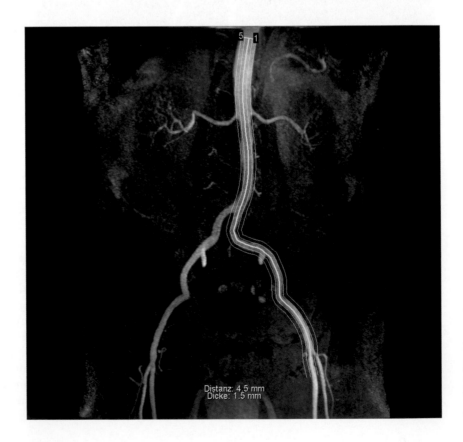

□ Fig. 21.7. Curved multiplanar reconstruction

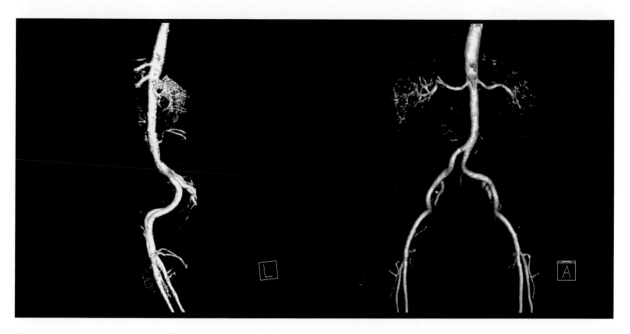

Fig. 21.8. Surface-shaded display (SSD)

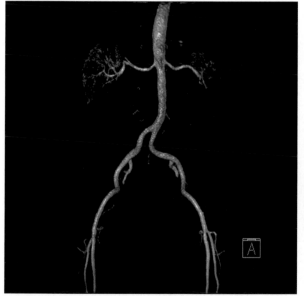

Fig. 21.9. Volume rendering technique (VRT)

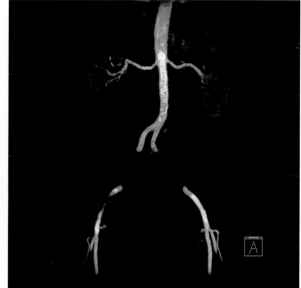

Fig. 21.10. Thin-slice VRT

which can be stored and loaded. Analogous to the other techniques, free projections or radial series can be generated for further documentation and diagnosis.

Similar to the MIP presentation over a freely defined thin-volume region, thin-slice VRT (thin VRT) is especially advantageous for MR data (■ Fig. 21.10), as it allows masking of superficially bright areas. The data can be scrolled interactively, or parallel series are calculated and stored.

Another new software module such as syngo Inspace 4D allows the dynamic viewing of the first pass and steady state series in an interactive mode. The user can move the 3D volumes as VRT or MIP in space and time. Switching between two or more datasets helps for the differentiation between arteries and veins on the high-resolution series, as shown in ■ Fig. 21.11. Arterial and venous series are shown side by side, whereas on the workstation they are stacked together on one screen.

21

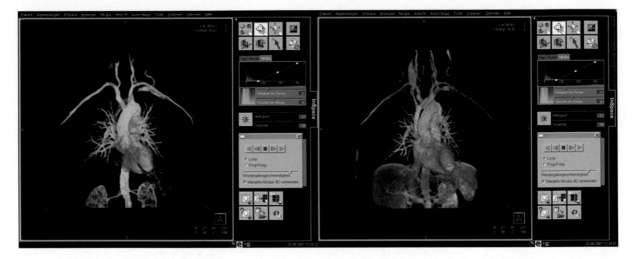

Fig. 21.11. Inspace 4D dynamic viewing showing two phases side by side

21.2.6   Quantitative Analysis, Vesselview

The determination of the degree of stenosis is essential for further treatment. In addition to the visual semi-quantitative assessment, direct measurement of the diameter (d) or still better the area (A) of the stenosed region of the vessel in relation to the post-stenotic values is the most accurate technique [4]. As a result of the frequently curved path of the vessels, an evaluation perpendicular to the path is essential for the accuracy of the measurement. This can be performed with double-tilted MPR sections or semi-automatically in an evaluation program, such as Vesselview (Fig. 21.12), which determines the path of the vessel and maps in the plane automatically once the section is entered by the user. This presentation allows superposition-free rotation of the diseased vessel around its longitudinal axis and determination of the cross-sectional areas at interactively defined vessel positions.

21.2.7   A-V Separation

The special feature of using a blood pool contrast agent, in addition to the purely arterial accentuated first pass data-set, is the late high-resolution series acquired, which depicts arteries and veins to the same extent. Segmentation of the two-vessel systems for the purpose of reducing venous superposition is desirable, especially in the region of the lower extremities. Various approaches and algorithms have been discussed in numerous publications [5– 7]. All techniques share the fact that the user has to set manual starting points and partly also end points in the arteries and the veins (A-V) as »seed points«, such that a trained

algorithm can find the path of the vessels automatically (Fig. 21.13). Simple criteria for the progression in the respective vascular system include the form (round, elliptical), linear dimensional orientation, and the intensity profiles of the vessel margins. The main challenge is the process of discriminating neighboring arteries and veins; new algorithms solve this problem adequately [8, 9]. High spatial resolution and good contrast simplify the process of segmentation. Additional measurements, such as phase contrast, can deliver differentiation criteria for A-V separation from the directional information contained in the previously acquired data. Once segmentation is completed, the intensity of the veins can be suppressed or cut out to improve assessment of the arterial system. In this technique, it is always the smaller and larger stenosed sections that cause problems which cannot be overcome by the algorithm. Further manual intervention into the segmentation process is unavoidable in such cases.

21.2.8   Virtual Intraluminal Endoscopy (Fly Through)

The technique of a virtual flight through a vessel lumen is used more frequently for initial diagnosis. Nevertheless, this tool delivers impressive films, which can be used for training purposes or for presentation to the patient. The automatic flight through the center of the vessel with variable field of view is based on the SSD threshold value setting. The transition from light vessel lumen to the dark tissue surroundings is interpreted as a vessel wall and is depicted in perspective with lustrous shadowing (Fig. 21.14). The technique lives from its interactive presentation.

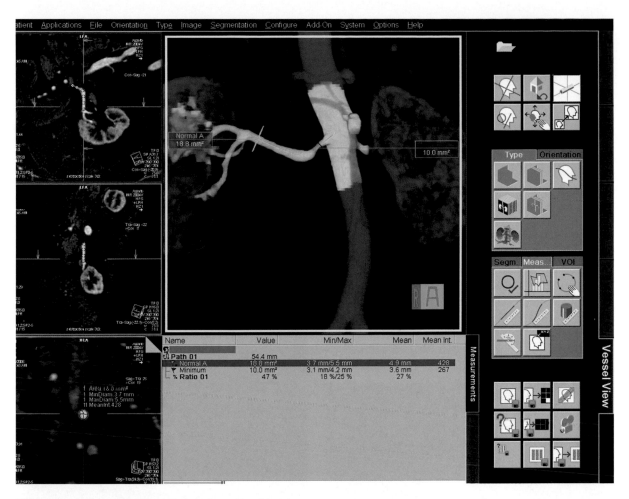

◨ Fig. 21.12. Quantitative analysis with the program Vesselview

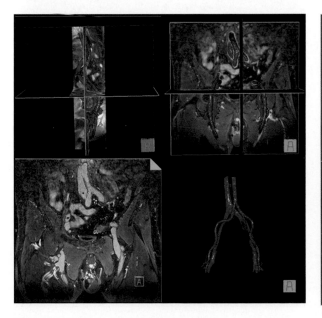

◨ Fig. 21.13. Different displays of A-V separation

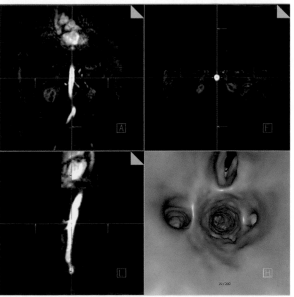

◨ Fig. 21.14. Virtual fly mode view above the renal arteries in caudal direction

21

21.2.9 Composing

The term composing describes joining several overlapping datasets with the same contrast originating from various table positions with the purpose of joint visualization for diagnosis and documentation. Coronally or sagittally acquired datasets or post-processed MIP are combined in this process. The holistic view of the vascular system and detail detection with the magnifying glass function (◻ Fig. 21.15) simplify diagnosis based on a large quantity of data.

21.2.10 Fusion of Image Series

Image data fusion is generally used to combine functional and morphological data, for example to register a PET dataset on a volume dataset from CT or MR. This enables improved assessment of the position of functional hotspots relative to anatomical landmarks. For MR angiography, improvements in depiction may be achieved in some cases if the subtraction data from the first pass measurements are registered on the blood pool data or morphological volume data (◻ Fig. 21.16). The process of registering the two datasets over each other takes place automatically and can still be optimized manually. The differentiation of the arteries (*blue*) from the neighboring veins is easily done; the first pass overlay can be blended up and down.

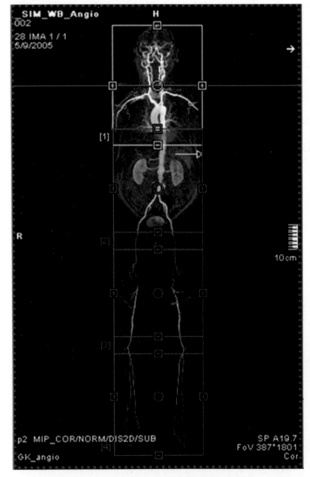

◻ **Fig. 21.15.** Composing of MIP images from various stations displaying the four measured stages

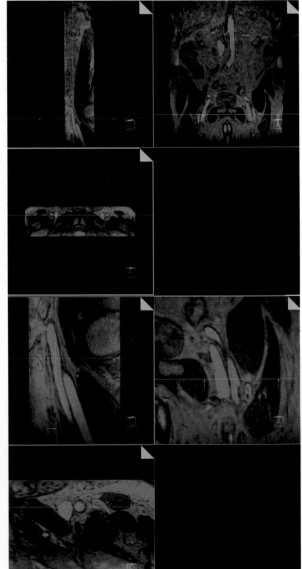

◻ **Fig. 21.16.** Fusion of a first pass (*blue*) and blood pool dataset (*blow-up, right*)

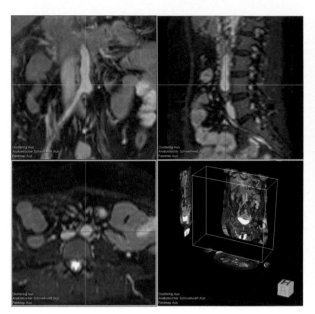

Fig. 21.17. Correlated orientations in different planes

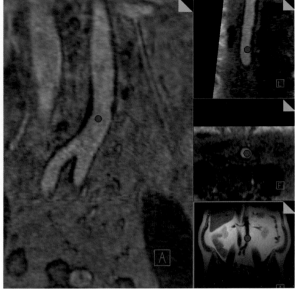

Fig. 21.18. Cross-referencing of various series (*red dot*)

21.3   Summary

The original measured data (source images) still represent the most important source of information for evaluation. Viewing in a correlated screen layout (■ Figs. 21.17, 21.18) of one or more series along with the MIP and thin-slice MIP analysis is the basic structure for diagnosis. The blood pool images support the diagnostic process for the first pass images with additional detailed information [10].

Lesion markers are automatically set in the MIP, MPR, and/or VRT display by automatically scrolling to the slice position or projection in the respective orientation, and they provide for greater diagnostic assurance by correlating the results in different series.

Take home messages

- Viewing of the source images remains basic and essential.
- Appropriate use of marketed post-processing tools can be helpful to achieve higher confidence in diagnosis, for both first pass and steady state MRA datasets.
- As is well-known from first pass MRA using conventional, extracellular MRI contrast media, 3D datasets are often best viewed as maximum intensity projections (MIP) in an overview.
- In particular for investigating 3D datasets from steady state images, a reduced number of se-

lected (coronal) slices leads to thin MIPs and often makes it possible to better visualize a selected region of interest.
- Multiplanar reconstruction/reformatting (MPR) in many cases provides a particularly accurate view for the evaluation of diseased vascular territory, including high-resolution steady state images in axial reformats.
- In specific cases, curved planar reconstruction (curved MPR) can be supportive to provide an extensive overall display of (single) vessels with otherwise hidden areas, for example, with complex geometry or within a disturbing vascular environment.

References

1. Douek PC (2005) Image processing in contrast-enhanced MR angiography. In: Schneider G, Prince MR, Meaney JFM, Ho VB (eds) Magnetic resonance angiography. Springer, Milan Berlin Heidelberg New York, pp 55–64
2. Rossnick S, Laub G, Braeckle R (1986) Three-dimensional display of blood vessels in MRI. In: Proceedings of the IEEE computers in cardiology conference, New York, pp 193–195
3. Laub GA, Kaiser WA (1988) MR angiography with gradient motion refocusing. J Comput Assist Tomogr 12:377–382
4. O'Donnell T, Tek H, Jolly M-P, Rasch M, Setser R (2006) Comprehensive cardiovascular image analysis using MR and CT at Siemens Corporate Research. Int J Comput Vision 70:165–178
5. Chen J, Amini AA (2004) Quantifying 3D vascular structures in MRA images using hybrid PDE and geometric deformable models. IEEE on Medical Imaging 23:1251–1262
6. Lei T, Udapa JK, Saha PK, Odhner D (2001) Artery-vein separation via MRA – an image processing approach. IEEE on MEDICAL Imaging 20:689–703
7. Bemmel van CM, Spreeuwers LJ, Viergever MA, Niessen WJ (2003) Level-set-based artery-vein separation in blood pool agent CE-MR angiograms. IEEE on Medical Imaging 22:1224–1234
8. Tek H, Ayvaci A, Comaniciu D (2005) Multi-scale vessel boundary detection. Computer vision for biomedical image applications, Springer, Berlin Heidelberg, pp 388–398
9. Tek H, Akova F, Aycaci A (2005) Region competition via local watershed operators. CVPR Conference on Computer Vision and Pattern Recognition, IEEE Computer Society. 2:361–368
10. Vogt F, Herborn C, Parsons E, Kröger K, Barkhausen J, Goyen M (2007) Diagnostic performance of contrast-enhanced MR angiography of the aortoiliac arteries with the blood pool agent Vasovist®: initial results in comparison to intra-arterial DSA. Rofo 179:412–420

Part VI   Pharmacoeconomic Impact

22

22.1   Introduction

Research on cost and outcomes has grown to become an integral part of radiology since the first controlled randomized studies in lung and breast cancer were carried out in the 1960s and 1970s. New diagnostic procedures and methods may reduce costs and generate benefits for patients simultaneously, as the introduction of noninvasive magnetic resonance (MR) or computer tomographic (CT) angiography [1] did. However, new methods often increase costs, as they tend not to replace but rather function as an adjunct to existing methods, or their initial costs are higher than those of the methods replaced, or the threshold for the new method is lowered due to a better convenience for the patient or operator [2].

Cost and outcomes research is fundamentally different in diagnostics from other areas of medicine because of the time distance between cause and effect, i.e., the efficacy regarding diagnosis and the effect on patient management. The main aim of radiologists is to provide an accurate diagnosis. The goal of the diagnostic procedure itself is to guide the diagnostician towards an accurate diagnosis, usually with the main focus on a distinction between normal and abnormal tissue. Subsequently, patient management, which is usually not controlled by the radiologist, could be altered by the change in working diagnosis. Health economics is the discipline that aims to find the answer to the question of whether changes in therapy are beneficial to the patient and whether the overall net costs of diagnosis and patient management are justified by improvements in the health and life expectancy of the patient. Hollingworth [2] pointed out that if any of the events not controlled by the radiologist fails, then this undermines the effectiveness and value of every new diagnostic procedure, regardless of its accuracy (efficacy). According to Drummond et al. [3], Efficacy is the ability of the new diagnostic procedure »to do more good than harm« [3], whereas effectiveness assesses the procedure's »performance in actual clinical use« [3].

To establish the cost-effectiveness of a new product or procedure, the effectiveness has to be evaluated for the relevant patient population. Efficacy alone is not sufficient to judge the clinical utility of a new contrast agent; effectiveness also has to be investigated.

In general, cost-effectiveness measures the costs and effects of new procedures, interventions, or technologies in health care. In other words, it establishes whether the new approach is economically worthwhile. When costs and outcomes, such as life-years gained, are evaluated in monetary terms, then this is expressed by cost-benefit analyses [4]. The evaluation of direct costs of the diagnostic procedure and patient management only is called cost-identification study. The comparison of two diagnostic procedures in such studies is a cost-minimization analysis according to Hunink [5]. Nevertheless, Hunink

[6] pointed out that the economic evaluation of diagnostic procedures differs significantly from that of other health care programs. The diagnostic procedure provides an immediate result. The outcome itself is driven by the treatment which is chosen according to the test result, and not a direct effect of the diagnostic procedure.

For the economic evaluation of new technologies, so-called health technology assessment (HTA) reports are prepared. Sources of HTAs can be found on several websites [7]:

- http://www.dimdi.de (Deutsches Institut für Medizinische Dokumentation und Information)
- http://nhscrd.york.ac.uk/htahp.htm (Health Technology Assessment Database, NHS Centre for Reviews and Dissemination, University of York)
- http://www.hta.nhsweb.nhs.uk/ (National Coordination Center for Health Technology Assessment

Best practice in undertaking and writing HTA reports is described in Busse et al. [8]. The book by Drummond et al. [3] is recommended as a standard textbook for further reading on the topic of health economics.

The health economic evaluation of the new MR contrast agent Vasovist® (Gadofosveset, Bayer Schering Pharma AG, Berlin, Germany) not only focuses on the economic modeling and the outcome cost-effectiveness and budget impact, but also stresses other benefits resulting in cost savings and advantages in patient comfort and management. As the first blood pool agent on the European market, Vasovist®-MRA offers advantages over magnetic resonance angiography with conventional extracellular contrast media (ECCM-MRA) and digital subtraction angiography (DSA) and provides increased diagnostic confidence in diagnosis by increasing the spatial resolution and extending the imaging window. This major advantage over current procedures was chosen to investigate the cost-effectiveness of this new contrast agent. The evaluation was performed using a health economic model based on probabilities derived from an expert panel and German cost data. Different diagnostic strategies were investigated to show whether starting with Vasovist®-MRA may prove to be beneficial over conventional ECCM-MRA and standard DSA. In addition, the technical abilities and the clinical development program were discussed in the light of health economics.

22.2   Objective of the Health Economic Evaluation for Vasovist®-MRA

The objective of this health economic evaluation is to provide economic evidence for the use of the new MRA contrast agent Vasovist® and to demonstrate the monetary benefits for payers when the new agent is used in clinical routine to diagnose peripheral arterial obstructive disease (PAOD).

22.3 Health Economic Evaluation: Technical Abilities

As the first blood pool agent, Vasovist® has been specifically developed for vascular imaging by optimizing the physicochemical properties for this requirement. The relaxivity is more than fivefold that of ECCM-MRA agents. By reversibly binding to albumin in the blood, the intravascular half-life is longer (29 min), leading to an extended imaging window. Higher resolution images and the possibility of steady state imaging are now available and allow for parallel assessment of the arterial and venous systems. With a missed bolus in first pass imaging there is no need for an additional injection of contrast agent. Also, re-imaging of regions with difficult anatomy or pathology is possible with higher focus and resolution, and imaging of multiple vessels in different body parts, functional MRA and peripheral as well as whole-body MRA (»moving bed imaging«), and imaging of vessel walls and plaque morphology are possible, allowing not only visualization of the vessel lumen (luminography) but a comprehensive view of the vascular system.

In addition to these technical abilities, and as one of the key advantages, Vasovist® allows for non-invasive angiography, avoiding side effects associated with the invasiveness of DSA. Other benefits of Vasovist®-MRA over ECCM-MRA are the prolonged imaging window (steady state) and higher resolution images which may reduce the number of artifacts and the risk of a »missed bolus« due to imperfect synchronization of bolus injection and image acquisition. These benefits can be obtained without software updates and without new or additional technical equipment and scanner hardware, so that no additional investments are required. As no bolus is needed for Vasovist® steady state MRA, injection with a simple syringe may be sufficient [9].

Resource utilization has not been evaluated in detail yet, but there is assumed potential to decrease costs when Vasovist®-MRA is used instead of DSA because of reduced examination time, personnel, and equipment resources. However, this assumed potential has to be confirmed by cost calculations on real resource utilization. A first evaluation was performed by Visser et al. [10], who showed that when PAOD was treated with angioplasty instead of more invasive treatments such as bypass surgery, MRA required similar costs for diagnosis compared with the combination of duplex ultrasound and DSA. When bypass surgery is one of the treatment options, a false diagnosis has a higher impact on costs, so that the costs for DSA were found to be slightly lower with higher effectiveness.

Further descriptions of the technical advantages of Vasovist®-MRA can be found in ▶ Chap. 1.

22.3.1 Health Economic Evaluation: Clinical Development

Challenges of Using Clinical Studies for Health Economic Evaluations

The clinical development of Vasovist® was carried out under the current guidelines at the time the clinical studies were being performed. Clinical studies on new diagnostic procedures follow not only the respective guidelines of the International Conference on Harmonisation on Good-Clinical-Practice (ICH-GCP) but also specific guidelines for diagnostic studies of the European Medicines Agency (EMEA) [11] and the US Food and Drug Administration (FDA) [12].

These requirements lead to settings to objectively evaluate the new contrast agent with regard to efficacy and safety. On the other hand, certain aspects in state-of-the-art studies for regulatory purposes may complicate the health economic evaluation of a new product. New diagnostic procedures may require a learning curve for an optimal performance, especially with regard to steady state imaging. Clinical studies and the regulatory process to receive market approval usually take years, and the technical equipment available at the start of the study is often outdated when the agent enters the market.

The standard of reference in clinical studies, which is defined as being the truth, may be imperfect but is still regarded as being correct in 100% of cases. Advantages of the new procedure may therefore be missed, e.g., any potential superiority of Vasovist®-enhanced MRA over the standard of reference DSA.

Also the clinical development program is focused on direct and relevant diagnostic parameters for the measurement of efficacy, such as sensitivity and specificity in detecting/excluding PAOD. Health economically relevant outcomes such as customer satisfaction are usually not part of studies, as these are not needed for the regulatory submission and lead to a more complex study design as well as to higher costs. Other outcomes, such as diagnostic confidence or quality-of-life parameters, are at most secondary end points in studies, as they are subjective and therefore not accepted as primary objectives in pivotal studies (i.e., phase III studies needed for submission).

Benefits of Vasovist®-MRA over ECCM-MRA and DSA

The results of the Vasovist® pivotal studies are presented in detail in the chapters by Brix (safety) and Goyen (efficacy).

Hadizadeh et al. [13] found that steady state imaging was more accurate than first pass imaging and increased diagnostic confidence. In addition, steady state was found to correspond highly with DSA and to be more reliable than first pass imaging. Further work by the same group [14] found that ultra-high resolution of the upper legs and lower legs with Vasovist®-MRA showed added diagnostic value and an increased level of diagnostic confidence in the assessment of PAOD as compared with first pass imaging alone. In a recently published study by Klessen et al. [14], Vasovist®-MRA was found to serve well for first pass imaging of whole-body MRA compared with ECCM-MRA, despite the much lower dose. The qualitative evaluation regarding arterial contrast, venous overlay, and overall image quality was evaluated in consensus by two blinded readers, leading to higher values in all areas of investigation. Significant superiority for Vasovist® with low volume and standard dose was found in the supra-aortic/throracic and abdominal/pelvic regions compared with double-dose Gd-DTPA. Also the accuracy in depiction of vessels and the visualization is increased in steady state Vasovist®-MRA, as shown by Wang et al. [15]. Nikolaou et al. [16] found sensitivities of 100% and 97% and specificities of 96% and 97%, respectively for Vasovist®-MRA in the detection of significant disease in the carotid and lower extremities. As another advantage, they reported easy separation of veins and arteries when the resolution is high enough in steady state imaging.

22.3.2   Health Economic Evaluation: Real-world Experience

The real-world experience is based on a Delphi panel of expert radiologists who were interviewed to provide their experience in comparing the performance of Vasovist®-MRA and ECCM-MRA. The Delphi panel itself is part of the Delphi method and a tool for extracting information from a multidisciplinary group of experts on a topic of interest. The name »Delphi« was first given to a Rand Corporation study in defense research in the USA, starting in the early 1950s. The aim of this study was to »obtain the most reliable consensus of opinion of a group of experts … by a series of intensive questionnaires interspersed with controlled opinion feedback [17]. The book by Linstone and Turoff [17] from 1975 can be regarded as the standard textbook on the Delphi method. A good introduction to the Delphi method can be found in Linstone [18]. The Delphi method is still under development. Newer approaches can be found in Rowe and Wright [19], for example.

Setup and Aim of the Delphi Panel

The primary objective of the Delphi panel was to collect and compare opinions of radiology experts on the confidence in diagnosis when using one of four diagnostic

modalities for the diagnosis of PAOD: Vasovist®-MRA, ECCM-MRA, and standard as well as selective DSA. These data were also used in the economic modeling (▶ chapter 22.4) and were published by Kienbaum et al. [24]. The expert knowledge was collected by interviews in a group meeting.

Diagnostic confidence is a subjective parameter for measuring the performance of diagnostic procedures. On the other hand, it reflects the main topic of diagnostics, which is to change the a-priori probability of a suspected disease towards a higher a-posteriori probability, leading to the diagnosis »diseased« or »non-diseased« after application of a diagnostic procedure. To reduce the subjectivity, six expert radiologists were invited to share their expertise and experience with regard to the four diagnostic procedures mentioned above.

The diagnostic confidence is often measured by a five-point (no, poor, moderate, good, or excellent confidence) or binary (no confidence, confidence) scale. The binary scale may be more applicable to the »real-world«, where a radiologist also has to make a »No/Yes« decision about whether to state a diagnosis or whether to order a second procedure. In the clinical development program, the diagnostic confidence was not obtained, so that a Delphi panel was initiated to obtain data on the confidence on a binary scale for the diagnosis of PAOD.

Results of the Delphi Panel

Six expert radiologists were invited to provide their expertise and experience on the confidence in diagnosing PAOD with Vasovist®-MRA, ECCM-MRA, and standard and selective DSA. All panel members with personal experience using Vasovist® agreed – although this was not proven by clinical trials – that the diagnostic confidence in both proximal and distal PAOD with Vasovist-MRA is clearly higher compared with ECCM-MRA and standard DSA and not worse compared with selective DSA.

The comparison of Vasovist®-MRA, ECCM-MRA, and DSA led to several points of agreement between the experts regarding the usefulness of Vasovist®-MRA. They agreed that differences in the modalities can be observed only in specific subgroups of PAOD, especially in distal disease. In distal critical limb ischemia (CLI), an advantage in diagnostic confidence of Vasovist®-MRA (95–99%) over ECCM-MRA (30–50%) and standard DSA (<50%) was reported. One reason may be that the whole vasculature is affected in distal CLI, leading to decreased image quality in ECCM-MRA and standard DSA.

In distal CLI, the advantages in diagnostic confidence were less distinct but still present (99% for Vasovist®-MRA, 70–80% for ECCM-MRA and >90% for standard DSA), whereas similar diagnostic confidence was seen for Vasovist®-MRA and selective DSA. Nevertheless, in the absence of supportive clinical trial data, all experts would still prefer selective DSA for legal reasons. These results were based on clinical experience with the four diagnostic procedures, and the experts agreed that appropriately designed clinical studies are needed to confirm their »real-world« experiences with respect to diagnostic confidence.

22.4   Health Economic Modeling

The aim of health economic modeling is to evaluate the cost-effectiveness of a new diagnostic procedure compared with the standards for the respective indications. As a new procedure, Vasovist®-MRA is to be compared with MRA using conventional extracellular contrast agents but also with the current standard of reference, DSA. For further reading on health economic evaluation, please refer to the book by Kobelt [20].

22.4.1   Methods

Health economic parameters for diagnostic procedures

Health economic modeling is used to compare new procedures with existing ones. The added clinical benefits over the existing procedure (the comparator) are to be compared with the societal willingness-to-pay (the so-called threshold barrier) to assess the acceptability of the new procedure. The comparator should be the next best available procedure; for Vasovist®, these are extracellular MRI contrast agents, as no other blood pool agent is currently on the market.

The threshold barrier is usually given by reimbursement agencies or payers and is often set to $50,000 per quality-adjusted-life-year (QALY). QALYs are years of complete health and are calculated as the health status (on a scale from 0 to 100%) multiplied by the time in this status.

The evaluation of costs of a new diagnostic procedure can be performed analogous to other interventions. The evaluation of the effects, on the other hand, is more challenging, because not only the direct effect, the diagnostic ability of the new procedure, but also indirect effects such as the kind of patient management chosen according to the diagnosis, have to be taken into account. The chosen patient management and its effectiveness has direct impact on the patient's outcome of the and therefore also on the effectiveness of the new diagnostic procedure.

In 1977, Fineberg et al. [21] proposed a framework for evaluating new diagnostic procedures on six levels (Fig. 22.1). The diagnostic performance is measured by levels 1–3. Level 1 describes the technical abilities

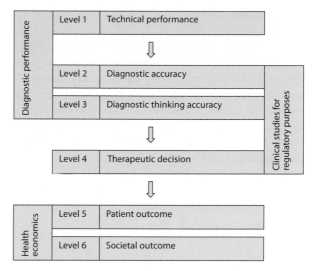

Fig. 22.1. Framework for measuring diagnostic procedures according to Fineberg et al.

of the new procedure, level 2 the diagnostic accuracy in terms of sensitivity and specificity. Level 3 describes the diagnostic thinking accuracy and measures how the diagnostic procedure changes the thinking of physicians. Levels 2 and 3 can be measured in clinical studies if the technical performance is adequate. In addition, the therapeutic decision, level 4, may be measured in clinical studies for regulatory purposes. The health economic evaluation is based on the results of clinical studies and measured in levels 5 and 6. Level 5 is the patient outcome measurement (following diagnosis and patient management) which could be obtained in randomized clinical studies but usually requires high sample sizes. Level 6 is the societal outcome measured by economic models and other aproaches.

Certain characteristics of clinical studies for regulatory purposes may bias the efficacy and therefore the effectiveness of a new diagnostic imaging procedure in a health economic evaluation. Users of a new procedure often show a learning curve when they obtain high-quality images, read images adequately, or feel confident in diagnosis, whereas these are assumed to be constant for procedures in clinical routine [22, 23]. The image quality itself is dependent on the equipment and acquisition parameters used in the clinical studies and is usually outdated by the time a new contrast agent reaches market authorization. The chosen standard of reference (SOR) in the studies has a major impact on the efficacy of a new test. When the SOR is imperfect, the true diagnostic ability may be higher than is found in the clinical studies. On the other hand, the interobserver agreement can be measured, as generally more than one reader assesses the images of the new procedure.

22

The health economic evaluation often depends on patient outcomes which may be difficult to capture, e.g., harm to the patient due to the invasiveness of an existing procedure in relation to its benefits. Also, the results of the diagnostic procedure are in any case only intermediate outcomes; cost savings, however, are most often the effect of the patient management chosen on the basis of the diagnosis and not a direct effect of the new procedure. Therefore, not only such tangible outcomes as survival or life expectancy may be collected to evaluate a diagnostic procedure, but also intangible outcomes which are related to the diagnostic procedure itself. Examples of intangible outcomes are customer satisfaction or confidence in the diagnosis.

Health Economic Modeling

The health economic model was based on a decision tree approach and was developed by Kienbaum et al. [24].

The learning curve of users is a major confounding factor in the health economic modeling of new diagnostic procedures. Hunink and Krestin [23] therefore proposed, ideally, replacement of an old by a new diagnostic procedure instead of simply adding it to the existing procedures. In clinical routine, however, Eisenberg [25] found that four of five new procedures do not replace an old one but are added, resulting in better diagnoses but also additional costs for diagnosing. Here, the aim is to replace extracellular contrast agents by Vasovist® for MRA.

For the health economic evaluation of Vasovist®, economic models for the management of PAOD were developed in two subgroups, CLI and intermittent claudication (IC), based on costs in Germany. The aim of the models was to gain cost-utility information of the initial use of Vasovist®-MRA compared with ECCM-MRA and standard DSA when diagnosing CLI and IC. Vasovist®-MRA, ECCM-MRA, and selective DSA were modeled as additional second procedures when the first method was inconclusive. Patient management options were percutaneous transluminal angioplasty (PTA) in the same session with selective DSA or in a second DSA session, bypass surgery, and finally amputation as the last possible intervention.

One basecase – i.e., a case close to the expected use in clinical routine – was defined according to the current German guidelines requiring confirmatory DSA in all cases where amputation is considered. A second basecase was defined assuming that these guidelines do not apply, i.e., where not only DSA but also Vasovist®-MRA or ECCM-MRA was considered sufficient. The PAOD decision-tree modeling was performed with the software Data Treeage® (Treeage Software, Inc, Williamstown, MA, USA).

Model Input

The model input – data on resource use, probabilities, and utilities – was defined in the model and gained mainly from the literature, as described by Kienbaum et al. [24]. Lifetime costs for dialysis and/or amputation due to CLI were based on assumed remaining life expectancies (literature) or on the DEALE (Declining Exponential Approximation of Life Expectancy) method [26]. Data which were not found in the literature were obtained by the Delphi panel as described above, especially data on diagnostic confidence and proportions of in-patient and out-patient procedures for the different indications.

Costs were evaluated from both the payer and the hospital perspective. In the payer perspective, all relevant costs for statutory health insurance in Germany were considered, taking into account legally required discounts and patients' co-payments. For the hospital perspective, Kienbaum et al. [24] assumed that all diagnostic procedures and the patient management occur within the hospital sector as event costs, summing the relevant costs incurred by hospitals, i.e., costs for the procedures and a single stay. In-patient therapies for CLI were bypass and amputation in all cases and MRA, DSA and PTA in 80%. For CLI, MRA was assumed to be an out-patient procedure in 100%, DSA and PTA in 50% of cases.

Model Structure

The model developed by Kienbaum et al. [24] started after ultrasound and clinical investigation were performed, resulting in a suspected stenosis in a vessel at a certain location. Subsequently, the physician, according to the model, had to choose between Vasovist®-MRA, ECCM-MRA, and standard DSA to confirm the initially suspected diagnosis. If the physician felt confident to confirm the diagnosis, he or she decided on patient management. In case of weak confidence, further diagnostic procedures were to be applied to decide on the patient management. The treatment options after MRA were PTA in combination with selective DSA, bypass surgery, or no intervention. The option amputation was valid only for suspected CLI. PTA and DSA may have caused renal failure requiring lifelong dialysis. If the confidence was not sufficient, a confirmatory selective DSA (basecase 1) or Vasovist®-MRA (basecase 2) was to be conducted, followed by the same treatment options. Only for ECCM-MRA may amputation have been chosen; however, it was not to be conducted immediately but required confirmation. If DSA was performed as the first procedure, the patient management was to be chosen without considering another diagnostic procedure.

Utility Values and Cost Data

Kienbaum et al. [24] derived the utility values mainly from the analysis by Holler [27] with annual discount rates of 5%. These were aggregated over the respective lifetimes. Long-term effects such as amputation and life-long dialysis were regarded as crucial for patients from a health economic perspective, whereas complications of invasive diagnostic procedures were regarded as negligible for the modeling.

The cost data for the payer perspective were obtained from appropriate tariffs and doctor's fee scales of the German statutory health insurance plans, whereas the costs from the hospital perspective were derived from the German Diagnosis-Related Groups (DRGs) [28] and tariff scheme of the German Hospital Federation (Deutsche Krankenhausgesellschaft Nebenkostentarif, DKG-NT) [29].

Further details on utility values and cost data of the model can be found in Kienbaum et al. [24].

22.4.2 Results: Cost-effectiveness Calculations

Modeling was based not only on the standard efficacy parameters for diagnostic procedures but also, and mainly, on diagnostic confidence. One reason for this is that the SOR used in the clinical studies for regulatory purposes is the imperfect standard of DSA. On the other hand, verification bias cannot be excluded in diagnostic testing when the diagnostic procedure is used in real life, outside of well-controlled clinical trials. Verification bias is present when only positive test results are verified by a second procedure or the standard of reference, so that the proportion of true-positive results increases and the proportion of false-negative results decreases, leading to an overestimation of the sensitivity and an underestimation of the specificity [5].

Critical Limb Ischemia

From both the payer and the hospital perspective, patient management of PAOD based on Vasovist®-MRA was found to be less expensive compared with ECCM-MRA or standard DSA. For basecase 1, the costs per QALY for patient management with Vasovist®-MRA from the payer perspective were €2571, leading to cost savings of €63 and €141 compared with ECCM-MRA and standard DSA, respectively. For basecase 2, i.e., where also Vasovist®-MRA is allowed as a final decision tool for amputation, the costs were very similar, leading to savings of €78 and €144. Also from the hospital perspective, costs were lower with initial use of Vasovist®-MRA (◘ Table 22.1).

The robustness of the model was tested by sensitivity analyses varying several pivotal parameters, showing that the ranking of the diagnostic alternatives did not change. The diagnostic confidence, however, was found to impact costs. From a payer perspective, Vasovist®-MRA was always found the least costly option, whereas from the hospital perspective, this dominance was found to change, with proportions of diagnostic confidence for Vasovist®-MRA lower than 0.58 and 0.55 for basecase 1 and 2, respectively.

The proportion of expected amputations in basecase 1 was 8.7% with initial standard DSA and 8.5% for ECCM-MRA and Vasovist®-MRA, whereas in basecase 2, all three procedures showed a proportion of 8.5%.

Intermittent Claudication

From both perspectives, that of the payer and that of the hospital, patient management of IC based on the diagnosis of Vasovist®-MRA was also found to be less expensive than ECCM-MRA or standard DSA with similar utility. For basecase 1, the costs per QALY for patient management with Vasovist®-MRA from the payer perspective were €270, leading to cost savings of €10 and €74 compared with ECCM-MRA and standard DSA, respectively. For basecase 2, the costs were very similar, leading to savings of €4 and €76, respectively, compared with ECCM-

◘ **Table 22.1.** Costs of patient management of CLI per QALY for Vasovist®-MRA compared with ECCM-MRA and standard DSA

	Vasovist®-MRA (2.158 QALYs)	Difference in costs per QALY	
	Costs per QALY	vs. ECCM-MRA (2.165 QALYs)	vs. standard DSA (2.169 QALYs)
Payer perspective			
Basecase 1	€2571	- €63	- €141
Basecase 2	€2561	- €78	- €144
Hospital perspective			
Basecase 1	€623	- €40	- €39
Basecase 2	€600	- €159	- €53

22

◻ Table 22.2. Costs of patient management of IC per QALY for Vasovist®-MRA compared with ECCM-MRA and standard DSA

	Vasovist®-MRA (6.658 QALYs)	Difference in costs per QALY	
	Costs per QALY	vs. ECCM-MRA (6.658 QALYs)	vs. standard DSA (6.655 QALYs)
Payer perspective			
Basecase 1	€270	- €10	- €74
Basecase 2	€270	- €4	- €76
Hospital perspective			
Basecase 1	€68	- €1	- €16
Basecase 2	€68	+ €8	- €16

MRA and standard DSA. From the hospital perspective, a similar result was found on a lower level, except for ECCM-MRA, which was found to be €8 less costly in basecase 2 (◻ Table 22.2).

Also for IC, the sensitivity analyses showed that the results were robust in general. The scenarios from a hospital perspective were found to be more sensitive to variations of parameters such as proportion of bypass surgeries or PTAs.

From the payers' perspective, a diagnostic confidence lower than 0.85 for Vasovist®-MRA in basecase 1 would lead to a change in advantage of Vasovist® compared with ECCM-MRA and standard DSA. For basecase 2, ECCM-MRA is to be preferred when the diagnostic confidence for ECCM-MRA is higher than 0.83 and for Vasovist®-MRA lower than 0.94.

From a hospital perspective, the results were found to be robust with a diagnostic confidence in more than 68% of cases for Vasovist®-MRA in basecase 1. In basecase 2, the model was very sensitive to variations of diagnostic confidence. Nevertheless, the costs per QALY for Vasovist®-MRA were found to be higher than for ECCM-MRA in most scenarios.

22.5   Conclusions

Advantages of Vasovist®-MRA were found in several areas, technically, clinically, and economically. Several technical advantages of Vasovist®-MRA are obvious and self-evident. These include a longer intravascular half-life, allowing for higher spatial resolution and extended imaging, and do not require further evidence. Clinical superiority was demonstrated for Vasovist®-MRA over non-enhanced MRA in the clinical development program with respect to DSA as SOR. In addition, recent publications have demonstrated a performance of Vasovist®-MRA equivalent

to that of ECCM-MRA with regard to first pass imaging (whole-body imaging) [14] and superiority of steady state imaging over first pass imaging [15]. First pass imaging with Vasovist® was found to be at least as good as first pass ECCM-MRA and revealed higher ratings in the qualitative evaluation of MRA images [14].

These advantages often cannot be directly translated into monetary advantages in the health economic sense. The clinical efficacy parameters such as sensitivity or specificity are not sufficient to evaluate a new diagnostic procedure but require further assessments according to the framework defined by Fineberg et al. [21] and Hunink [30]. For the assessment of Vasovist®-MRA, diagnostic confidence was chosen as the primary factor to evaluate its health economic impact and to calculate such health economic parameters as QALY and costs per QALY. Kienbaum et al. [24] published such a model based on diagnostic confidence and compared Vasovist®-MRA with ECCM-MRA and standard DSA with regard to the diagnoses CLI and IC in PAOD patients.

For the patient management of CLI, Kienbaum et al. [24] found Vasovist®-MRA to be cost-effective compared with both ECCM-MRA and standard DSA, leading to lower costs per QALY. This result was confirmed in the sensitivity analyses, except for the hospital perspective, where the diagnostic confidence for Vasovist®-MRA is very low. The proportions of proposed amputations were found to be similar for the three diagnostic procedures.

For IC, the picture was less straightforward. From the payers' perspective Vasovist®-MRA was more cost-effective than ECCM-MRA and standard DSA; this was confirmed in the sensitivity analyses. From the hospital perspective, however, the model was very sensitive to changes of the diagnostic confidence. Nevertheless, ECCM-MRA was found to be superior to Vasovist®-MRA in most scenarios.

Take home messages

- Vasovist®-MRA can deliver improved images compared with ECCM-MRA due to technical advantages, with no extra costs in terms of additional investments. These benefits allow more practitioners than only those at highly specialized centers to undertake high-quality MRA.
- Vasovist®-MRA showed superiority in diagnostic accuracy compared with non-enhanced MRA with respect to DSA as standard of reference. Recent publications support the value of Vasovist®-MRA. First pass imaging is at least as good with Vasovist® as with extracellular agents. Furthermore, steady state imaging enables ultra-high-resolution imaging, with increased accuracy in depiction of vessels and visualization of walls. In addition, high accuracy values were reported for the detection of significant disease in the carotids and lower extremities.
- Experts agree that the diagnostic confidence of Vasovist® MRA is higher compared with ECCM-MRA and standard DSA, especially in distal CLI and CI, and is similar to selective DSA in CI.
- Vasovist®-MRA was shown to be cost-effective in patient management of CLI compared with ECCM-MRA and standard DSA, leading to lower costs per QALY. This result was confirmed in the sensitivity analyses except for the hospital perspective,

where the diagnostic confidence for Vasovist®-MRA is very low. The proportions of proposed amputations were found to be similar for the three diagnostic procedures.
- Vasovist®-MRA proved to be cost-effective from a payer perspective with regard to the patient management of IC, compared with ECCM-MRA and standard DSA. This result was confirmed in the sensitivity analyses. From the hospital perspective, the costs per QALY were found to be lower for ECCM-MRA than for Vasovist® MRA in most scenarios, but this depended heavily on the assumed diagnostic confidence, as the model was found very sensitive to variations of diagnostic confidence.
- Overall, Vasovist®-MRA was found to be a solid and effective diagnostic procedure for evaluating the arterial and venous systems. Technical advantages of Vasovist®-MRA over ECCM-MRA were clearly shown. Also, the clinical value was demonstrated with respect to unenhanced and ECCM-MRA. Cost-effectiveness was evaluated for CLI and IC from the perspective of German payers and hospitals, leading to the overall conclusion that – except for the hospital perspective in some scenarios – in most scenarios Vasovist®-MRA was found to be less costly than ECCM-MRA and standard DSA relative to the efficacy.

References

1. Budoff MJ, Achenbach S, Duerinckx A (2003) Clinical utility of computed tomography and magnetic resonance techniques for noninvasive coronary angiography. J Am Coll Cardiol 42:1867–1878
2. Hollingworth (2005) Radiology cost and outcomes studies: Standard practice and emerging methods. AJR Am J Roentgenol 185:833–839
3. Drummond MF, Sculpher MJ, Torrance GW, O'Brian B, Stoddart GL (2005) Methods for the economic evaluation of health care programmes, 3rd edn. Oxford Medical Publications, Oxford
4. Phillips C, Thompson G (2003) What is cost-effectiveness. www.evidence-based-medicine.co.uk; volume 1, number 3, http://www.evidence-based-medicine.co.uk/ebmfiles/Whatiscosteffect.pdf (accessed 2007, August 10)
5. Hunink MGM (1996) Outcomes research and cost-effectiveness analysis in radiology. Eur Radiol 6:615–620
6. Hunink MGM (1996) Cost-effectiveness research in radiology. Acad Radiol 3:S13–S16
7. Leidl R (2003) Der Effizienz auf der Spur: Eine Einführung in die ökonomische Evaluation. In: Schwartz FW, Badura B, Busse R, Leidl R, Raspe H, Siegrist J, Walter U (eds) Das Public Health Buch, 2nd edn. Urban & Fischer, Munich
8. Busse R, Orvain J, Valesco M, Perleth M, Drummond M, Gürtner F, Jorgensen T, Jovell A, Malone J, Rüther A, Wild C (2002) Best prac-

tice in undertaking and reporting health technology assessments. Int J Techn Assessm Health Care 18:361–422
9. Bock M (2006) Artifacts and limitations of MR angiography. In: Goyen M (ed) MR angiography with blood pool agents. Vasovist® – the first blood pool contrast agent for MR angiography. ABW Wissenschaftsverlag GmbH, pp 38–53
10. Visser K, Kuntz KM, Donaldson MC, Gazelle GS, Hunink MGM (2003) Pretreatment imaging workup for patients with intermittent claudication: a cost-effectiveness analysis. J Vasc Interv Radiol 14:53–62
11. CPMP Points to consider (2001) Points to consider on the evaluation of diagnostic agents, CPMP/EWP/1119/98
12. FDA Draft Guideline (2000) Developing medical imaging drugs and biological Products
13. Hadizadeh DR, Gieseke J, Bayer T, Voth M, Loetsch R, Verrel F, Schild HH, Willinek WA (2007) MR Angiographie der Beingefäße mittels Vasovist: Intra-individueller Vergleich bei Verwendung von arterieller Phase- und Steady State- Bildgebung. Presentation at Röfo 2007, Rofo S1, vol 179
14. Klessen C, Hein PA, Huppertz A, Voth M, Wagner M, Elgeti T, Kroll H, Hamm B, Taupitz M, Asbach P (2007) First pass whole-body magnetic resonance angiography (MRA) using the blood-pool contrast medium gadofosveset trisodium: comparison to gadopentetate dimeglumine. Invest Radiol 42:659–664
15. Wang MS, Haynor DR, Wilson GJ, Leiner T, Maki JH (2007): Maximizing contrast-to-noise ratio in ultra-high resolution peripheral

22

MR angiography using a blood pool agent and parallel imaging. J Magn Reson Imaging 26:580–588

16. Nikolaou K, Kramer H, Grosse C, Clevert D, Dietrich O, Hartmann M, Chamberlin P, Assmann S, Reiser MF, Schoenberg SO (2006) High-spatial-resolution multistation MR angiography with parallel imaging and blood pool contrast agent: initial experience. Radiology 241:861–872

17. Linstone HA, Turoff M (eds) (1975) The Delphi method. Techniques and applications. Reading/Mass. (Electronic Version: Turoff M and Linstone H (2002) at http://www.is.njit.edu/pubs/delphibook/, accessed September 23, 2007)

18. Linstone HA The Delphi technique. In: Fowles J (1978). Handbook of futures research. Westport/Connecticut, London, pp 273–300

19. Rowe G, Wright G (1999) The Delphi technique as a forecasting tool: issues and analysis. Int J Forecasting 15:377–379

20. Kobelt G (2002) Health Economics: An introduction to economic evaluation. 2. Edition, Office of Health Ecomomics (www.OHE. org), London

21. Fineberg HV, Baumann R and Sosman M (1977): Computerized cranial tomography: effect on diagnostic and therapeutic plans. JAMA; 238: 224-227

22. Gazelle GS, McMahon PM, Siebert U and Beinfeld MT (2005): Cost-effectiveness analysis in the assessment of diagnostic imaging technologies. Radiology 235: 361-370

23. Hunink MG and Krestin GP (2002): Study design for concurrent development, assessment, and implementation of new diagnostic imaging technology. Radiology 222: 604-614

24. Leiner T, Kienbaum S (2008) Cost-effectiveness of Gadofosveset in the management of patients with symptomatic peripheral arterial occlusive disease, TouchBriefings, European Cardiovascular Disease, (in press)

25. Eisenberg JM (1999) Ten lessons for evidence-based technology assessment. JAMA 282:1865–1869

26. Beck JR, Kassirer JP, Pauker SG (1982) A convenient approximation of life expectancy (the »DEALE«) I. Validation of the method. Am J Med 73:883–888

27. Holler D (2004) Gesundheitsökonomische Aspekte der Versorgung chronischer Kranker am Beispiel der peripheren arteriellen Verschlusskrankheit. Eine Analyse aus Sicht der Gesellschaft und der Krankenversicherung. Versicherungswissenschaft in Hannover. [Health-economic aspects of care of the chronically ill: the example of peripheral arterial occlusive disease. An analysis from the perspectives of society and the hospital. Actuarial science in Hanover.] Hannoveraner Reihe (Band 23). Graf von der Schulenburg JM (ed) Verlag Versicherungswissenschaft GmbH, Karlsruhe

28. Institut für das Entgeltsystem im Krankenhaus (InEK) gGmbH (2006) [Institute for the Reimbursement Sytem in Hospitals.] German Diagnosis-Related Groups (G-DRG) Version (V2.4) 2006

29. Deutsche Krankenhausgesellschaft. Tarif der Deutschen Krankenhausgesellschaft für die Abrechnung erbrachter Leistungen und für die Kostenerstattung vom Arzt an das Krankenhaus (DKG-NT). [German Hospital Society. Tariff of the German Hospital Society for the accounting of services performed and for the reimbursement of the hospital by the doctor.] Stuttgart: W. Kohlhammer Verlag, 2005

30. Hunink MGM (2007) Whole body imaging: Who does and who does not benefit? Presentation at ECR, 2007

Patient Management and Referrals: The Impact of High-resolution Steady state MRA with Vasovist®

Winfried A. Willinek, Dariusch R. Hadizadeh

252 **Chapter 23** · Patient Management and Referrals: The Impact of High-resolution Steady state MRA with Vasovist®

23

23.1 Introduction

Since its introduction in 1993, three-dimensional contrast-enhanced MR angiography (3D CEMRA) has made tremendous progress and now is routinely used in the assessment of arterial stenosis of the vasculature in many centers as an alternative to digital subtraction angiography (DSA) [1-4]. However, DSA still is considered the standard of reference due to its superior spatial resolution, even though it does not provide the advantages of a 3D data set in post-processing.

While spatial resolution was limited in standard 3D CEMRA with non-blood pool (»extracellular«) contrast agents because of the limited acquisition window for imaging, i.e., first pass imaging during the arterial bolus passage, the introduction of an intravascular (»blood pool«) contrast agent offers for the first time the opportunity to virtually increase scan duration indefinitely in order to greatly increase spatial resolution in 3D CEMRA. Vasovist® (Gadofosveset, Bayer Schering Pharma AG, Berlin, Germany) is the first intravascular contrast agent which has been approved for use with magnetic resonance angiography in the European Union. Vasovist® reversibly binds to albumin, providing extended intravascular enhancement compared with existing extracellular magnetic resonance contrast agents [5, 6]. The albumin binding prolongs the intravascular phase of the contrast agent to a steady state that may last for more than 1 h [7] and leads to the highest relaxivity of currently available contrast agents [8].

The prolonged available acquisition time can be exploited to acquire additional high-resolution images during the equilibrium phase, yielding submillimeter 3D CEMRA datasets, e.g., of the calf region, with enhanced vascular delineation compared with standard-resolution 3D CEMRA. In this chapter, the known added value to date of high-resolution MRA in the steady state over first pass with extracellular contrast agents is summarized, and implications for clinical patient management are presented.

23.2 Technical Considerations

In order to perform high-resolution steady state 3D CEMRA of peripheral arteries, existing protocols need to be modified to take advantage of the prolonged available imaging time to obtain higher spatial resolution datasets. However, as compared with standard first pass 3D CEMRA protocols only minor modifications are required for steady state imaging. All images from cases that are presented in this chapter were acquired with a 1.5-T whole-body MR scanner (Achieva; Philips Medical Systems, Best, The Netherlands) with the following protocol parameters: coronal T1-weighted gradient echo sequences during the first pass (arterial bolus passage): Upper legs: TR/TE, 2.8/0.94 ms;

flip angle, 25°; RFOV, 100%; slab thickness, 90 mm; image matrix, 336 x 252 over a 451-mm field of view; 60 thin partitions of 1.5 mm yielding a reconstructed voxel size of 0.88 x 0.88 x 1.50 mm³ after zero-filling; acquisition time was 13.4 s. Lower legs: TR/TE, 4.8/1.36 ms; flip angle, 25°; RFOV, 100%; slab thickness, 88 mm; image matrix, 400 x 300 over a 451-mm field of view; 80 thin partitions of 1.1 mm yielding a reconstructed voxel size of 0.88 x 0.88 x 1.1 mm³ after zero-filling; the acquisition time was 35.9 s. Steady state 3D CEMRA acquisitions were started 4 min after administration of contrast medium. The acquisition parameters for the coronal T1-weighted gradient echo sequences during the steady state were as follows: Upper legs: TR/TE, 4.9/1.44 ms; flip angle, 25°; RFOV, 100%; slab thickness, 94.05 mm; image matrix, 416 x 312 over a 451-mm field of view; 95 thin partitions of 0.99 mm yielding a reconstructed voxel size of 0.88 x 0.88 x 0.99 mm³ after zero-filling; acquisition time of 1:50 min. Lower legs: TR/TE, 5.8/1.68 ms; flip angle, 25°; RFOV, 100%; slab thickness, 83.3 mm; image matrix, 464 x 348 over a 451-mm field of view; 170 thin partitions of 0.49 mm yielding a reconstructed voxel size of 0.52 x 0.52 x 0.49 mm³ after zero-filling; the acquisition time was 2:54 min.

A 4-channel phased array flexible surface coil (Philips Medical Systems, Best, The Netherlands) was used for imaging of the lower legs. Images of the upper legs were acquired with the integrated quadrature body coil. A biphasic injection protocol was implemented with automatic power injection of contrast medium (Spectris; Medrad Europe, Beek, The Netherlands). Vasovist® was injected at a flow rate of 1.2 ml/s, followed by 25 ml saline at a flow rate of 0.6 ml/s.

23.3 Peripheral Arterial Disease Detection and Treatment

Peripheral arterial disease (PAD) is a highly prevalent atherosclerotic syndrome that affects up to 15% of the general population depending on age, gender, race, and cardiovascular risk factors and is associated with significant morbidity and mortality [9, 10]. Treatment options for patients with PAD include risk factor reduction, exercise training, antiplatelet therapy, and surgical and/or interventional revascularization. In order to select the optimal treatment for each individual patient, correct classification of the disease is of the utmost importance. Hence, high spatial resolution imaging of the vasculature is clinically required, especially from the perspective of the referring physicians. However, not only the characterization of the diseased vessel segment itself, but also information about the distal outflow is needed in this interdisciplinary approach, as it determines the success and the functional outcome of the revascularization therapy, including success of primary arterial reconstruction, long-term patency, and limb salvage. Non-invasive imaging methods such as MR angiography play a pivotal role in the preoperative workup of patients with critical limb ischemia and have been shown to be a powerful diagnostic tool in the evaluation of PAD. Furthermore, MRA was reported to be powerful and often superior in comparison to duplex ultrasound for treatment planning and to DSA in the depiction of distal vessel patency in patients with proximal long-distance vessel segment occlusion [11, 12].

23.4 Rationale for High-resolution MRA in the Steady State

3D CEMRA of the arteries of the lower extremities at standard spatial resolution during the first pass of gadolinium-based contrast agents has been shown to be highly accurate in the assessment of stenosis grading as compared with DSA [13, 14] and has been proposed as the first-line diagnostic tool in arterial vessel imaging [15]. The administration of intravascular contrast agents has been shown to allow for safe and effective MRA studies during arterial bolus passage [5, 6]. The use of dedicated protocols for first pass and steady state imaging at the recommended dosage for Vasovist®-enhanced MRA of 0.03 mmol/kg [16] offers numerous advantages over standard-resolution first pass MRA alone. Among the most important are the following: increased robustness of MRA procedures, increased diagnostic confidence of MRA reports, improved grading of stenosis in peripheral arterial occlusive disease, improved diagnostic value due to additional findings, and expansion of diagnostic options for MRA, including venous imaging as an add-on to standard arterial-only imaging of the lower extremities [17–19].

Increased robustness of MRA procedures is achieved for the following reasons: Conventional first pass 3D CEMRA requires exact bolus timing. In practice, this cannot always be achieved. In at least 15% of the procedures bolus timing is not optimal for technical reasons. Moreover, vascular pathology in patients with peripheral occlusive disease and concomitant ulcers and/or diabetes is often obscured by early and heavy venous enhancement. In addition, because of different bolus arrival times in the two legs depending on the severity of the disease and the vascular involvement, arterial enhancement can be inhomogeneous. This drawback can be overcome with the use of blood pool contrast agents. In case of a missed bolus during first pass, a second acquisition can always be performed with steady state imaging without a second injection. This option also exists in case of patient movement. Furthermore, if diseased segments are discovered during first pass, it is possible to acquire additional very high resolution images of the specific region of interest without injection of additional contrast agent

within one single comprehensive scan during a time window of at least 1 h.

23.5 Patient Management and Clinical Cases

Superiority of steady state MRA over first pass MRA with a blood pool contrast agent was found in an initial prospective intra-individual comparative study of more than 25 patients with PAD grades IIb-IV. In more than 60% of the patients, the grade of stenosis of at least one of the evaluated vessels differed in steady state MRA as compared with first pass MRA alone. The grade of stenosis in steady state MRA matched with the reference standard DSA in all of the cases, demonstrating the excellent diagnostic performance of the non-invasive technique [17, 18].

The improved diagnostic accuracy of high spatial resolution MRA in the steady state also had an impact on therapeutic decision-making and patient management. A 78-year-old female patient with critical limb ischemia, amputation of the left lower extremity, and non-healing ulcers on the right foot presented at the emergency room. Because of a history of allergic reaction to iodinated contrast agent she was referred first to MRA. First pass MRA images did not allow reliable depiction of the right lower leg arteries (◻ Fig. 23.1). Nevertheless, the vascular surgeon specifically asked for patency of the calf arteries to decide on the option of distal bypass graft surgery to salvage the remaining right leg. A curved multiplanar reformat of the steady state high-resolution images allowed for clear depiction of a patent right anterior tibial artery, resulting in the possibility of distal origin bypass graft surgery for revascularization. The preserved distal blood supply of the calf and foot by the anterior tibial artery as diagnosed by high spatial resolution MRA was later confirmed by DSA (◻ Fig. 23.1). Whereas results of first pass imaging alone would have led to the diagnosis of no persistent distal vessel or potential bypass graft recipient, reading of the high spatial resolution images changed the patient management from possible contralateral leg amputation to lower limb salvage by bypass graft surgery. After surgery, the patient was rescheduled for follow-up 3D CEMRA with Vasovist®, and bypass patency to the anterior tibial artery was demonstrated (◻ Fig. 23.1).

Increased diagnostic confidence of MRA with Vasovist® has been reported in initial results of prospective studies using the first pass and steady state [17, 18]. In an intra-individual analysis of a sub-population of routine patients at the University of Bonn, more vessel segments could be evaluated on steady state MRA of the peripheral arteries with Vasovist® compared with first pass MRA alone. Fifty-three patients with suspected PAOD were included in a comparison of first pass imaging only and combined first pass and steady state imaging. The number of visible segments and the grade of stenosis were evalu-

23

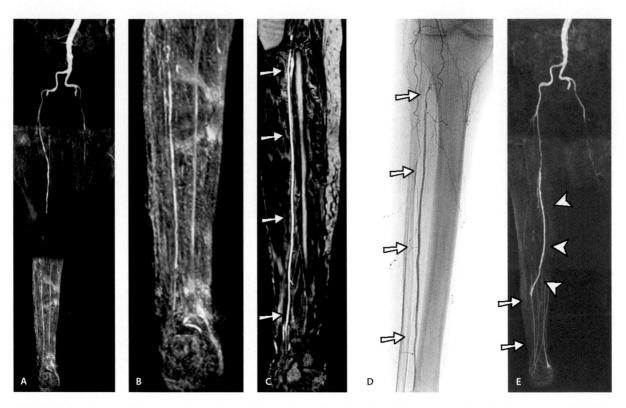

■ **Fig. 23.1A–E.** A 78-year-old female patient with critical limb ische-mia, amputation of the left lower extremity, and non-healing ulcers on the right foot. **A** (Detail: **B**) Maximum intensity projections of a contrast-enhanced T1-weighted GRE scan (TE, 2.8 ms/TR, 0.94 ms) do not allow reliable depiction of right lower leg arteries. **C** A curved multiplanar reformat of the steady state high-resolution contrast-enhanced T1-weighted GRE scan (TE, 4.9 ms/TR, 1.44 ms) obtains suf-ficiently high spatial resolution to allow for clear depiction of the right anterior tibial artery (*arrows*). **D** The anterior view of selective DSA of the right superficial femoral artery confirms the patency of the right anterior tibial artery (*arrows*). **E** The maximum intensity projection of the contrast-enhanced T1-weighted GRE scan (TE, 2.8 ms/TE, 0.94 ms) after distal bypass graft surgery shows the patency of the implanted bypass graft (*arrowheads*) and the right anterior tibial artery (*arrows*)

ated in a consensus by two experienced radiologists. In addition, the diagnostic confidence was evaluated for each patient on a three-point scale. The results demonstrated that for 85% of the patients either additional segments were depicted with steady state imaging or the grade of stenosis differed after evaluation of steady state MRA. The diagnostic confidence of the readers was increased in steady state imaging as compared with first pass imaging alone for 20% of the evaluated vessel segments [17, 18].

The performance of peripheral MRA with Vasovist® also had an impact on patient management, as highlighted by clinical case studies. An 80-year-old male patient with MR-compatible stent in the right common iliac artery was referred to MRA for follow-up of the intervention. In first pass MRA using gadolinium-DTPA, a significant in-stent stenosis was suspected even after careful reading of the source images. As a consequence, the patient was scheduled for re-intervention. Before undergoing the in-vasive procedure, a second MRA study using Vasovist® as the contrast agent was performed. High spatial resolution MRA in the steady state revealed a normal vessel segment

without in-stent stenosis. DSA of the iliac arteries con-firmed the patency of the stent in the right common iliac artery and, hence, the findings of steady state MRA. The better match between MRA with Vasovist® and DSA may be explained by the smaller voxel size implemented in steady state MRA, including a reduction of slice thickness by 50%. This may result in significant reduction of partial volume effects, as seen in ■ Fig. 23.2. One can hypothesize that the performance of high-resolution steady state MRA as the first-line diagnostic tool may have prevented the patient in this situation from undergoing an invasive and potentially harmful procedure.

More accurate grading of stenosis in peripheral arterio-occlusive disease was documented in a comparative study, as mentioned earlier. The classification of atherosclerotic disease was compared intra-individually with the use of first pass and steady state MRA and DSA. In 22 patients, 221 segments were available for intra-individual compari-son. In 82% of the patients, the grade of stenosis differed between the steady state and first pass. Furthermore, in 100% of the segments the grade of stenosis according to

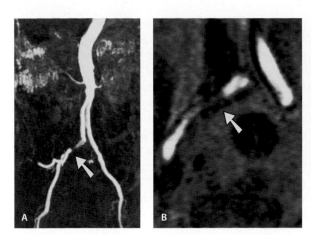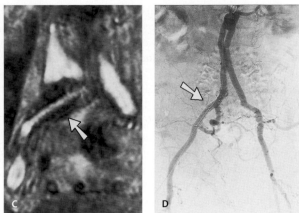

■ **Fig. 23.2A–D.** An 80-year-old male patient with an MR-compatible stent in the right common iliac artery. **A** Maximum intensity projections of a contrast-enhanced T1-weighted GRE scan (TE, 2.8 ms/TE, 0.94 ms) show an in-stent stenosis of the right common iliac artery (*arrow*). **B** A curved multiplanar reformat of the same dataset as in A confirms the suspected in-stent stenosis (*arrow*). **C** A curved multiplanar reformat of the steady state high-resolution contrast-enhanced T1-weighted GRE scan (TE, 4.9 ms/TE, 1.44 ms) allows for the correct diagnosis: exclusion of in-stent stenosis of the right common iliac artery (*arrow*). **D** The anterior view of DSA of the iliac arteries confirms the patency of the stent in the right common iliac artery (*arrow*)

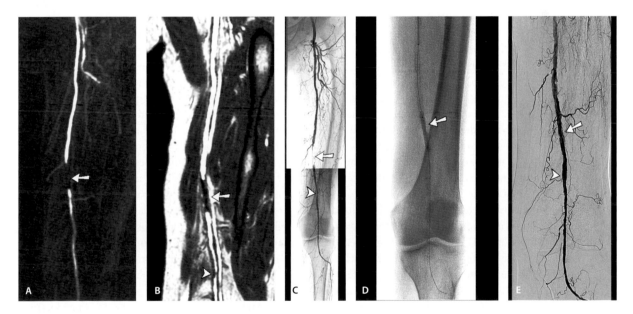

■ **Fig. 23.3A–E.** An 81-year-old female patient with absolute arrhythmia and acute leg pain. **A** The maximum intensity projection of a contrast-enhanced T1-weighted GRE scan (TE, 2.8 ms/TR, 0.94 ms) displays a focal occlusion of the left superficial femoral artery (*arrow*). **B** A curved multiplanar reformat of the high-resolution contrast-enhanced T1-weighted GRE scan during the steady state (TE, 4.9 ms/TR, 1.44 ms) shows the same focal arterial occlusion (*arrow*) and, in addition, atherosclerotic plaques distal to the occluded segments (*arrowhead*). **C** The anterior view of selective DSA of the left superficial femoral artery corresponds to steady state 3D CEMRA (**B**). **D, E** Percutaneous transluminal balloon angioplasty of the diseased segments was performed both to recanalize the occluded segment (*arrow*) and to dilate the distal stenotic segments (*arrowhead*)

steady state imaging corresponded to the findings on DSA. However, when determined on first pass MRA, both over- and underestimation of the grade of stenosis occurred in an almost equal number of cases in comparison to higher spatial resolution steady state MRA and DSA [19]. These findings might be explained by the increased number of pixels available within the vessel lumen in the high spatial resolution acquisition, yielding a more accurate classification of the disease especially on orthogonal cross-sectional images as has been reported previously [20, 21].

■ Figure 23.3 displays the case of an 81-year-old female patient with arrhythmia and acute leg pain. The patient had a history of hyperthyroidism and cardiac arrest during previous surgery. An arterial embolus was suspected on the basis of clinical signs and symptoms. Because of the patient's medical history and her age, she was taken to peripheral MRA first to avoid exposition to an iodinated contrast agent. The clinical diagnosis of an acute peripheral embolus was confirmed by first pass MRA with a segmental occlusion of the left superficial femoral artery (◘ Fig. 23.3). The high spatial resolution steady state images revealed underlying atherosclerotic vascular disease with multiple stenosed vessel segments that were not clearly depicted on first pass alone. The vascular surgeon was involved in the reading and decision-making at this point. As a result of the cardiac problems during previous surgery, the vascular surgeon hesitated to take the patient to the operating room for embolectomy. In addition, the results of the high-resolution steady state MRA supported the diagnosis of atherosclerosis as primary cause of disease, superimposed by an acute embolus; the application of a Fogarty catheter alone by the vascular surgeon would only have removed the thrombus but would not have ameliorated the steno-occlusive disease. Based on the findings on the high-resolution steady state images, the clinical workflow was changed after initiation of natrium-perchlorate and methimazole therapy in order to perform endovascular aspiration of the thrombus followed by transluminal angioplasty and stent placement in the stenosed vessel segments. The diagnosis made on the basis of the high-resolution steady state images was confirmed during the interventional procedure (◘ Fig. 23.3). The case demonstrates well the added value of high spatial resolution steady state imaging for the correct diagnosis of vascular disease and its potential implication for therapeutic decision-making.

The added diagnostic value of high spatial resolution steady state MRA with a blood pool contrast agent includes the depiction of incidental findings that are prevalent in other vascular beds, taking into account that atherosclerosis is a systemic disease and not limited to a specific region (peripheral occlusive disease, renal artery stenosis, carotid stenosis, coronary artery disease, etc.). In contrast to most protocols for whole-body MRA during the first pass [2], a single injection of contrast medium and standard MR equipment are sufficient for the acquisition of high spatial resolution 3D CEMRA of any arterial segment that needs to be evaluated for clinical decision-making.

Furthermore, 3D CEMRA in the steady state with Vasovist® enables the expansion of the clinical indications for MRA, including the diagnosis of venous disease, i.e., the performance of MR phlebography in routine clinical practice. It is inherent in the properties of an intravascular contrast agent that the venous system can be investigated in the steady state images in a similar manner as the arterial system with the same high spatial resolution. 3D CEMRA with Vasovist® performed during the equilibrium phase has been reported to be a reliable and easy method of venous imaging [22]. The resulting image quality and the diagnostic performance were comparable to those with conventional phlebography and Doppler-ultrasound. The latter is still regarded as the standard of reference in daily practice, but it is inherently associated with the disadvantages of ultrasound procedures in general (e.g., operator dependency, small field of view, depth dependence, and examination time). Indications beyond the arterial system have gained increasing importance in daily clinical practice, including the identification of bypass-suitable vessels and the depiction of the most appropriate locations for distal origin bypass (DOB) surgery. Moreover, reliable determination of the localization and extent of plaque and/or thrombi are often insufficient in luminographic procedures with standard spatial resolution. In the case of deep venous thrombosis, a complete checkup including lung perfusion, detection of pulmonary emboli by means of high-resolution pulmonary artery imaging, and diagnosis of underlying deep vein thrombosis (DVT) is of pivotal interest and is now feasible in a single comprehensive protocol using a blood pool contrast agent [23].

Concomitant arterial and venous disease is frequent in patients with PAD and may have an impact on the outcome of revascularization [10]. In addition, the diagnosis of subclinical DVT has an impact on patient management and requires anticoagulation therapy. A 49-year-old female patient with acute leg pain, a cold foot, and edema of the same presented to the emergency department. The patient had a history of an allergic reaction to iodinated contrast agents and was referred to peripheral MRA because of suspected PAD. Curved multiplanar reformats (MPR) of high spatial resolution 3DCEMRA with Vasovist® that were acquired in the steady state displayed a focal occlusion of the right anterior tibial artery, most likely due to an embolus (◘ Fig. 23.4). Axial MPR reformats of the same patient revealed incidental DVT with thrombi in the right fibular veins. The MRA diagnosis was subsequently confirmed by Doppler ultrasound, and anticoagulation therapy was initiated. The most likely underlying cause, i.e., open foramen ovale, was later excluded by echocardiography. As the venous system is displayed in the high spatial resolution steady state images without the need of a second injection or extra acquisition, peripheral MRA with Vasovist® may allow for diagnosis of relevant concomitant and even subclinical arterial and venous disease; this will simplify the diagnostic workup and influence patient management.

23.6 Referrers

Added diagnostic value, improved diagnostic confidence, and improved diagnostic work flow are of the utmost interest to referring physicians. In over 1 year of Vasovist®

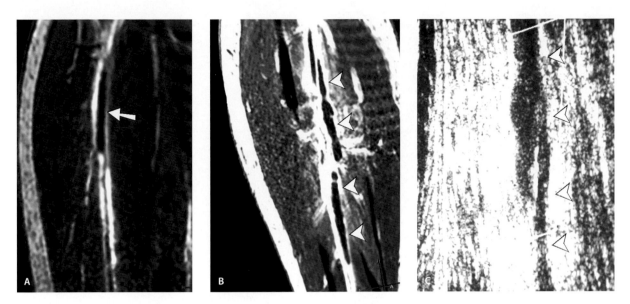

Fig. 23.4A–C. A 49-year-old female patient with leg pain, a cold foot, and edema. **A** A curved multiplanar reformat of the steady state high-resolution contrast-enhanced T1-weighted GRE scan (TE, 4.9 ms/ TR, 1.44 ms) displays a focal occlusion of the right anterior tibial artery (*arrow*). **B** Another curved multiplanar reformat of the same scan shows the additional finding of thrombi in the right fibular veins (*arrowheads*). **C** A Doppler-ultrasound study confirmed the occlusion of the right fibular veins by large thrombi (*arrowheads*)

use in a specialized vascular center at the University of Bonn, the application of a blood pool contrast agent with the previously summarized advantages in 3D CEMRA not only improved the diagnostic performance but also had a significant influence on the number of referrals: A mean increase of 30% in the number of referrals was seen following the introduction of the blood pool contrast agent, reflecting the acceptance of this approach by the referring clinicians, in addition to the impact on patient management and treatment. Furthermore, broader indications for MRA including MR phlebography and preoperative »one-stop-shop imaging« were noted.

Take home messages

- Steady state MRA, when used as an adjunct to standard first pass sequences, yields images with much higher spatial resolution. These images are easy to interpret with higher confidence.
- Steady state MRA with the blood pool contrast agent Vasovist® improves the diagnostic performance and the robustness of 3D CEMRA.

- The current level of evidence and the initial results of ongoing studies lead to the conclusion that steady state imaging not only provides added diagnostic value, but also influences patient management and the numbers of referrals.

References

1. Lenhart M, Finkenzeller T, Paetzel C, Strotzer M, Mann S, Djavidani B, et al (2002) Contrast-enhanced MR angiography in the routine work-up of the lower extremity arteries [in German]. Rofo 174:1289–1295
2. Nikolaou K, Kramer H, Grosse C, Clevert D, Dietrich O, Hartmann M, et al (2006) High-spatial-resolution multistation MR angiography with parallel imaging and blood pool contrast agent: initial experience. Radiology 241:861–872
3. Prince MR, Yucel EK, Kaufman JA, Harrison DC, Geller SC (1993) Dynamic gadolinium-enhanced three-dimensional abdominal MR arteriography. J Magn Reson Imaging 3:877–881
4. Willinek WA, von Falkenhausen M, Born M, Gieseke J, Holler T, Klockgether T, et al (2005) Noninvasive detection of steno-occlu-

sive disease of the supra-aortic arteries with three-dimensional contrast-enhanced magnetic resonance angiography: a prospective, intra-individual comparative analysis with digital subtraction angiography. Stroke 36:38–43
5. Goyen M, Edelman M, Perreault P, O'Riordan E, Bertoni H, Taylor J, et al (2005) MR angiography of aortoiliac occlusive disease: a phase III study of the safety and effectiveness of the blood-pool contrast agent MS-325. Radiology 236:825–833
6. Rapp JH, Wolff SD, Quinn SF, Soto JA, Meranze SG, Muluk S, et al (2005) Aortoiliac occlusive disease in patients with known or suspected peripheral vascular disease: safety and efficacy of gadofosveset-enhanced MR angiography--multicenter comparative phase III study. Radiology 236:71–78

7. Grist TM, Korosec FR, Peters DC, Witte S, Walovitch RC, Dolan RP, et al (1998) Steady state and dynamic MR angiography with MS-325: initial experience in humans. Radiology 207:539–544

8. Corot C, Violas X, Robert P, Gagneur G, Port M 2003) Comparison of different types of blood pool agents (P792, MS325, USPIO) in a rabbit MR angiography-like protocol. Invest Radiol 38:311–319

9. Hirsch AT, Criqui MH, Treat-Jacobson D, Regensteiner JG, Creager MA, Olin JW, et al (2001) Peripheral arterial disease detection, awareness, and treatment in primary care. JAMA 286:1317–1324

10. Hirsch AT, Murphy TP, Lovell MB, Twillman G, Treat-Jacobson D, Harwood EM, et al (2007) Gaps in public knowledge of peripheral arterial disease. The First National PAD Public Awareness Survey. Circulation

11. Leiner T, Tordoir JH, Kessels AG, Nelemans PJ, Schurink GW, Kitslaar PJ, et al (2003) Comparison of treatment plans for peripheral arterial disease made with multi-station contrast medium-enhanced magnetic resonance angiography and duplex ultrasound scanning. J Vasc Surg 37:1255–1262

12. Nelemans PJ, Leiner T, de Vet HC, van Engelshoven JM (2000) Peripheral arterial disease: meta-analysis of the diagnostic performance of MR angiography. Radiology 217:105–114

13. Hany TF, Debatin JF, Leung DA, Pfammatter T (1997) Evaluation of the aortoiliac and renal arteries: comparison of breath-hold, contrast-enhanced, three-dimensional MR angiography with conventional catheter angiography. Radiology 204:357–362

14. Koelemay MJ, Lijmer JG, Stoker J, Legemate DA, Bossuyt PM (2001) Magnetic resonance angiography for the evaluation of lower extremity arterial disease: a meta-analysis. JAMA 285:1338–1345

15. Ruehm SG, Goyen M, Debatin JF (2002) MR angiography: first choice for diagnosis of the arterial vascular system [in German]. Rofo 174:551–561

16. Perreault P, Edelman MA, Baum RA, Yucel EK, Weisskoff RM, Shamsi K, et al (2003) MR angiography with gadofosveset trisodium for peripheral vascular disease: phase II trial. Radiology 229:811–820

17. Hadizadeh D, Gieseke J, Loetsch R, Verrel F, Schild H, Willinek WA (2007) Peripheral MR angiography with Vasovist: intraindividual comparison of first pass and steady state imaging of the upper and lower legs. Eur Radiol 17(S1):317

18. Hadizadeh D, Gieseke J, Bayer T, Voth M, Loetsch R, Verrel F, et al (2007) MR Angiographie der Beingefäße mittels Vasovist: Intraindividueller Vergleich bei Verwendung von arterieller Phase- und Steady State-Bildgebung. Rofo 179(S1):S171

19. Hadizadeh D, Gieseke J, Loetsch R, Verrel F, Schild H, Willinek WA (2007) High resolution steady state imaging of peripheral arteries with a blood pool agent compared with standard first pass imaging and DSA: assessing the clinical benefit. Proc Intl Soc Mag Reson Med 15:2498

20. Hoogeveen RM, Bakker CJ, Viergever MA (1998) Limits to the accuracy of vessel diameter measurement in MR angiography. J Magn Reson Imaging 8:1228–1235

21. Schoenberg SO, Rieger J, Weber CH, Michaely HJ, Waggershauser T, Ittrich C, et al (2005) High-spatial-resolution MR angiography of renal arteries with integrated parallel acquisitions: comparison with digital subtraction angiography and US. Radiology 235:687–698

22. Sharafuddin MJ, Stolpen AH, Sun S, Leusner CR, Safvi AA, Hoballah JJ, et al (2002) High-resolution multiphase contrast-enhanced three-dimensional MR angiography compared with two-dimensional time-of-flight MR angiography for the identification of pedal vessels. J Vasc Interv Radiol 13:695–702

23. Fink C, Goyen M, Lotz J (2007) Expanding role of MR angiography in clinical practice. Eur Radiol 17 [Suppl 2]:B38–B44

Subject Index